Complexities Involving the Ankle Sprain

Editor

ALEXANDRE LEME GODOY-SANTOS

FOOT AND ANKLE CLINICS

www.foot.theclinics.com

Consulting Editor
CESAR DE CESAR NETTO

June 2023 • Volume 28 • Number 2

ELSEVIER

1600 John F. Kennedy Boulevard • Suite 1800 • Philadelphia, Pennsylvania, 19103-2899

http://www.theclinics.com

FOOT AND ANKLE CLINICS Volume 28, Number 2
June 2023 ISSN 1083-7515, ISBN-978-0-443-18290-7

Editor: Megan Ashdown
Developmental Editor: Arlene B. Campos

Foot and Ankle Clinics (ISSN 1083-7515) is published quarterly by Elsevier, Inc., 360 Park Avenue South, New York, NY 10010-1710. Months of issue are March, June, September, and December. Periodicals postage paid at New York, NY, and additional mailing offices. Subscription price per year is $362.00 (US individuals), $635.00 (US institutions), $100.00 (US students), $389.00 (Canadian individuals), $762.00 (Canadian institutions), $100.00 (Canadian students), $504.00 (international individuals), $762.00 (international institutions), and $215.00 (international students). To receive student/resident rate, orders must be accompanied by name of affiliated institution, date of term, and the *signature* of program/residency coordinator on institution letterhead. Orders will be billed at individual rate until proof of status is received. Foreign air speed delivery is included in all *Clinics* subscription prices. All prices are subject to change without notice. **POSTMASTER:** Send address changes to *Foot and Ankle Clinics*, Elsevier Health Sciences Division, Subscription Customer Service, 3251 Riverport Lane, Maryland Heights, MO 63043. **Customer Service: 1-800-654-2452 (US and Canada). From outside of the United States and Canada, call 314-447-8871. Fax: 314-447-8029. E-mail: JournalsCustomerService-usa@ elsevier.com (for print support); JournalsOnlineSupport-usa@elsevier.com (for online support).**

Reprints. For copies of 100 or more, of articles in this publication, please contact the Commercial Reprints Department, Elsevier Inc., 360 Park Avenue South, New York, NY 10010-1710. Tel.: 212-633-3874; Fax: 212-633-3820; E-mail: reprints@elsevier.com.

Contributors

CONSULTING EDITOR

CESAR DE CESAR NETTO, MD, PhD
Assistant Professor, Director of the Orthopedic Functional Imaging Research Laboratory
(OFIRL), Department of Orthopedics and Rehabilitation, University of Iowa, Carver College
of Medicine, Iowa City, Iowa, USA; Duke University Medical Center, Durham, North
Carolina, USA

EDITOR

ALEXANDRE LEME GODOY-SANTOS, MD, PhD
Professor at Lab. Prof. Mario Manlio Marco Napoli, Instituto de Ortopedia e
Traumatologia, Hospital das Clínicas HCFMUSP, Faculdade de Medicina da Universidade
de São Paulo, Professor at Programa Aparelho Locomotor, Hospital Israelita Albert
Einstein, São Paulo, Brazil

AUTHORS

AYYOUB A. AL-DOLAYMI, MD, FIBMS (Ortho)
Aspetar Orthopaedic and Sports Medicine Hospital, Doha, Qatar

KEPLER ALENCAR MENDES DE CARVALHO, MD
Department of Orthopedics and Rehabilitation, University of Iowa, Carver College of
Medicine, Iowa City, Iowa, USA

MOHAMMAD T. AZAM, BS
Orthopedic Surgery Research Fellow, Foot and Ankle Division, Department of Orthopedic
Surgery, NYU Langone Health, New York, New York, USA

VISHNU BABURAJ, MS (Orthopaedic Surgery)
Senior Resident, Department of Orthopedic Surgery, PGIMER, Chandigarh, India

KERRI LYNNE BELL, MD
Orthopaedic Surgery, Henry Ford Health, Detroit, Michigan, USA

ALESSIO BERNASCONI, MD, PhD
FEBOT, Federico 2 University of Napoli, Napoli, Italy

ANDRZEJ BOSZCZYK, MD, PhD
Idea Ortopedia, Warsaw, Poland

ANDREW I. BRASH, MD
Orthopedic Surgery Resident, Foot and Ankle Division, Department of Orthopedic
Surgery, NYU Langone Health, New York, New York, USA

JAMES J. BUTLER, MB, BCh
Orthopedic Surgery Research Fellow, Foot and Ankle Division, Department of Orthopedic Surgery, NYU Langone Health, New York, New York, USA

JAMES CALDER, OBE, TD, MD, PhD, FRCS (Tr & Orth) FFSEM (UK)
Fortius Clinic (FIFA Medical Centre of Excellence), Department of Bioengineering, Imperial College London, London, United Kingdom

PIETER D'HOOGHE, MD, PhD, MBA
Aspetar Orthopaedic and Sports Medicine Hospital, Doha, Qatar

MIKI DALMAU-PASTOR, PhD
Laboratory of Arthroscopic and Surgical Anatomy, Department of Pathology and Experimental Therapeutics (Human Anatomy Unit), University of Barcelona, Barcelona, Spain; MIFAS by GRECMIP, Merignac, France

CESAR DE CESAR NETTO, MD, PhD
Assistant Professor, Director of the Orthopedic Functional Imaging Research Laboratory (OFIRL), Department of Orthopedics and Rehabilitation, University of Iowa, Carver College of Medicine, Iowa City, Iowa, USA; Duke University Medical Center, Durham, North Carolina, USA

BRITTANY DECLOUETTE, MD
Orthopedic Surgery Resident, Foot and Ankle Division, Department of Orthopedic Surgery, NYU Langone Health, New York, New York, USA

MANDEEP S. DHILLON, MS (Orthopaedic Surgery)
Professor and Head, Department of Orthopedic Surgery, PGIMER, Chandigarh, India

TANIA DIAZ, PhD
Department of Anatomy and Human Embryology, Faculty of Medicine, University of Barcelona, Barcelona, Spain

ADHAM DO AMARAL E CASTRO, MD, PhD
Hospital Israelita Albert Einstein, Universidade Federal de São Paulo, São Paulo, São Paulo, Brazil

ERIC I. FERKEL, MD
Attending Orthopaedic Surgeon, Southern California Orthopedic Institute, In Affiliation with UCLA Health, Los Angeles, California, USA; Southern California Orthopedic Institute, Van Nuys, California, USA

JAN FRITZ, MD, PD, RMSK
Division of Musculoskeletal Radiology, Department of Radiology, NYU Grossman School of Medicine, New York, New York, USA

ALEXANDRE LEME GODOY-SANTOS, MD, PhD
Professor at Lab. Prof. Mario Manlio Marco Napoli, Instituto de Ortopedia e Traumatologia, Hospital das Clínicas HCFMUSP, Faculdade de Medicina da Universidade de São Paulo, Professor at Programa Aparelho Locomotor, Hospital Israelita Albert Einstein, São Paulo, Brazil

TIAGO MOTA GOMES, MD, PhD
Adjunct Professor, Researcher, Foot and Ankle Unit, Department of Anatomy and Human Embryology, Faculty of Medicine, University of Barcelona, Barcelona, Spain

CHOON CHIET HONG, MBBS, MMed (Ortho), FRCSED
Fortius Clinic (FIFA Medical Centre of Excellence), London, United Kingdom; Department of Orthopaedic Surgery, National University Hospital, Singapore

JOHN G. KENNEDY, MD, MCh, FFSEM, FRCS (Orth)
Chief, Foot and Ankle Surgery, Foot and Ankle Division, Department of Orthopedic Surgery, NYU Langone Health, New York, New York, USA

BRANDON WILLIAM KING, MD
Orthopaedic Surgery, Henry Ford Health, Detroit, Michigan, USA

FRANÇOIS LINTZ, MD, MS, FEBOT
UCP Foot and Ankle Center, Ramsay Healthcare Clinique de L'Union, Saint-Jean, Toulouse, France

NACIME SALOMÃO BARBACHAN MANSUR, MD, PhD
University of Iowa, Carver College of Medicine, Iowa City, Iowa, USA; Escola Paulista de Medicina – Universidade Federal de São Paulo, São Paulo, Brazil

THEODORAKYS MARÍN FERMÍN, MD
Aspetar Orthopaedic and Sports Medicine Hospital, Doha, Qatar

XAVIER MARTIN OLIVA, MD, PhD
Orthopedic Surgeon, Department of Orthopedics, Clinica Del Remei, Professor, Department of Anatomy and Human Embryology, Faculty of Medicine, University of Barcelona, Barcelona, Spain

EUN HAE PARK, MD, PhD
Division of Musculoskeletal Radiology, Department of Radiology, NYU Grossman School of Medicine, New York, New York, USA; Department of Radiology, Jeonbuk National University Medical School, Jeonju, Republic of Korea

SANDEEP PATEL, MS (Orthopaedic Surgery)
Associate Professor, Department of Orthopedic Surgery, PGIMER, Chandigarh, India

PATRICK PFLÜGER, MD
Department of Orthopedics, Balgrist University Hospital, University of Zurich, Zurich, Switzerland

STEFAN RAMMELT, MD, PhD
Professor, Head, Foot and Ankle Center, University Center for Orthopaedic, Trauma and Plastic Surgery, University Hospital Carl Gustav Carus at the TU Dresden, Dresden, Germany

BRUCE J. SANGEORZAN, MD
Orthopaedic Surgery, Harborview Medical Center, University of Washington, Seattle, Washington, USA

TIM SCHEPERS, MD, PhD
Trauma Unit, Department of Surgery, Amsterdam UMC Location Melbergdreef, Amsterdam, the Netherlands

SÉRGIO SOARES, MD, PhD(c)
Researcher, PhD Student, Foot and Ankle Unit, Department of Anatomy and Human Embryology, Faculty of Medicine, University of Barcelona, Barcelona, Spain; Department of Orthopaedics, Hôpital Fribourgeois, Villars-sur-Glâne, Switzerland

PANAGIOTIS D. SYMEONIDIS, MD, PhD
St. Luke's Hospital, Thessaloniki, Greece

ATUL K. TANEJA, MD, PhD
Hospital Israelita Albert Einstein, São Paulo, São Paulo, Brazil; Department of Radiology, UT Southwestern Medical Center, Dallas, Texas, USA

VICTOR VALDERRABANO, MD, PhD
Swiss Ortho Center, University of Basel, Schmerzklinik Basel, Swiss Medical Network, Hirschgässlein, Basel, Switzerland

JORDI VEGA, MD
Laboratory of Arthroscopic and Surgical Anatomy, Department of Pathology and Experimental Therapeutics (Human Anatomy Unit), University of Barcelona, Foot and Ankle Unit, iMove Traumatology-Clinica Tres Torres, Barcelona, Spain; MIFAS by GRECMIP, Merignac, France; Foot and Ankle Consultant, Clinique Montchoisi, Lausanne, Switzerland

JOSE ANTONIO VEIGA SANHUDO, MD, PhD
Foot and Ankle Department, Hospital Moinhos de Vento, Porto Alegre, Brazil

ELSA VIRIDIANA SANCHEZ, MD
Department of Anatomy and Human Embryology, Faculty of Medicine, University of Barcelona, Barcelona, Spain

Editorial Advisory Board

Contents

Lateral ankle sprain (LAS) is not as simple as it was believed to be as it has substantial negative impacts on the active sporting population. The negative impact on physical function, quality of life (QoL) and economic burden is significant with increased risk of reinjury, development of chronic lateral ankle instability and posttraumatic ankle osteoarthritis resulting in functional deficits, decreased QoL and chronic disabilities. Economic burden from a societal perspective demonstrated notably higher indirect costs from productivity loss. Preventative interventions with early surgery for a selective cohort of active sporting population may be considered to mitigate morbidities associated with LAS.

Understanding of the ankle and subtalar joint ligaments is essential to recognize and manage foot and ankle disorders. The stability of both joints relies on the integrity of its ligaments. The ankle joint is stabilized by the lateral and medial ligamentous complexes while the subtalar joint is stabilized by its extrinsic and intrinsic ligaments. Most injuries to these ligaments are linked with ankle sprains. Inversion or eversion mechanics affect the ligamentous complexes. A profound knowledge of the ligament's anatomy allows orthopedic surgeons to further understand anatomic or nonanatomic reconstructions.

Lateral ankle ligament sprains and syndesmotic injuries are two different entities. However, they may be combined under the same spectrum depending on the arch of violence during the injury. Currently, the clinical examination has a limited value in the differential diagnosis between an acute anterior talofibular ligament rupture and a syndesmotic high ankle sprain. However, its use is indispensable for raising a high index of suspicion for detecting these injuries. Based on the mechanism of injury, clinical examination plays an essential role in guiding further imaging and early diagnosis of low/high ankle instability.

ultimate goal of bringing the individual back to preinjury level of activity. This protocol of conservative treatment should always be offered before considering any surgical intervention.

Despite the high frequency of ankle sprains, the ideal management is controversial, and a significant percentage of patients sustaining an ankle sprain never fully recover. There is strong evidence that residual disability of ankle joint injury is often caused by an inadequate rehabilitation and training program and early return to sports. Therefore, the athlete should start their criteria-based rehabilitation and gradually progress through the programmed activities, including cryotherapy, edema relief, optimal weight-bearing management, range of motion exercises for ankle dorsiflexion improvement, triceps surae stretching, isometric exercises and peroneus muscles strengthening, balance and proprioception training, and bracing/taping.

Lateral ligament attenuation may occur after repetitive ankle sprains, creating instability. Management of chronic ankle instability requires a comprehensive approach to mechanical and functional instability. Surgical treatment, however, is indicated when conservative treatment is not effective. Ankle ligament reconstruction is the most common surgical procedure to resolve mechanical instability. Anatomic open Broström-Gould reconstruction is the gold standard for repairing affected lateral ligaments and returning athletes to sports. Arthroscopy may also be beneficial for identifying associated injuries. In severe and long-standing instability, reconstruction with tendon augmentation could be necessary.

Ankle microinstability results from the superior fascicle of anterior talofibular ligament (ATFL) injury and is a potential cause of chronic pain and disability after an ankle sprain. Ankle microinstability is usually asymptomatic. When symptoms appear, patients describe a subjective ankle instability feeling, recurrent symptomatic ankle sprains, anterolateral pain, or a combination of them. A subtle anterior drawer test can usually be observed, with no talar tilt. Ankle microinstability should be initially treated conservatively. If this fails, and because superior fascicle of ATFL is an intra-articular ligament, an arthroscopic procedure is recommended to address.

Lateral ankle ligament complex injuries are most commonly managed non-operatively. If no improvements have been made following conservative management, surgical intervention is warranted. Concerns have been raised regarding complication rates following open and traditional arthroscopic anatomical repair. In-office needle arthroscopic anterior talo-fibular ligament repair provides a minimally invasive arthroscopic approach to the diagnosis and treatment of chronic lateral ankle instability. The limited soft tissue trauma facilitates rapid return to daily and sporting activities making this an attractive alternative approach to lateral ankle ligament complex injuries.

Injuries of the medial ankle ligament complex (MALC; deltoid and spring ligament) are more common following ankle sprains than expected, especially in eversion-external rotation mechanisms. Often these injuries are associated with concomitant osteochondral lesions, syndesmotic lesions, or fractures of the ankle joint. The clinical assessment of the medial ankle instability together with a conventional radiological and MR imaging is the basis for the definition of the diagnosis and therefore the optimal treatment. This review aims to provide an overview as well as a basis to successfully manage MALC sprains.

Probably one of the most controversial subjects in the orthopedic field is the distal tibiofibular articulation. Even though its most primary knowledge can be a matter of enormous debate, it is in the diagnosis and treatment most of the disagreements reign. Distinguishing between injury and instability remains challenging as well as an optimal clinical decision regarding surgical intervention. The last years presented technology and that was able to bring body to an already well-developed scientical rationale. In this review article, we aim to demonstrate the current data behind syndesmotic instability in the ligament scenario, whereas using few fracture concepts.

Not all ankle sprains are the same and not all ankles behave the same way after an injury. Although we do not know the mechanisms behind an injury producing an unstable joint, we do know ankle sprains are highly underestimated. While some of the presumed lateral ligament lesions might eventually heal and produce minor symptoms, a substantial number of patients will not have the same outcome. The presence of associated injuries, such as additional medial chronic ankle instability, chronic syndesmotic instability, has been long discussed as a possible reason behind this. To explain multidirectional chronic ankle instability, this article aims to present the literature surrounding the condition and its importance nowadays.

Acute and chronic subtalar instability and commonly coexistent with other hindfoot pathology but can be difficult to diagnose. A high degree of clinical suspicion is required as most imaging modalities and clinical maneuvers are poor at detecting isolated subtalar instability. The initial treatment is similar to ankle instability, and a wide variety of operative interventions have been presented in the literature for persistent instability. Outcomes are variable and limited.

The contribution of Lauge-Hansen to the understanding and treatment of ankle fractures cannot be underestimated, an unquestionable merit being the analysis of the ligamentous component of these injuries that are considered as equivalent to the respective malleolar fractures. In numerous clinical and biomechanical studies, the lateral ankle ligaments are ruptured either together with or instead of the syndesmotic ligaments, as predicted by the Lauge-Hansen stages. A ligament-based view on malleolar fractures may deepen the understanding of the mechanism of injury and lead to a stability-based evaluation and treatment of the 4 osteoligamentous pillars (malleoli) at the ankle.

FOOT AND ANKLE CLINICS

RELATED SERIES

Orthopedic Clinics
Clinics in Sports Medicine
Physical Medicine and Rehabilitation Clinics

THE CLINICS ARE NOW AVAILABLE ONLINE!
Access your subscription at:
www.theclinics.com

Preface

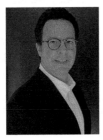

Alexandre Leme Godoy-Santos, MD, PhD
Editor

Ankle ligament injuries represent one of the most common injuries in orthopedic practice. It affects nonathletes, active athletes, and elite athletes of different ages. It is a musculoskeletal injury that is still neglected. Epidemiologically, the numbers are large, and it is indeed a major health problem worldwide.

In the general population, incidence rates reported range from 2.15 to 7 per 1000 person-years. Studies have reported an incidence rate of approximately 3.2 to 6 per 1000 player-hours in elite athletes. Regarding professional athletes, for example, in the UEFA Champions League, 1080 ankle injuries were recorded out of 8029 injuries during 1,057,201 exposure hours, constituting 13% of all injuries.

Without proper treatment, a high proportion of ankle sprains may not heal, resulting in chronic instability, loss of joint range of motion, decreased athletic performance, and ankle osteoarthritis.

Therefore, it is necessary to accurately diagnose and differentiate medial and lateral injuries from high ankle sprain observe subtalar ligaments injuries, and understand the role of ligament injuries associated with fractures.

In this remarkable issue of *Foot and Ankle Clinics of North America*, a special group of experts have joined forces to provide an accurate, literature-based view of ankle ligament injuries.

The specific epidemiologic findings include the detailed and modern knowledge of the ankle and hindfoot topographic anatomy, the precise physical examination, the complementary diagnostic investigation based on traditional and innovative methods (MRI, WBCT, needle arthroscopy), the diagnoses of subtalar instability, microinstability of the ankle, the role of ligament injuries associated with fractures; in addition to nonsurgical treatment, open and arthroscopic surgical procedures for acute and chronic injuries to the lateral, medial, and high ligaments of the ankle.

Foot Ankle Clin N Am 28 (2023) xv–xvi
https://doi.org/10.1016/j.fcl.2023.01.010
1083-7515/23/© 2023 Published by Elsevier Inc.

We hope this reading provides increased knowledge on the subject, in order to allow the best clinical outcomes for patients.

Alexandre Leme Godoy-Santos, MD, PhD
Lab. Prof. Mario Manlio Marco Napoli
Instituto de Ortopedia e Traumatologia
Hospital das Clínicas HCFMUSP
Faculdade de Medicina da Universidade de São Paulo
São Paulo, Brazil

Programa Aparelho Locomotor
Hospital Israelita Albert Einstein
Sào Paulo, Brazil

E-mail address:
alexandrelemegodoy@gmail.com

*Corresponding author. Rua Barão de Capanema, 112, Sao Paulo 01411010, Brazil.

The Burden of the "Simple Ankle Sprains"

A Review of the Epidemiology and Long-Term Impact

Choon Chiet Hong, MBBS, MMed (Ortho), FRCSEd[a,b,]*,
James Calder, OBE, TD, MD, PhD, FRCS (Tr & Orth) FFSEM (UK)[a,c]

KEYWORDS

- Ankle sprains • Burden • Impact • Epidemiology • Consequences
- Long-term impact • Sequela

KEY POINTS

- Lateral ankle sprain is very common and more prevalent in the active sporting population.
- It is not as simple as it was thought to be because it has substantial negative influence on physical function, quality of health, and economic burden.
- Specifically, significant sequela such as high rates of reinjury and development of chronic lateral ankle instability leading to negative economic consequences and long-term impact of posttraumatic ankle osteoarthritis adds on to the burden of ankle sprain.
- Preventative interventions are recommended and early surgery for a selective cohort of active sporting population may be considered to mitigate morbidities associated with lateral ankle sprains.

INTRODUCTION

Ankle sprain is one of the commonest musculoskeletal injuries with more than 75% of them affecting the lateral ligament complex[1–9] with the others being deltoid ligament injuries and syndesmosis injuries.[9,10] The lateral ligament complex consists of the anterior talofibular ligament (ATFL), calcaneofibular ligament (CFL), and the posterior talofibular ligament, with the ATFL and CFL most commonly injured during supination-inversion sprains.[7–9] The ATFL, which is the main restraint for anterior talar translation,

a Fortius Clinic (FIFA Medical Centre of Excellence), 17 Fitzhardinge Street, London, W1H 6EQ, UK; b Department of Orthopaedic Surgery, National University Hospital of Singapore, 1E, Kent Ridge Road, Singapore 119228, Singapore; c Department of Bioengineering, Imperial College London, London, SW7 2AZ, UK
* Corresponding author. Department of Orthopaedic Surgery, National University Hospital of Singapore, 1E, Kent Ridge Road, Singapore 119228, Singapore.
E-mail address: choonchiet@gmail.com

Foot Ankle Clin N Am 28 (2023) 187–200
https://doi.org/10.1016/j.fcl.2022.12.002
1083-7515/23/© 2022 Elsevier Inc. All rights reserved.
foot.theclinics.com

is the most commonly injured ligament in a lateral ankle sprain, whereas the CFL, which limits excessive ankle inversion, is the second most common structure injured.[7–9,11] Notably, the ATFL is often injured in isolation in approximately two-thirds of ankle sprains[7,11] with combined injuries of both ATFL and CFL was observed in 20% to 40% of ankle sprains.[7,9,12] Therefore, this review will focus on the more common supination-inversion ankle sprains affecting the lateral ligament complex.

The lateral ligament complex injury from ankle sprain is often considered an innocuous injury that heals after a short period of rest. However, up to 40% of individuals with such injuries may experience residual symptoms such as recurrent instability, pain, and swelling during sporting activities, and a significant proportion have a reinjury with subsequent missed time from training and competition for athletes.[13] Studies have reported that chronic lateral ankle instability (CLAI) can develop in up to 70% of individuals with acute ankle sprains resulting in long-term disability.[2,8,14–16] CLAI is also associated with the development of ankle osteoarthritis (OA).[2,8,17,18] Therefore, lateral ankle sprains are not simple and harmless but rather, strongly associated with residual functional deficits and chronic disabilities. As a result, we concur and echo both van Dijk and Vuurberg's conclusion in their editorial commentary that "there is no such thing as a simple ankle sprain."[19]

EPIDEMIOLOGY

In the general population, between 3% and 5% of the population presenting to the emergency department (ED) are for acute ankle sprains giving rise to an approximate 5600 injuries daily in the United Kingdom (UK).[2,20,21] Similarly, close to 2 million acute ankle sprains occur annually in the United States of America (USA).[8,22] Waterman and colleagues[22] used data from the National Electronic Injury Surveillance System (NEISS) between 2002 and 2006 and found that an incidence rate of 2.15 per 1000 person-years for acute ankle sprains. Another study by Lambers and colleagues[23] using data from NEISS on 119,815 patient presentation to ED in 2009 reported that ankle sprains are the commonest cause of acute presentation to ED with an estimate incidence rate of 2.06 ankle sprains per 1000 person-years. Similarly, a review by Herzog and colleagues[8] on incidence of ankle sprains in the general population reviewed 6 studies (UK, USA, and Denmark), which used large ED databases reported that the incidence rate ranges from 2.15 to 7 per 1000 person-years.

In the active sporting population, a study used data from the National Collegiate Athletic Association Injury Surveillance Program (NCAA-ISP) and reported the incidence rate of lateral ligament complex sprains to be 0.495 per 1000 elite athletic exposures (AEs) in 25 NCAA sports from the 2009 to 2010 through 2014 to 2015 academic years in the USA.[3,8] An AE was defined as 1 student-athlete participating in 1 NCAA-sanctioned practice or competition in which he or she was exposed to the possibility of an athletic injury regardless of the time spent in that participation.[3] The highest lateral ligament complex sprain rates were in men's basketball (1.196/1000 AEs), women's basketball (0.95/1000 AEs) and women's soccer (0.836/1000 AEs).[3] This is in line with a recent meta-analysis of 181 studies, which reported that lateral ankle sprain is one of the most frequent musculoskeletal injuries sustained by athletes with an incidence of 0.93 per 1000 elite AEs, which is defined as 1 athlete participating in 1 competition or practice when compared with medial ankle or syndesmosis sprains at 0.06 and 0.38 per 1000 elite AEs, respectively.[24]

Correspondingly, professional athletes playing in the Premiership Rugby reported incidence rate of ankle injuries at around 6 per 1000 player hours and the lateral ankle ligament injury was ranked as the third most common injury with an incidence rate of

4.5 per 1000 player-hours.[25] In addition, foot and ankle injuries account for 20% of all football injuries in an English Premier League club, with injury to the lateral ligament ankle complex being most common accounting for 31% of all injuries.[26] In an 11-year follow-up of UEFA Champions League injury study, 1080 ankle injuries out of 8029 injuries were recorded during 1,057,201 exposure hours constituting 13% of all injuries.[27] This translates to an incidence rate of 1 per 1000 hour equating to approximately 7 ankle injuries in each season for a 25-player squad in a professional football club.[27] Lateral ligament ankle sprain was found to be commonest injury sub-type accounting for 51% in all ankle injuries with an incidence rate of 0.7 per 1000 hours, which means a professional 25-player squad will suffer an average of 4 to 5 ankle sprains in each season.[27] In the USA, elite basketball players in the National Basketball Association had an incidence rate of approximately 3.2 to 3.5 per 1000 player-games.[8,28,29] Similarly, players from the National Football League (NFL) reported a cumulative incidence of 11.2% for ankle injuries sustained over 3 seasons from 2015 to 2017.[30]

Acute ankle sprains are also frequently reported in the military where intensive training and high-demand physical activities are required. A study from the United States Military Academy reviewing a large cohort of military academy cadets reported the incidence rate of ankle sprain to be 58.4 per 1000 person-years.[31] They also found that women (96.4/1000) compared with men (52.7/1000) had a significantly elevated rate ratio for ankle sprain of 1.83.[31] Furthermore, a systematic review and meta-analysis of 181 prospective epidemiology studies on incidence and prevalence of ankle sprains demonstrated a pooled cumulative incidence rate of 11.55 per 1000 exposures (injuries) and pooled prevalence period of 11.88% for high-quality studies.[24] This review included 174 studies on sporting populations and 7 studies involving military populations. Meta-analysis for sex reported a higher incidence rate of acute ankle sprains for women with 13.6 per 1000 exposures when compared with 6.94 per 1000 exposures for men. The incidence rate was also noted to decrease with age from children to adolescent and finally adults (2.85 > 1.94 > 0.72 per 1000 exposures).[24] Additionally, the risk of lateral ankle sprains was reported to be 3.8 ankle sprains per 1000 parachute jumps in the 7 studies with entirely military-related results.[24]

IMPACT OF LATERAL ANKLE SPRAIN ON PHYSICAL FUNCTION AND QUALITY OF LIFE

Lateral ankle sprain typically results in a short duration of functional deficit due to the acute inflammatory phase from the trauma, which will resolve after a short period of immobilization.[2,32,33] Following that, functional rehabilitation with removable semirigid brace to prevent inversion during the proliferative phase of ligament healing helps to promote proper collagen fiber orientation.[21,33] However, it has been observed that some patients continued to have residual symptoms such as pain, subjective instability, and reinjury.[2,8,13–16,34] Gerber and colleagues[13] reviewed a group of military cadets with ankle sprains and found that 40% of them still had residual symptoms with dysfunction at 6 months after the injury. At 7 years after ankle inversion injury, Konradsen and colleagues[10] evaluated 648 patients with 32% of them still troubled by chronic pain, swelling, and recurrent sprains, whereas 72% reported that they were functionally impaired by residual disabilities. Similarly, Anandacoomarasamy and Barnsley reported 74% of their patients with acute inversion ankle injury continued to have residual symptoms such as instability, pain, weakness, and swelling at 1.5 to 4 years after the acute injury.[14] Van Rijn and colleagues[34] performed a systematic review of 31 studies where they demonstrated that 15% to 64% still had residual symptoms such as pain, reinjury, and subjective instability at 3 years after lateral ankle sprain. Additionally, lateral ankle sprain have been shown to negatively affect mental health and quality of life where studies have shown that patients with ankle sprains have poorer quality of life and disability even after they have recovered from the acute symptoms of the injury.[2,35–37] A recent cross-sectional study in Australia reported that individuals with ankle instability reported greater disability, poorer function and worse quality of life compared with asymptomatic individuals (270 symptomatic vs 124 asymptomatic).[35]

These residual symptoms could be explained by incompetent or weakened stabilizing structures[2,8,9,38–40] and neuromuscular function such as altered postural stability, foot positioning during gait and prolonged time to stabilization after a jump as demonstrated by a systematic review of 55 studies that included patients with recurrent ankle sprains (≥ 2 sprains).[2,41] Besides, multiple studies have reported abnormal coordination and balancing during gait due to sensorimotor deficits after acute lateral ankle sprains.[42–47] Notably, Wikstrom and colleagues[43] reported in their systematic review and meta-analysis of 12 studies that balance is actually bilaterally impaired after an acute lateral ankle sprain, and the authors suggested that this is due to centrally mediated changes such as spinal-level motor control deficits. Several studies on abnormal balance and movement after lateral ankle sprain was performed by Doherty and colleagues, which the authors concluded that lateral ankle sprain often result in sensorimotor deficits that may not resolve completely even up to 1 year, which may then lead to residual disabilities.[2,44–47]

Risk of Reinjury

One of the most frequently cited risk factors for lateral ankle sprain is a history of previous lateral ankle sprain.[2,8,48–51] The reinjury rate of lateral ankle sprain after the acute episode have been reported to be relatively high.[2,3,5,8,34,48–52] At 1 year after acute lateral ankle sprain, a systematic review of 31 studies reported 34% of patients sustained at least another 1 resprain.[34] Roos and colleague analyzed data from NCAA-ISP in 25 NCAA sports demonstrated that 11.9% of lateral ligament complex sprains were recurrent injuries where the majority involved women's sports such as basketball (21.1%), outdoor track (21.1%), field hockey (20%), and men's basketball (19.1%).[3] Verhagen and colleagues[52] in their analysis of 116 volleyball teams reported that players with history of ankle sprains have twice the odds of reinjury at 1 year after the initial ankle sprain. Herzog and colleagues[8] reported the proportion of reinjuries after ankle sprains to range from 12% to 47% in their review of 6 studies on epidemiology of ankle sprains. Up to 9% of professional soccer player may sustain a reinjury the same season and 34% within 3 years.[5,34] A large prospective cohort study of 9811 military cadets from the 3 largest military academies in the USA reported that cadets with a history of ankle sprains were at 3.5 times increased risk of experiencing another sprain even after adjusting for age, high school sports participation, distance running index, academy, cohort year, and participation in an injury-prevention course.[53] This risk was found to be similar for both men and women cadets.[53] Therefore, it has been suggested that the increased risk of reinjury after acute lateral ankle sprain is a significant contributor to CLAI.[2,8,48,51,54]

Chronic Lateral Ankle Instability

CLAI is defined as the perception by the patient of an abnormal ankle with a constellation of symptoms including recurrent sprains, pain and swelling, or avoidance of activities.[40,51,54] It can be further classified into mechanical instability and functional instability. Mechanical instability is also known as the actual anatomical instability where the ankle range of motion exceeds the physiological limit of the joint motion due to laxity caused by incompetent stabilizing structures such as lax or ruptured ligaments, whereby this laxity can be demonstrated clinically or radiological.[40,51,54] The high reinjury rate after acute lateral ankle sprain had been reported as the single most important cause for CLAI as recurrent injury adds on further damage to the already weakened lateral ankle stabilizers[2,8,38–40] including causing a greater fatigue-induced changes to the dynamic posture control.[2,55,56] Functional instability was defined by Freeman in 1965 as a subjective feeling of the ankle or foot giving way without objectively demonstrable clinical or radiological deviation of ankle joint motion beyond physiological range of motion of the talus.[42] In contrast to mechanical instability, altered neuromuscular recruitment patterns such as abnormal peroneal muscle spindle activities and mechanoreceptor activity, increased peroneal response time, and impaired reflex response to inversion/supination had been reported to lead to functional instability of the ankle.[2,8,40–47]

There is a spectrum of disease in CLAI, and it is not entirely based on the concept of mechanical or functional instability in isolation that cause symptoms but rather interactions between them both. Recent publications have explored the likelihood that the diagnosis of functional instability may actually be an isolated injury of the superior ATFL fascicle, which can lead to subtle instability and chronic anterolateral ankle pain known as "microinstability."[57–59] This isolated tear of the superior ATFL fascicle tear, which is intra-articular, is difficult to recognize with physical examination.[57,59] Vega and colleagues[57] reviewed ankle arthroscopy video records from 232 patients with suspected ankle microinstability and demonstrated 4 different injury patterns affecting the superior ATFL fascicle, which was only confirmed arthroscopically. Similarly, Takao and colleagues[60] described a case series of 14 patients diagnosed with apparent functional ankle instability due to no demonstrable abnormal ligament laxity but noted to have morphologic ligamentous abnormality on arthroscopic assessment. These patients underwent anatomical ATFL reconstruction with good outcomes at 2 years.[60]

CLAI may occur after inadequate rehabilitation following an acute ankle sprain due to the repetitive trauma causing damage to the already injured stabilizing structures leading to insufficiency of the lateral ligament complex mechanically and functionally as described earlier. In the same vein, a prospective cohort study of 70 patients with acute first-time lateral ankle reported that 40% of the cohort were diagnosed with CLAI at 1 year.[61] The authors also showed that certain predictive factors identified at 6 months postinjury were able to correctly predict 84.8% of the CLAI cases at 1 year, and these predictive factors include deficits during movement task in Star Excursion Balance Test and poorer scores on the activities of daily living subscale of the Foot and Ankle Ability Measure (FAAM) score.[61] Lin and colleagues[62] in a recent systematic review of CLAI reviewed 9 studies with 3804 subjects using criteria from the International Ankle Consortium demonstrated the overall prevalence of CLAI at 25% ranging between 7% and 53%, whereas the prevalence of CLAI in patients with previous history of ankle sprain was higher at 46% ranging between 9% and 76%. Donovan and colleagues[63] performed a cross-sectional study of 1002 healthy adolescent athletes (mean age; 15.6 ± 1.6 years) and found a CLAI prevalence of 20%, and the presence of CLAI negatively affected these athletes with significantly lower ankle functional and quality of life scores.

Posttraumatic Ankle Osteoarthritis

Long-term impact of ankle sprains includes the development of posttraumatic ankle OA, which has been associated with both single and recurrent lateral ankle sprains.[2,8,17,18,64–66] Saltzman and colleagues[64] reported that recurrent ankle sprains (14.6%) and a single ankle sprain (13.7%) are among the prevalent subcauses of post-traumatic ankle OA. Valderrabano and colleagues[66] reported 60 out of 313 patients with posttraumatic ankle OA had ankle ligamentous lesions in their study on etiology of ankle arthritis. Up to 50% of patients with ankle OA were reported to have sustained at least a single ankle sprain or recurrent sprains and/or CLAI.[2,64,66,67]

The association of posttraumatic ankle OA and ankle instability are not unfounded because studies have shown that acute lateral ankle sprain does not always result in isolated lateral ligament injury but also causes damage to other structures. Khor and Tan performed MRI for 64 consecutive patients with acute inversion injury to the ankle (median time from injury to MRI: 6 weeks, range 4 days to 12 weeks) and found only 22% had isolated lateral ligament complex injuries, whereas others have concomitant pathologic conditions such as bone bruising, syndesmosis injury, deltoid ligament injuries, and other injuries.[68] They also reported 14% had osteochondral lesions while 22% had fractures such as avulsion-type fractures that led the authors to conclude that ankles sprains may not be as simple as thought to be.[68] In addition, Takao and colleagues[69] demonstrated the importance of arthroscopic assessment for residual ankle pain after sprains and found 40.3% of 72 patients with residual ankle disability lasting for more than 2 months after the initial injury (mean 7 months) had osteochondral lesions. Similarly, intra-articular pathologic condition such as chondral lesions were found in 89% of acute ankle sprains while 95% were found in those with chronic ankle sprains.[70] In a recent study on return to play for 41 patients after lateral ligament reconstruction for CLAI, May and colleagues[71] reported that 32% had concomitant osteochondral lesions of the talus. As illustrated by Gribble and colleagues,[2] the presence of cartilage damage after ankle sprains was only reported in patients who were surgically treated rendering potential underestimation of the true prevalence of patients with cartilage damage after ankle sprains. This is further corroborated by the findings from Hiller and colleague's study in which they found that up to 60% of the general population with ankle sprain did not seek formal medical care.[15] Hence, it is very likely that the lack of early and appropriate medical evaluation and treatment can contribute to the development of cartilage degeneration after ankle sprains.[2,8,15,19,54]

In the general population, the prevalence of ankle OA is estimated to be 3.4% in people aged older than 50 years.[72] Notably, the prevalence of ankle OA is significantly higher at 12% to 19% after a professional football career of 16 to 22 years.[17,73–75] A recent cross-sectional study on 553 former professional football (n = 401) and rugby (n = 152) reported prevalence of ankle OA at 9.2% and 4.6% for football and rugby, respectively.[17] Notably, when comparing football players with ankle OA and those without (94% vs 54%) had history of 1 or more ankle injury and (62% vs 14%) had undergone 1 or more ankle surgery.[17] They have also showed that football players with history of severe ankle injury were 30% more likely to report ankle OA (OR 1.3; 95% CI 1.1 to 1.6, $P < .001$), whereas those with ankle surgery were 2 times more likely to report ankle OA (OR 2.1; 95% CI 1.4 to 3.1, $P < .001$) adjusted for both age and BMI.[17] Similarly, Song and colleagues[18] examine the association of ankle-injury history with OA prevalence in retired NFL players and found that prevalence of OA was higher among those with a history of ankle injury (40.8% in those with history of ankle injury vs 33.1% in those without history of ankle injury).

Despite that, the exact etiology of ankle OA following single ankle sprain or CLAI is unknown although mechanical and sensorimotor deficits leading to instability after ligamentous injury have been suggested to cause damage to articular cartilage surfaces due to changes in joint surface contact stresses.[76,77] Several studies have provided evidence that CLAI leads to the development of osteochondral lesions of the talus and early arthritis due to altered joint biomechanics and repetitive trauma to cartilage.[78–81] Caputo and colleagues[79] performed an in vivo kinematic study of the tibiotalar joints in patients with CLAI and reported increased anterior translation, internal rotation, and superior translation of the talus. Similarly, Bischof and colleagues[78] showed that in vivo peak cartilage contact strains increased at the anteromedial of the ankle joint with significant anterior translation and medial translation at 100% body weight. Interestingly, an in vivo kinematic study of the tibiotalar joints in patients with CLAI preoperatively and postoperatively by Wainright and colleagues[81] reported statistically significant improvement in the aberrant ankle joint motion after a modified Broström-Gould repair, which was similar to the uninjured ankle. Despite that, there are no prospective cohort studies to date that have provided clinically evidence of the advantage of surgical stabilization of single ankle sprains or CLAI at mitigating early ankle joint degeneration.

ECONOMIC IMPACT OF ANKLE SPRAIN

The negative impacts of ankle sprain on physical function and quality of life are very concerning and are frequently considered as the primary burden of injury although an equally important but often forgotten consequence is the economic sequela of ankle sprain. As clinicians, our focus is always on the clinical and functional outcomes without considering the economic impact on the health-care system and patients. This economic impact is significant because it includes not only the direct medical cost of the injury but also the indirect medical cost such as lost productivity (sports time lost, missing school due to disability and work absenteeism).[2] Although a thorough economic evaluation such as cost-effectiveness analysis would be appropriate to provide accurate quantification of the cost involved, we shall only focus the discussion on rough description of economic cost from the societal perspective, which describes the direct and indirect medical cost of ankle sprain for the society in this review.

In the USA, Shah and colleagues[82] reported the direct cost of ankle sprains in EDs to be at a median of US$1029 (IQR: US$723 to US$1457) and after propensity score adjustment, lateral ankle sprains incurred the greatest amount of charges compared with other types of ankle sprain at a median of US$1008 (IQR: US$702 to US$1408) with statistical significance when directly compared with medial ankle sprains at US$914 (IQR: US$741 to US$1108). Gribble and colleagues in their review on direct medical costs of injury including consultation costs, operational costs, medications, and those directly related to treatment of ankle sprain showed that the direct costs of standard care for ankle sprains to the ED in UK to be £135, whereas 2 studies from the Netherlands reported direct costs of €43 and €61, respectively.[2] They also reinforced that it is difficult to provide exact breakdowns due to differences in market prices, inflation, valuation of costs and effectiveness of health-care systems although a large component of the direct costs covers the consultation with physiotherapist in most studies.[2]

Indirect medical costs due to productivity loss are much more significant because it considers the perspective from the society, which is often not considered from a health-care system point of view. In the Netherlands where an estimated 520,000 ankle sprains occur annually, an estimated annual €35.88 million is required for health-care costs and productivity loss.[83] It was also reported that approximately 50% of all ankle injuries needs medical treatment, and the average sick leave was 2.5 weeks with 90% reporting back to work by 6 weeks.[84,85] Hupperets and colleagues[83] reported the importance of measuring costs attributable to productivity loss because up to 86% of all indirect cost per injured athlete were costs due to sick leave. The authors also showed that an average of €385 indirect cost was incurred compared with the €61direct cost per athlete when the costs of productivity loss are considered.[83] Similarly, Verhagen and colleagues[52] analyzed data from Dutch recreational volleyball players and found that the indirect costs from ankle sprain was €318 when productivity loss was considered (average 2.3 days work absenteeism, 29.8 hours of unpaid leisure time lost per injury) compared with direct medical costs of €43. In the UK, Cooke and colleagues[86] reported an average of 6.9 days of lost paid work due to ankle sprains costing an additional £805 due to loss of productivity compared with direct health-care costs of £135. In professional athletes, this is even more pertinent because productivity loss affect their function and livelihood. Our own data demonstrated that 147 elite athletes with early surgical repair for acute grade III lateral ligament injuries provided early return to sports with a median of 69 days (range 58–132 days).[90] White and colleagues[87] demonstrated a median downtime of 77 days (range: 56 to 178 days) after an acute grade III lateral ligament repair for professional athletes. In addition, Lee and colleagues[88] reported outcomes on 18 elite athletes with surgical lateral ligament repair after failure of 3 to 6 months of conservative management where the average return to play was 3.9 ($\pm$1.4) months after the initial period of nonsurgical treatment resulting in an even longer downtime after the index injury. Although both the authors (White and colleagues & Lee and colleagues) did not translate the downtime to monetary value for the estimation of productivity loss in elite athletes, one can easily postulate that the estimated productivity loss in monetary terms would be exponentially high considering the nature of these professional athletes' career.[7,9,19,40,54,87,89,90] This was corroborated by JLT Specialty Limited (insurance broker) that the cost of injuries increased by 21% for the Premier League football with £217 million paid out to footballers while injured in the 2017/18 season.[91] Nevertheless, there is insufficient data on costs incurred with recurrent sprains and most of these estimations are approximations because less than half of patients with lateral ankle sprains seek formal medical attention.[2,15,49,54] With all things considered, one can agree that a lateral ankle sprain does not just affect the physical function and quality of life but adds on to the economic burden from a societal cost perspective involving the general population to professional athletes.

SUMMARY

Acute lateral ankle sprains are very common musculoskeletal injuries, and it can affect everyone from the general population to sporting athletes, although it is more prevalent in the active sporting population. Even though it is a common injury, the negative impact on physical function, quality of life, and economic burden is significant with an increased risk of reinjury, development of CLAI and posttraumatic ankle OA resulting in functional deficits, decreased quality of life, and chronic disabilities. The high reinjury rate after acute lateral ankle sprain contributes to the development of CLAI while chronic and repetitive injuries to the ankle joint in patients with CLAI give rise to cartilage damage and degeneration, which culminates in posttraumatic ankle OA. Interestingly, the economic consequences of ankle sprain provide a new viewpoint in analyzing the burden of ankle sprain on top of the conventional functional and quality of life impairments. Costs were described in direct and indirect costs allowing a differentiation between the relatively low direct medical cost with the much higher indirect costs consisting of productivity loss from paid (sick leave) and unpaid (leisure time) activities reflecting the societal economic perspective. As a result, lateral ankle sprain has a substantial negative effect on physical function, quality of life, and economic consequences.

Therefore, the prevention of recurrent sprains with proprioceptive training program,[83] neuromuscular training, and bracing[92] are important because they have been shown in cost-effectiveness analysis that these interventions are cost-effective for the prevention of ankle sprain recurrences. In professional athletes with lateral ligament injuries especially those with grade III injury, early surgical intervention in the form of acute lateral ligament repair has been recommended to mitigate the risk of nonsurgical treatment failure resulting in increased downtime while providing a predictable recovery and high rate of return to sports.[7,9,19,40,54,87,89,90] Perhaps, early surgery should also be considered for a certain subset of active sporting population besides professional athletes because lateral ankle sprains have been shown to be more prevalent in this cohort of athletic individuals in order to mitigate the significant morbidities from lateral ankle sprain because there is no such thing as a simple ankle sprain.

CLINICS CARE POINTS

- Lateral ankle sprain is very common especially in the active sporting population.
- The negative impact on physical function, quality of life, and economic burden is significant with an increased risk of reinjury, development of CLAI, and posttraumatic ankle OA, resulting in functional deficits, decreased quality of life, and chronic disabilities.
- Economic burden from a societal perspective illustrated the notably higher indirect costs consisting of productivity loss from paid (sick leave) and unpaid (leisure time) activities compared with the relatively lower direct medical cost.
- Therefore, lateral ankle sprain is not as simple as it was thought to be because it has substantial negative impact on physical function, quality of health, and economic burden.
- Preventative interventions are recommended, and early surgery for a selective cohort of active sporting population may be considered to mitigate morbidities associated with lateral ankle sprains.

DISCLOSURE

CC Hong has nothing to disclose. J. Calder received remuneration for speaking in educational program by Arthrex unrelated to this review article.

REFERENCES

1. Fong DT, Hong Y, Chan LK, et al. A systematic review on ankle injury and ankle sprain in sports. Sports Med 2007;37(1):73–94.
2. Gribble PA, Bleakley CM, Caulfield BM, et al. Evidence review for the 2016 International Ankle Consortium consensus statement on the prevalence, impact and long-term consequences of lateral ankle sprains. Br J Sports Med 2016;50(24): 1496–505.
3. Roos KG, Kerr ZY, Mauntel TC, et al. The epidemiology of lateral ligament complex ankle sprains in national collegiate athletic association sports. Am J Sports Med 2017;45(1):201–9.
4. Ekstrand J, Gillquist J. Soccer injuries and their mechanisms: a prospective study. Med Sci Sports Exerc 1983;15(3):267–70.
5. Woods C, Hawkins R, Hulse M, et al. The Football Association Medical Research Programme: an audit of injuries in professional football: an analysis of ankle sprains. Br J Sports Med 2003;37(3):233–8.

6. Hawkins RD, Hulse MA, Wilkinson C, et al. The association football medical research programme: an audit of injuries in professional football. Br J Sports Med 2001;35(1):43–7.

7. Hunt KJ, Fuld RS III, Sutphin BS, et al. Return to sport following lateral ankle ligament repair is under-reported: a systematic review. J ISAKOS 2017;2:234–40.

8. Herzog MM, Kerr ZY, Marshall SW, et al. Epidemiology of ankle sprains and chronic ankle instability. J Athl Train 2019;54(6):603–10.

9. D'Hooghe P, Cruz F, Alkhelaifi K. Return to play after a lateral ligament ankle sprain. Curr Rev Musculoskelet Med 2020;13(3):281–8.

10. Waterman BR, Belmont PJ Jr, Cameron KL, et al. Risk factors for syndesmotic and medial ankle sprain: role of sex, sport, and level of competition. Am J Sports Med 2011;39(5):992–8.

11. Boardman DL, Liu SH. Contribution of the anterolateral joint capsule to the mechanical stability of the ankle. Clin Orthop Relat Res 1997;341:224–32.

12. Broström L. Fotleds- vrickning [Ankle sprains]. Lakartidningen 1967;64(16): 1629–44. Swedish.

13. Gerber JP, Williams GN, Scoville CR, et al. Persistent disability associated with ankle sprains: a prospective examination of an athletic population. Foot Ankle Int 1998;19(10):653–60.

14. Anandacoomarasamy A, Barnsley L. Long term outcomes of inversion ankle injuries. Br J Sports Med 2005 Mar;39(3):e14 [discussion: e14].

15. Hiller CE, Nightingale EJ, Raymond J, et al. Prevalence and impact of chronic musculoskeletal ankle disorders in the community. Arch Phys Med Rehabil 2012;93(10):1801–7.

16. Konradsen L, Bech L, Ehrenbjerg M, et al. Seven years follow-up after ankle inversion trauma. Scand J Med Sci Sports 2002;12(3):129–35.

17. Paget LDA, Aoki H, Kemp S, et al. Ankle osteoarthritis and its association with severe ankle injuries, ankle surgeries and health-related quality of life in recently retired professional male football and rugby players: a cross-sectional observational study. BMJ Open 2020;10(6):e036775.

18. Song K, Wikstrom EA, Tennant JN, et al. Osteoarthritis prevalence in retired national football league players with a history of ankle injuries and surgery. J Athl Train 2019;54(11):1165–70.

19. van Dijk CN, Vuurberg G. There is no such thing as a simple ankle sprain: clinical commentary on the 2016 International Ankle Consortium position statement. Br J Sports Med 2017;51(6):485–6.

20. Cooke MW, Lamb SE, Marsh J, et al. A survey of current consultant practice of treatment of severe ankle sprains in emergency departments in the United Kingdom. Emerg Med J 2003;20(6):505–7.

21. Lamb SE, Marsh JL, Hutton JL, et al. Collaborative Ankle Support Trial (CAST Group). Mechanical supports for acute, severe ankle sprain: a pragmatic, multi-centre, randomised controlled trial. Lancet 2009;373(9663):575–81.

22. Waterman BR, Owens BD, Davey S, et al. The epidemiology of ankle sprains in the United States. J Bone Joint Surg Am 2010;92(13):2279–84.

23. Lambers K, Ootes D, Ring D. Incidence of patients with lower extremity injuries presenting to US emergency departments by anatomic region, disease category, and age. Clin Orthop Relat Res 2012;470(1):284–90.

24. Doherty C, Delahunt E, Caulfield B, et al. The incidence and prevalence of ankle sprain injury: a systematic review and meta-analysis of prospective epidemiological studies. Sports Med 2014;44(1):123–40.

25. Brooks JH, Fuller CW, Kemp SP, et al. Epidemiology of injuries in English professional rugby union: part 1 match injuries. Br J Sports Med 2005;39(10):757–66.
26. Jain N, Murray D, Kemp S, et al. Frequency and trends in foot and ankle injuries within an English Premier League Football Club using a new impact factor of injury to identify a focus for injury prevention. Foot Ankle Surg 2014;20(4):237–40.
27. Waldén M, Hägglund M, Ekstrand J. Time-trends and circumstances surrounding ankle injuries in men's professional football: an 11-year follow-up of the UEFA Champions League injury study. Br J Sports Med 2013;47(12):748–53.
28. Deitch JR, Starkey C, Walters SL, et al. Injury risk in professional basketball players: a comparison of Women's National Basketball Association and National Basketball Association athletes. Am J Sports Med 2006;34(7):1077–83.
29. Drakos MC, Domb B, Starkey C, et al. Injury in the national basketball association: a 17-year overview. Sports Health 2010;2(4):284–90.
30. Desai SS, Dent CS, Hodgens BH, et al. Epidemiology and outcomes of ankle injuries in the national football league. Orthop J Sports Med 2022;10(6). 23259671221101056.
31. Waterman BR, Belmont PJ Jr, Cameron KL, et al. Epidemiology of ankle sprain at the United States Military Academy. Am J Sports Med 2010;38(4):797–803.
32. Bleakley CM, McDonough SM, MacAuley DC, et al. Cryotherapy for acute ankle sprains: a randomised controlled study of two different icing protocols. Br J Sports Med 2006;40(8):700–5 [discussion: 705].
33. Petersen W, Rembitzki IV, Koppenburg AG, et al. Treatment of acute ankle ligament injuries: a systematic review. Arch Orthop Trauma Surg 2013;133(8):1129–41.
34. van Rijn RM, van Os AG, Bernsen RM, et al. What is the clinical course of acute ankle sprains? A systematic literature review. Am J Med 2008;121(4):324–31.e6.
35. Al Mahrouqi MM, MacDonald DA, Vicenzino B, et al. Quality of life, function and disability in individuals with chronic ankle symptoms: a cross-sectional online survey. J Foot Ankle Res 2020;13(1):67.
36. Kosik KB, Johnson NF, Terada M, et al. Health-related quality of life among middle-aged adults with chronic ankle instability, copers, and uninjured controls. J Athl Train 2020;55(7):733–8.
37. Houston MN, Van Lunen BL, Hoch MC. Health-related quality of life in individuals with chronic ankle instability. J Athl Train 2014;49(6):758–63.
38. Delahunt E, Coughlan GF, Caulfield B, et al. Inclusion criteria when investigating insufficiencies in chronic ankle instability. Med Sci Sports Exerc 2010;42(11):2106–21.
39. Hiller CE, Kilbreath SL, Refshauge KM. Chronic ankle instability: evolution of the model. J Athl Train 2011;46(2):133–41.
40. Hong CC, Tan KJ. Concepts of ankle instability: A review. OA Sports Medicine 2014;2(1):3.
41. Hiller CE, Nightingale EJ, Lin CW, et al. Characteristics of people with recurrent ankle sprains: a systematic review with meta-analysis. Br J Sports Med 2011;45(8):660–72.
42. Freeman MA, Dean MR, Hanham IW. The etiology and prevention of functional instability of the foot. J Bone Joint Surg Br 1965;47(4):678–85.
43. Wikstrom EA, Naik S, Lodha N, et al. Bilateral balance impairments after lateral ankle trauma: a systematic review and meta-analysis. Gait Posture 2010;31(4):407–14.

44. Doherty C, Bleakley C, Delahunt E, et al. Treatment and prevention of acute and recurrent ankle sprain: an overview of systematic reviews with meta-analysis. Br J Sports Med 2017;51(2):113–25.

45. Doherty C, Bleakley C, Hertel J, et al. Dynamic balance deficits in individuals with chronic ankle instability compared to ankle sprain copers 1 year after a first-time lateral ankle sprain injury. Knee Surg Sports Traumatol Arthrosc 2016;24(4):1086–95.

46. Doherty C, Bleakley C, Hertel J, et al. Single-leg drop landing movement strategies in participants with chronic ankle instability compared with lateral ankle sprain 'copers. Knee Surg Sports Traumatol Arthrosc 2016;24(4):1049–59.

47. Doherty C, Bleakley C, Hertel J, et al. Coordination and symmetry patterns during the drop vertical jump, 6-months after first-time lateral ankle sprain. J Orthop Res 2015;33(10):1537–44.

48. Beynnon BD, Murphy DF, Alosa DM. Predictive factors for lateral ankle sprains: a literature review. J Athl Train 2002;37(4):376–80.

49. McKay GD, Goldie PA, Payne WR, et al. Ankle injuries in basketball: injury rate and risk factors. Br J Sports Med 2001;35(2):103–8.

50. Milgrom C, Shlamkovitch N, Finestone A, et al. Risk factors for lateral ankle sprain: a prospective study among military recruits. Foot Ankle 1991;12(1):26–30.

51. Hertel J. Functional anatomy, pathomechanics, and pathophysiology of lateral ankle instability. J Athl Train 2002;37(4):364–75.

52. Verhagen EA, van Tulder M, van der Beek AJ, et al. An economic evaluation of a proprioceptive balance board training programme for the prevention of ankle sprains in volleyball. Br J Sports Med 2005;39(2):111–5.

53. Kucera KL, Marshall SW, Wolf SH, et al. Association of injury history and incident injury in cadet basic military training. Med Sci Sports Exerc 2016;48(6):1053–61.

54. Guillo S, Bauer T, Lee JW, et al. Consensus in chronic ankle instability: aetiology, assessment, surgical indications and place for arthroscopy. Orthop Traumatol Surg Res 2013;99(8 Suppl):S411–9.

55. Gribble PA, Hertel J, Denegar CR, et al. The effects of fatigue and chronic ankle instability on dynamic postural control. J Athl Train 2004;39(4):321–9.

56. Gribble PA, Hertel J, Denegar CR. Chronic ankle instability and fatigue create proximal joint alterations during performance of the Star Excursion Balance Test. Int J Sports Med 2007;28(3):236–42.

57. Vega J, Malagelada F, Dalmau-Pastor M. Ankle microinstability: arthroscopic findings reveal four types of lesion to the anterior talofibular ligament's superior fascicle. Knee Surg Sports Traumatol Arthrosc 2021;29(4):1294–303.

58. Vega J, Malagelada F, Manzanares Céspedes MC, et al. The lateral fibulotalocalcaneal ligament complex: an ankle stabilizing isometric structure. Knee Surg Sports Traumatol Arthrosc 2020;28(1):8–17.

59. Vega J, Peña F, Golanó P. Minor or occult ankle instability as a cause of anterolateral pain after ankle sprain. Knee Surg Sports Traumatol Arthrosc 2016;24(4):1116–23.

60. Takao M, Innami K, Matsushita T, et al. Arthroscopic and magnetic resonance image appearance and reconstruction of the anterior talofibular ligament in cases of apparent functional ankle instability. Am J Sports Med 2008;36(8):1542–7.

61. Doherty C, Bleakley C, Hertel J, et al. Recovery from a first-time lateral ankle sprain and the predictors of chronic ankle instability: a prospective cohort analysis. Am J Sports Med 2016;44(4):995–1003.

62. Lin CI, Houtenbos S, Lu YH, et al. The epidemiology of chronic ankle instability with perceived ankle instability- a systematic review. J Foot Ankle Res 2021; 14(1):41.
63. Donovan L, Hetzel S, Laufenberg CR, et al. Prevalence and impact of chronic ankle instability in adolescent athletes. Orthop J Sports Med 2020;8(2). 2325967119900962.
64. Saltzman CL, Salamon ML, Blanchard GM, et al. Epidemiology of ankle arthritis: report of a consecutive series of 639 patients from a tertiary orthopaedic center. Iowa Orthop J 2005;25:44–6.
65. Valderrabano V, Hintermann B, Horisberger M, et al. Ligamentous posttraumatic ankle osteoarthritis. Am J Sports Med 2006;34(4):612–20.
66. Valderrabano V, Horisberger M, Russell I, et al. Etiology of ankle osteoarthritis. Clin Orthop Relat Res 2009;467(7):1800–6.
67. Saltzman CL, Zimmerman MB, O'Rourke M, et al. Impact of comorbidities on the measurement of health in patients with ankle osteoarthritis. J Bone Joint Surg Am 2006;88(11):2366–72.
68. Khor YP, Tan KJ. The anatomic pattern of injuries in acute inversion ankle sprains: a magnetic resonance imaging study. Orthop J Sports Med 2013;1(7). 2325967113517078.
69. Takao M, Uchio Y, Naito K, et al. Arthroscopic assessment for intra-articular disorders in residual ankle disability after sprain. Am J Sports Med 2005;33(5): 686–92.
70. Taga I, Shino K, Inoue M, et al. Articular cartilage lesions in ankles with lateral ligament injury. An arthroscopic study. Am J Sports Med 1993;21(1):120–6 [discussion: 126-7].
71. May NR, Driscoll M, Nguyen S, et al. Analysis of return to play after modified broström lateral ankle ligament reconstruction. Orthop J Sports Med 2022;10(2). 23259671211068541.
72. Murray C, Marshall M, Rathod T, et al. Population prevalence and distribution of ankle pain and symptomatic radiographic ankle osteoarthritis in community dwelling older adults: a systematic review and cross-sectional study. PLoS One 2018;13(4):e0193662.
73. Drawer S, Fuller CW. Propensity for osteoarthritis and lower limb joint pain in retired professional soccer players. Br J Sports Med 2001;35(6):402–8.
74. Kuijt MT, Inklaar H, Gouttebarge V, et al. Knee and ankle osteoarthritis in former elite soccer players: a systematic review of the recent literature. J Sci Med Sport 2012;15(6):480–7.
75. Turner AP, Barlow JH, Heathcote-Elliott C. Long term health impact of playing professional football in the United Kingdom. Br J Sports Med 2000;34(5):332–6.
76. Wikstrom EA, Hubbard-Turner T, McKeon PO. Understanding and treating lateral ankle sprains and their consequences: a constraints-based approach. Sports Med 2013;43(6):385–93.
77. Hirose K, Murakami G, Minowa T, et al. Lateral ligament injury of the ankle and associated articular cartilage degeneration in the talocrural joint: anatomic study using elderly cadavers. J Orthop Sci 2004;9(1):37–43.
78. Bischof JE, Spritzer CE, Caputo AM, et al. In vivo cartilage contact strains in patients with lateral ankle instability. J Biomech 2010;43(13):2561–6.
79. Caputo AM, Lee JY, Spritzer CE, et al. In vivo kinematics of the tibiotalar joint after lateral ankle instability. Am J Sports Med 2009;37(11):2241–8.
80. Hintermann B, Boss A, Schäfer D. Arthroscopic findings in patients with chronic ankle instability. Am J Sports Med 2002;30(3):402–9.

81. Wainright WB, Spritzer CE, Lee JY, et al. The effect of modified Broström-Gould repair for lateral ankle instability on in vivo tibiotalar kinematics. Am J Sports Med 2012;40(9):2099–104.

82. Shah S, Thomas AC, Noone JM, et al. Incidence and cost of ankle sprains in united states emergency departments. Sports Health 2016;8(6):547–52.

83. Hupperets MD, Verhagen EA, Heymans MW, et al. Potential savings of a program to prevent ankle sprain recurrence: economic evaluation of a randomized controlled trial. Am J Sports Med 2010;38(11):2194–200.

84. Goudswaard AN, Thomas S, Van den Bosch WJHM, et al. NHG-Standaard enkel-distorsie. In: Wiersma TJ, Boukes FS, Geijer RMM, et al, editors. NHG-standaar-den voor de huisarts 2009. Houten: Bohn Staflen van Loghum; 2009. p. 1101–8.

85. Lin CW, Uegaki K, Coupé VM, et al. Economic evaluations of diagnostic tests, treatment and prevention for lateral ankle sprains: a systematic review. Br J Sports Med 2013;47(18):1144–9.

86. Cooke MW, Marsh JL, Clark M, et al. CAST trial group. Treatment of severe ankle sprain: a pragmatic randomised controlled trial comparing the clinical effective-ness and cost-effectiveness of three types of mechanical ankle support with tubular bandage. The CAST trial. Health Technol Assess 2009;13(13):1–121, iii, ix-x.

87. White WJ, McCollum GA, Calder JD. Return to sport following acute lateral liga-ment repair of the ankle in professional athletes. Knee Surg Sports Traumatol Ar-throsc 2016;24(4):1124–9.

88. Lee K, Jegal H, Chung H, et al. Return to play after modified broström operation for chronic ankle instability in elite athletes. Clin Orthop Surg 2019;11(1):126–30.

89. Kerkhoffs GM, Van Dijk CN. Acute lateral ankle ligament ruptures in the athlete: the role of surgery. Foot Ankle Clin 2013;18(2):215–8.

90. Hong C.C., Calder J. Ability to return to sports after early lateral ligament repair of the ankle in 147 elite athletes. Knee Surg Sports Traumatol Arthrosc. 2022. https://doi.org/10.1007/s00167-022-07270-2. Epub ahead of print.

91. JLT specialty Ltd – Football injury analysis. Available at: https://northern-assessors.co.uk/2018/08/14/jlt-reveals-premier-league-injury-bill/. Accessed 6th October, 2022.

92. Janssen KW, Hendriks MR, van Mechelen W, et al. The cost-effectiveness of mea-sures to prevent recurrent ankle sprains: results of a 3-arm randomized controlled trial. Am J Sports Med 2014;42(7):1534–41.

Anatomy of the Ankle and Subtalar Joint Ligaments
What We Do Not Know About It?

Tiago Mota Gomes, MD, PhD[a], Xavier Martin Oliva, MD, PhD[b,c],*,
Elsa Viridiana Sanchez, MD[c], Sérgio Soares, MD, PhD(c)[a,d],
Tania Diaz, PhD[c]

KEYWORDS

- Ankle anatomy • Ankle ligaments • Subtalar ligaments
- Lateral ligamentous complex • Medial ligamentous complex

KEY POINTS

- Ankle and subtalar joint ligaments play an essential role in foot and ankle biomechanics and stability.
- Understanding of the ankle and subtalar joint ligaments is essential to recognize and manage of foot and ankle disorders.
- Anatomic variability affects anatomic and nonanatomic ligament reconstructions.
- Failure to reconstruct ligamentous complexes may lead to progressive ankle deformities.

INTRODUCTION

Ankle sprains are one of the most common musculoskeletal injuries and consultation motive, which ensues a great social and health-care liability.[1,2] Most ankle sprains occur during physical activity, and the inversion of the foot is the most common injury mechanism.[3] Knowledge on ankle anatomy is of utmost importance to physicians who attend these issues because it is vital for a correct intervention on the healing process.

The ankle joint is mainly stabilized by the lateral ligamentous complex and MCL.[4]

The lateral collateral ligament is composed by 3 ligaments: posterior talofibular ligament (PTFL), anterior talofibular ligament (ATFL), and calcaneofibular ligament (CFL).[5] The ATFL and CFL are key structures in assuring lateral ankle stability.[5] ATFL's

[a] Foot and Ankle Unit, Department of Anatomy and Human Embryology, Faculty of Medicine, University of Barcelona, Barcelona, Spain; [b] Department of Orthopedics, Clinica Del Remei, Barcelona, Spain; [c] Department of Anatomy and Human Embryology, Faculty of Medicine, University of Barcelona, Barcelona, Spain; [d] Department of Orthopaedics, Hôpital Fribourgeois, Villars-sur-Glâne, Switzerland
* Corresponding author. Foot and Ankle Unit, Department of Anatomy and Human Embryology, Faculty of Medicine, University of Barcelona, Carrer de Casanova, 143, Barcelona 08036, Spain.
E-mail address: Xmoliva@icloud.com

Foot Ankle Clin N Am 28 (2023) 201–216
https://doi.org/10.1016/j.fcl.2022.12.003
1083-7515/23/© 2022 Elsevier Inc. All rights reserved.

isolated rupture is found in most ankle sprains (66%–80%). However, a combined rupture of ATFL and CFL only occurs in 20%.[6] Although most patients presenting an acute ankle sprain respond well to conservative treatment, about 20% to 40% develop some degree of ankle instability.[7]

Several surgical techniques have been described throughout the years fluctuating from ATFL and CFL direct repair to autograft or allograft reconstruction.[8] Anatomic stabilization techniques have demonstrated superiority to nonanatomic. The gold standard of this reconstruction is the modified Broström technique with excellent results reported.[9] However, poor outcomes have been reported in the literature with reports of recurrent instability in 16% of cases. In some cases, this technique is not available to surgeons due to ligament deficiency or low quality.[10] Therefore, anatomic reconstruction of these ligaments is indicated with tendon grafts.[11] Moreover, there is a widespread consensus among surgeons on anatomic placement of tunnels and grafts.[11]

It has been stated that the CFL has an important role in subtalar stability.[12] The precise concept and cause of subtalar instability remains uncertain and a topic of debate in the literature. Proposed theories include tears of different ligaments (CFL, cervical ligament [CL], or interosseous talocalcaneal). However, the association of CFL tears and subtalar instability is still not clear because different reports state that it only affects ankle stability.[13]

The medial ankle ligament complex is composed by the deltoid ligament. It was first described in the 1920s.[14] This complex is primarily responsible for stabilizing the medial side of the ankle anteriorly and posteriorly, limiting talar abduction and limiting hindfoot eversion.[15–21]

However, we must not forget in ankle instability the role of the anterior and posterior syndesmotic ligaments because they act as stabilizers of the joint.[4,22]

The objective of this report is to describe the anatomy of the ligamentous complexes of the ankle and subtalar joints.

ANATOMY
Tibiofibular or Syndesmotic Ligaments

The distal part of the tibia and fibula articulate through the tibiofibular syndesmosis. This syndesmosis is a true articulation fixated by the tibiofibular ligaments ensuring the stability between both bones resisting axial, rotational, and translation forces. The syndesmosis is composed of 3 ligaments: the anterior tibiofibular ligament (ATiFL), the interosseous ligament, and the posterior tibiofibular ligament (PTiFL).[23]

Anterior tibiofibular ligament
The ATiFL (**Fig. 1**) has a trapezoid form. Its origin is at the anterolateral tibial tubercle (Tillaux-Chaput tubercle) and describes a distal and lateral course up insertion at the anterior edge of the fibula, to the Wagstaffe tubercle. Its fibular insertion extends almost continuously with the proximal attachment at the fibula of the ATFL.[22] The ATiFL has a multifascicular structure. Between its fascicles runs the perforating branch of the peroneal artery. This is of clinical importance in case of a ligamentous torsion with ATiFL rupture associated. The injury of this blood vessel produces an important hematoma and local tumefaction that is very striking and guides toward the diagnosis of ATiFL tear.[24]

The distal portion of the ATiFL also known as the Baset ligament, which seems to be independent fibers of the rest of the ligament. It is separated by a small orifice full of adipose tissue that individualizes it. The Baset ligament covers the anterolateral angle formed by the tibia and fibula staying physiologically in contact with the lateral edge of

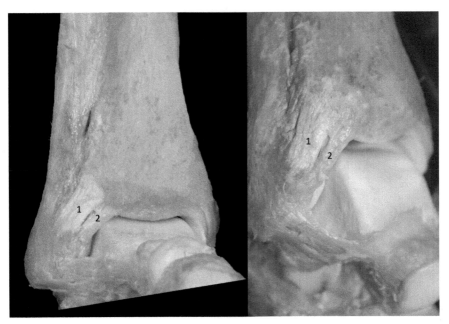

Fig. 1. Anterior ankle view. 1- ATiFL and 2- Baset ligament.

the talus when the ankle is in neutral position.[4] This anatomic detail must be known by surgeons performing ankle arthroscopy because it is a physiologic structure that under normal circumstances should not be resected because it is neither a cause of pain nor a pathology source. Moreover, Williams and colleagues,[25] in a cadaveric study, show the role of each syndesmotic ligament and state that the ATiFL is the one with the major contribution to the syndesmosis.

Interosseous ligament
The interosseous ligament represents the distal part of the interosseous membrane. It is short and thick, and we can identify it as a dense mass of fibers mixed with adipose tissue. Its vascularization is provided by branches of the peroneal artery.[26]

This ligament is located approximately 5 cm proximal to the center of the tibial pilon and approximately 7 cm proximal to the fibula tip and superior to the synovial recess. Most fibers have a lateral and distal direction from the tibia to the fibula. However, some of the superficial fibers run in the opposite direction (**Fig. 2**).[23,27]

The interosseous ligament may be considered the distal continuation of the interosseous membrane at the syndesmosis' level.[26]

There are authors who mention the interosseous ligament is not of great importance in the syndesmosis biomechanics.[28] However, it has been reported as an essential structure to ankle stability.[23]

Posterior tibiofibular ligament
The posterior tibiofibular ligament (PTiFL) is a historically controversial ligament about its description. Nonetheless, recent studies described it being formed by 2 independent components, superficial and deep layer; it is a multifascicular, compact, and strong ligament.[4,23] Furthermore, it has a trapezoid shape and a broad attachment to the lateral malleolus. This ligament mergers with the tibialis posterior tendon sheath medially and laterally with the peroneal tendon sheath.[24]

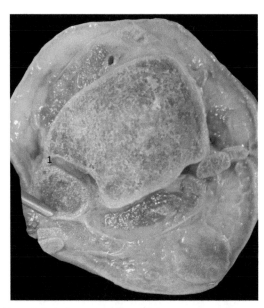

Fig. 2. Coronal ankle cut. 1- Interosseous ligament.

The superficial PiTFL fibers originate at the posterior edge of the lateral malleolus running proximal and medial obliquely to its insertion on the Volkman tubercle, located on the posterior and lateral aspect of the distal tibia.[29] The upper margin of the superficial PiTFL has approximately 17.3 mm of length while its lower margin has approximately 22.3 mm. Its tibial insertion width is approximately 17.5 mm while its lateral malleolus insertion is approximately 13.7 mm (**Fig. 3**).[4,23]

The deep PiTFL, also known as inferior transverse ligament, is denser compared with the superficial PiTFL and presents a condensed insertion site.[30] The deep layer has its origin on the posterior fibular fossa inserting in the margin of the posterior ridge of the tibia. Furthermore, it runs more horizontally than the superficial PiTFL (**Fig. 4**). This ligament has been described as a labrum-like extension of the posterior border of the tibial articular surface.[25] Its insertion is immediately posterior to the cartilaginous surface of inferior tibial articular surface because its fibers may reach the medial malleolus. This ligament increases the articular surface of the tibia apparently forming a true labrum. Moreover, it provides talocrural stability preventing mostly posterior translation of the talus.[4,23]

The length of the upper and lower margin of the deep PiTFL is approximately 25.3 mm and 26.2 mm, respectively. Its tibial insertion width is approximately 5.2 mm while its lateral malleolus insertion is approximately 3.2 mm.[25]

According to Martins and colleagues, the angle between the 2 components of the PiTFL is approximately 20.9°. The angle between the tibial articular surface with the superficial component is approximately 33.6° and with the deep component is approximately 13.1°.[23]

Intermalleolar Ligament

The intermalleolar ligament (IML) is located between the deep PiTFL and the PTFL running obliquely from lateral to medial and from distal to proximal (see **Fig. 3**).[4] Its shape varies from a thin fibrous band to a thick cordlike structure. This variation

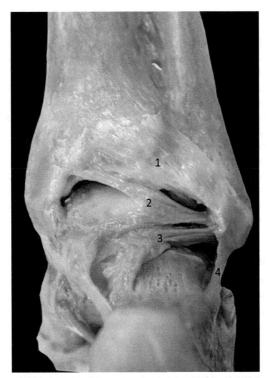

Fig. 3. Posterior ankle view. 1- Superficial PiTFL; 2- deep PiTFL; 3- IML; and 4- PTFL.

may be due to medial arising sites, the number of fiber bundles, and compactness of the bundle. The medial arising sites of the ligament have been located at the lateral border of the medial malleolar sulcus, the medial border of the medial malleolar sulcus through the septum between the flexor digitorum longus and posterior tibial tendons,

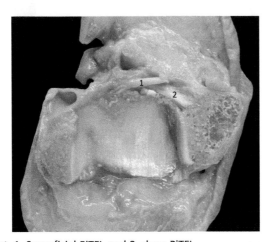

Fig. 4. Coronal cut. 1- Superficial PiTFL and 2- deep PiTFL.

the posterior distal margin of the tibia, the joint membrane covering the posterior process of the talus, and the floor of the flexor hallux longus' tunnel.[23,24,31]

The bundles of fibers are reported to converge laterally into a discrete cord on the PTFL near the lateral malleolus running into the medial fossa of the lateral malleolus alongside the PTFL.[26,27]

The IML has been reported with a prevalence up to 82.4%. However, its presence may vary from study-to-study existing conflicting reports in the literature stating this ligament may be an occasional finding.[28,32] Moreover, its nomenclature is also under some controversy because authors prefer using Paturet and colleagues[23,32,33] nomenclature, "posterior intermalleolar ligament."

This ligament has been proposed as a cause of soft tissue posterior impingement. This syndrome causes posterior ankle pain when plantar flexion occurs. Besides the ligament described, it is important to highlight the synovial recess. This recess has its anterior and posterior limits defined by the bony crests of the fibularis tibiae notch, which is concave, it is a space covered by synovial tissue with its origin in the tibiotalar articular line arriving proximal to the distal border of the IML.[23]

Lateral Ligamentous Complex

The lateral ligamentous complex (LLC) unites the fibula with the talus and calcaneus and provides stability on the lateral aspect of the ankle. It is the ligamentous complex most easily injured in the lower limb as ankle sprains (supination torsion) cause the rupture of this ligament.[34] The LLC is composed by 3 distinct ligaments: The ATFL, the CFL, and the PTFL.[35]

Anterior talofibular ligament

The ATFL is a flat, elongated ligament that controls anterior translation of the talus and is closely related to the ankle joint capsule.[36] It is the most easily injured ligament with supination torsion of the ankle.[37] In most cases, this ligament is composed of 2 bundles clearly differentiated.[38] Between them runs a branch of the peroneal artery that would be the responsible for the hematoma produced in the lateral side of the ankle when an injury of this ligament occurs (**Fig. 5**).[36,39]

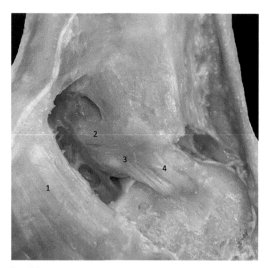

Fig. 5. Anterolateral ankle view. 1- IER; 2- ATFL; 3- connecting fibers; and 4- CFL.

The ATFL plays an important role in holding the tibia and fibula in place and prevent extraneous fibular displacement and external talar rotation (inversion in plantar flexion and anterolateral translation of the talus in the socket).[40–42]

The ATFL extends from the anteroinferior border of the fibula to the neck of the talus 45° to 90° to the longitudinal axis of the tibia.[41] Its origin is approximately 10 mm proximal to the tip of the fibula and insertion is directly distal to the articular cartilage of the talus with an approximately length of 13 to 29 mm and an approximate width of 6 to 10 mm.[43]

The ATFL has been reported being composed of a different number of bands/bundles (single, double, or triple). A band is considered as a collection of fascicles separated by an interval that would allow the passage of vascular branches. The prevalence of the different bands is reported as variable in the literature. Single bundle up to 60%, double bundle approximately 80%, and triple bundle approximately 9%. The double bundle is composed of the superior and inferior fascicles. The triple bundle is composed of the superior, median, and inferior fascicles (**Fig. 6**).[44]

It is important that surgeons are aware of the anatomic characteristics and differences between bundles of the ATFL because it is reported that the superior bundle is the most frequently injured and it can be repaired by completely intra-articular arthroscopy. This bundle is injured by fibular detachment while its fibers are kept intact. This is the reason why, in most cases, the repair may be done anchoring it to its original bony landmark.[32,38]

Calcaneofibular ligament

The CFL has been described as a cordlike or flat and fanning bundle.[45,46] It crosses the tibiotalar and subtalar articulations acting as a stabilizer for both. Most of the ligament is covered by the peroneal sheath with approximately 1 cm not covered.[28,47] It originates from below the insertion of the inferior bundle of the ATFL at the short tip of the lower segment of the deep aspect of the anterior border of the lateral malleolus. It has an oblique direction (posterior-inferior medial) inserting at the small tubercle at the

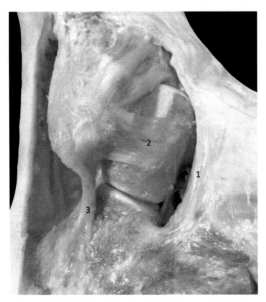

Fig. 6. Lateral ankle view. 1- IER; 2- double bundle ATFL; and 3- CFL.

posterior aspect of the lateral calcaneus surface with a reported length 1.85 to 3.58 cm (**Fig. 7**).[5]

Anatomic variations of the CFL have been reported in the literature. A single bundle (most frequent), a Y-shape double bundle, V-shape double bundle, and CFL associated with the lateral talocalcaneal ligament. The last 3 are reported as uncommon.[23]

The CFL and the inferior ATFL bundle are 2 different structures. However, they share a common fibular attachment and are connected by arciform fibers, forming an anatomic structure known as the lateral fibulotalocalcaneal ligamentous complex.[45,48] The arc-shaped fibers originate at the inferior border of the inferior ATFL bundle and the lateral portion of the talar body spanning distal and posteriorly to the anterior border of the CFL.[12] The isolated injury of this ligament is very rare. Its injury usually occurs concomitant with an ATFL injury during an ankle torsion in supination in 20% of lateral ankle sprains.[6] The CFL connection to the peroneal sheath conditionate the repair of this ligament, inflicting possible injuries to the peroneal vincula affecting the peroneal tendons vascularization.[47] The calcaneus extra-articular insertion increases the difficulty of its repair by arthroscopy because it is not always easy to visualize the footprint using the subtalar joint as a reference to find the CFL insertion.

Posterior talofibular ligament

The PTFL is the posterior component of the LLC. It has its origin in its articular pit in the posterior surface of the fibula and runs horizontally inserting on the posterior and lateral colliculus of the posterior tuberosity of the talus (see **Fig. 3**).[35] It has an approximately length of 25.8 to 27.3 mm and an approximate width of 6 mm.[19] The injury of this ligament is highly infrequent and usually occurs associated with high-energy mechanisms such as ankle luxation.[8,50] This ligament is responsible for the posterior translation of the fibula after a posterior malleolus fracture. It is clinically relevant because the anatomic reduction of the posterior malleolus facilitates the lateral malleolus fracture reduction.

A recent study by Kobaishi and colleagues revealed the presence of connecting fibers between the ATFL and PTFL at the articular tip of the fibula. They suggested this connection may be correlated with injury to the PTFL when an ATFL injury occurs. Moreover, they hypothesize that PTFL injury could exist in chronic ankle instability. These findings are relevant to surgeons because they should be careful with this ligament and could potentially improve surgical outcomes.[49]

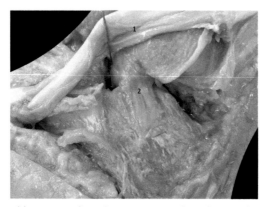

Fig. 7. CFL uncovered by peroneal tendons. 1- Peroneal tendons and 2- CFL.

Subtalar Ligaments

The subtalar joint consists of 2 bones: the talus and the calcaneus. The talus is located obliquely on the anterior surface of the calcaneus and has no muscle/tendinous insertions. The ligaments surrounding the subtalar joint can be divided into intrinsic and extrinsic ligaments (**Fig. 8**).[26]

The intrinsic ligaments are composed of the interosseous talocalcaneal ligament (ITCL), CL, and the anterior capsular ligament (ACaL).[13] The extrinsic ligaments are composed of the 3 components of the inferior extensor retinaculum (IER), lateral, medial, and intermediate. However, we must consider the CFL because it is the only ligament crossing both the tibiotalar and subtalar joints. Despite having a major role on the stability of the tibiotalar joint, this ligament is fundamental to the subtalar stability.[51]

The CL is the only subtalar ligament easily visualized in the anterior part of the tarsal sinus, whereas the ITCL, ACaL, and IER are difficult to assess because they remain in the posterior part of the tarsal sinus.[13] Perhaps, this may be the cause for the different descriptions, location, and nomenclature found in the literature about the subtalar ligaments.[52]

Intrinsic ligaments

The CL can be described as a thin structure in the tarsal sinus in front of the IER. This ligament has been found wider than the ATFL and ITFL and located anterior to the IER. This ligament has an intimate relation to the posterior surface of calcaneus-navicular joint capsule.[53]

Both footprints of the CL are in the tarsal sinus. The calcaneus footprint is located at the superior anterolateral surface of the calcaneus while the talus footprint is located at the medial surface of the talus neck approximately 2.8 mm posterior to the talonavicular joint cartilage.[13,53]

The ACaL runs vertical to the calcaneus surface. It has been described as a rectangular bundle when found in the anterior part of the posterior subtalar joint capsule, at the level of the anterior border of this joint.[26,54] However, conflicting reports of its prevalence remain in the literature.

The ITCL remains anterior to the ACaL has been described in a Y and V shape located in the tarsal canal running in an oblique direction with a length varying from 10.7 to 11 mm.[13]

Extrinsic ligaments

The CFL is the only ligament that crosses the tibiotalar and subtalar joint. The CFL acts to restraint to anterolateral ankle laxity with assistance of the lateral talocalcaneal

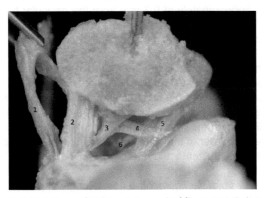

Fig. 8. Subtalar ligaments. 1- Lateral IER root; 2- cervical ligament; 3- intermediate IER root; 4- medial IER root; 5- ACaL; and 6- interosseous ligament.

ligament. The CFL provides stability to the subtalar joint when the ankle is neutral dorsiflexion-plantarflexion and restricts the adduction when the ankle is in neutral position and in dorsiflexion.[45]

The IER is found in the lateral surface of the Chopart joint. Three divisions of the IER can be described: medial, intermediate, and lateral root.[26]

The lateral root can be found attached to the lateral border of the tarsal sinus running to the calcaneus superolateral facet. Medial to the lateral root lays the intermediate root and medial to it lays the medial root.[13,53]

The medial root runs from the IER to the tarsal sinus, it penetrates the tarsal canal, and it finally inserts in the talus and calcaneus, almost in contact with the ITCL insertion on the talus and calcaneus.[13,26,53]

The medial root insertion on the calcaneus has a V-shape inside the tarsal canal. This insertion is reported as constant meanwhile the talus insertion has a 75% incidence. The layout described for this root is fundamental in stabilizing the subtalar joint as well as its dynamic roll due to the extensor tendons action.[13]

Medial Ligamentous Complex

The MCL consists of the deltoid ligament. This complex is responsible for stabilizing the medial side of the ankle anteriorly and posteriorly, limiting talar abduction and hindfoot eversion.[15–21]

Throughout the years, various anatomic descriptions of its components have been made.[15,55–59] Nonetheless, the most recent cadaveric studies about the anatomy of the deltoid ligament have become more consistent with their description. These components have been described as contiguous and very difficult to differentiate because they are covered by the ligamentous sheaths of the posterior tibialis and flexor digitorum tendons.[28,59] This components caracteristics are considered the main reason for the different nomenclature and identification of the deltoid ligament components.[60,61]

The deltoid ligament has been reported consistently to present up to 6 individual ligamentous bands.[26,55–57,59–63] These ligamentous bands are divided in 2 layers: a superficial and a deep one.

Superficial layer of the deltoid ligament

Tibionavicular ligament: It has its origin at the anterior border of the anterior colliculus approximately at 16.1 mm of the distal center of the intercollicular groove and extends to the dorsomedial side of the navicular closely anterior to the talonavicular articular cartilage border at approximately at 9.7 mm from the navicular tuberosity (**Fig. 9**).[15] This Ligament is the most anterior aspect of the superficial deltoid ligaments.

Tibiospring ligament: It has its origin at the anterior border of the anterior colliculus approximately at 13.1 mm of the distal center of the intercollicular groove, proximal and posterior to the tibionavicular ligament. Moreover, it inserts at the superomedial border of the calcaneonavicular (spring) ligament with a width of approximately 5.9 mm.[15] This ligament is the most superficial of the superficial deltoid ligaments.

Tibiocalcaneal ligament: It has its origin at the medial border of the anterior colliculus approximately at 6.0 mm of the distal center of the intercollicular groove. Moreover, it inserts at the posterior border of the sustentaculum tali at 8.0 mm approximately from the posterior point of the sustentaculum tali and at the superomedial calcaneonavicular ligament.[15]

Superficial posterior tibiotalar ligament: It has its origin approximately at 3.5 mm of the distal center of the intercollicular groove and inserts at the posteroinferior medial talar body at 10.4 mm approximately to the anterosuperior to the posterior medial talar

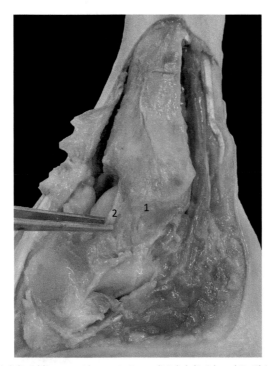

Fig. 9. Superficial deltoid ligament layer. 1- Superficial deltoid and 2- tibiocalcaneal bundle.

tubercle. This ligament is the most posterior aspect of the superficial deltoid ligaments.[15]

Deep layer of the deltoid ligament
Deep anterior tibiotalar ligament: It has its location immediately deep to the tibionavic-ular and tibiospring ligaments (**Fig. 10**). Its origin is located at the tip of the anterior col-liculus and the anterior part of the intercollicular groove approximately at 11.1 mm from the distal center of the intercollicular groove. Moreover, it inserts on the antero-superior portions of the medial talar body 12.2 mm posteroinferior to the anteromedial corner of the trochlea.[15]

    Deep posterior tibiotalar ligament: It has its location immediately deep to the tibion-calcaneal and superficial posterior tibiotalar ligaments. Its origin is located at the inter-collicular sulcus, the posterior colliculus, and the upper segment of the posterior surface of the anterior colliculus, 7.6 mm from the distal center of the intercollicular groove. Its insertion is located at the posterosuperior aspect of the medial talar body inferior to the trochlea articular cartilage, 17.9 mm anterosuperior to the poster-omedial talar body.[15]

    The prevalence of each ligamentous band has been reported in the literature as var-iable as well as anatomic variants reported.[60] The most noticeable variation concerns the tibiocalcaneal bundle because it could be the most important to be reconstructed in cases of medial ankle instability.

    A recent study by Guerra-Pinto and colleagues with a large sample assessed the morphology and prevalence of this bundle. The authors identified an anatomic variant where in absence of the tibiocalcaneal bundle, the tibiospring bundle would have a span of oblique fibers inserting in the *sustentaculum tali* (**Fig. 11**). This is particularly

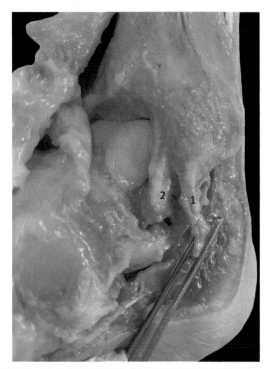

Fig. 10. Deep deltoid ligament layer. 1- Superficial deltoid and 2- deep deltoid.

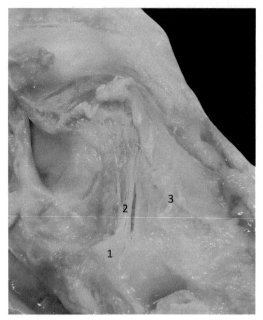

Fig. 11. Oblique deltoid ligament fibers running posteriorly from the tibiospring ligament to the sustentaculum tali anatomic variant. 1- Sustentaculum tali; 2- tibiocalcaneal bundle; and 3- tibiospring bundle.

relevant when reconstructing the deltoid ligament because the surgical technique should stabilize the tibiotalar and subtalar joints. Moreover, in cases of chronic medial instability, the reconstruction should obtain an alignment with the vertical axis of the tibia, which is the orientation of the tibiocalcaneal bundle. Besides, there is biomechanical data in the literature reporting a stabilizing effect of this ligament against supination in cases of concomitant lateral ligament injuries.[64,65]

The main reasons for the variability of the deltoid ligament complex might be author's own interpretation of what a band/bundle is, and the dissection method performed to visualize the complex. However, the growing consensus in the literature during the last years and a wide range of anatomic studies have been essential to uniformize a precise anatomic description of this ligament.

SUMMARY

Understanding of the ankle and subtalar joint ligaments is essential to recognize and manage foot and ankle disorders. The stability of both joints relies on the integrity of its ligaments. The ankle joint is stabilized by the lateral ligamentous complex and MCL while the subtalar joint is stabilized by its extrinsic and intrinsic ligaments. Most injuries to these ligaments are linked with ankle sprains. Inversion or eversion mechanics affect the ligamentous complexes. A profound knowledge of the ligament's anatomy allows orthopedic surgeons to further understand anatomic or nonanatomic reconstructions.

CLINICS CARE POINTS

- The CFL plays a fundamental role in the stability of both ankle and subtalar joints.
- Injuries of the subtalar joint ligaments, especially the interosseous and/or CLs, lead to subtalar instability; nonetheless, they play a major role in chronic ankle instability.
- The syndesmotic ligaments anatomy is fundamental to the stabilization of the talotibiofibular joint and plays a fundamental role in the malleolar fractures treatment.

DISCLOSURE

The authors have nothing to disclose.

REFERENCES

1. Fong DT-P, Man C-Y, Yung PS-H, et al. Sport-related ankle injuries attending an accident and emergency department. Injury 2008;39(10):1222–7.
2. Mulcahey MK, Bernhardson AS, Murphy CP, et al. The epidemiology of ankle injuries identified at the National Football League Combine, 2009-2015. Orthop J Sport Med 2018;6(7). 2325967118786227.
3. Gribble P, Bleakley C, Caulfield BM. 2016 consensus statement of the InternationalAnkle Consortium: prevalence, impact and long-termconsequences of lateral ankle sprains. Br J Sports Med 2016;50: 1493–5.
4. Hermans JJ, Beumer A, De Jong TAW, et al. Anatomy of the distal tibiofibular syndesmosis in adults: a pictorial essay with a multimodality approach. J Anat 2010; 217(6):633–45.
5. Matsui K, Takao M, Tochigi Y, et al. Anatomy of anterior talofibular ligament and calcaneofibular ligament for minimally invasive surgery: a systematic review. Knee Surg Sports Traumatol Arthrosc 2017;25(6):1892–902.

6. Fong DT-P, Hong Y, Chan L-K, et al. A systematic review on ankle injury and ankle sprain in sports. Sports Med 2007;37(1):73–94.
7. Drakos M, Hansen O, Kukadia S. Ankle instability. Foot Ankle Clin 2022;27(2): 371–84.
8. Bäcker H, Krause FG, Attinger MC. Treatment of chronic lateral ankle instability - a review, JSM Foot Ankle 2017;2(1):1–8.
9. Broström L. Sprained ankles. V. Treatment and prognosis in recent ligament ruptures. Acta Chir Scand 1966;132(5):537–50.
10. Cao Y, Hong Y, Xu Y, et al. Surgical management of chronic lateral ankle instability: a meta-analysis. J Orthop Surg Res 2018;13(1):159.
11. Glazebrook M, Eid M, Alhadhoud M, et al. Percutaneous ankle reconstruction of lateral ligaments. Foot Ankle Clin 2018;23(4):581–92.
12. Pereira BS, van Dijk CN, Andrade R, et al. The calcaneofibular ligament has distinct anatomic morphological variants: an anatomical cadaveric study. Knee Surg Sports Traumatol Arthrosc 2020;28(1):40–7.
13. Michels F, Matricali G, Vereecke E, et al. The intrinsic subtalar ligaments have a consistent presence, location and morphology. Foot Ankle Surg 2021;27(1): 101–9.
14. Toldt C, Hochstetter F. Anatomischer Atlas Für Studierende Und Ärzte: G. Die Nervenlehre; H. Die Sinneswerkzeuge. German: Urban Und Schwarzenberg.; 1921.
15. Campbell KJ, Michalski MP, Wilson KJ, et al. The ligament anatomy of the deltoid complex of the ankle: a qualitative and quantitative anatomical study. J Bone Joint Surg Am 2014;96(8):1–10.
16. Earll M, Wayne J, Brodrick C, et al. Contribution of the deltoid ligament to ankle joint contact characteristics: a cadaver study. Foot Ankle Int 1996;17(6):317–24.
17. Harper MC. An anatomic study of the short oblique fracture of the distal fibula and ankle stability. Foot Ankle 1983;4(1):23–9.
18. Harper MC. Deltoid ligament: an anatomical evaluation of function. Foot Ankle 1987;8(1):19–22.
19. Harper M. The deltoid ligament. An evaluation of need for surgical repair. Clin Orthop Relat Res 1988;(226):156–68.
20. Lauge-Hansen N. Ligamentous ankle fractures; diagnosis and treatment. Acta Chir Scand 1949;97(6):544–50.
21. Lee SH, Jacobson J, Trudell D, et al. Ligaments of the ankle: normal anatomy with MR arthrography. J Comput Assist Tomogr 1998;22(5):807–13.
22. Khambete P, Harlow E, Ina J, et al. Biomechanics of the distal tibiofibular syndesmosis: a systematic review of cadaveric studies. Foot Ankle Orthop 2021;6(2). 24730114211012700.
23. Jamieson MD, Stake IK, Brady AW, et al. The calcaneofibular ligament has distinct anatomic morphological variants: an anatomical cadaveric study. Knee Surg Sports Traumatol Arthrosc 2021;27(4). 232596712110472.
24. Littlechild J, Mayne A, Harrold F, et al. A cadaveric study investigating the role of the anterior inferior tibio-fibular ligament and the posterior inferior tibio-fibular ligament in ankle fracture syndesmosis stability. Foot Ankle Surg 2020;26(5): 547–50.
25. Williams BT, Ahrberg AB, Goldsmith MT, et al. Ankle Syndesmosis: a qualitative and quantitative anatomic analysis. Am J Sports Med 2015;43(1):88–97.
26. Kelikian A. Sarrafian's anatomy of the foot and ankle: descriptive, topographic, and functional. Philadelphia: Lippincott Williams & Wilkins; 2011.

27. Standring S, Neil RB. In: Livingstone C, editor. Gray's anantomy: the anatomical basis of clinical practice. 40th edition. Edinburgh (Scotland): Elsevier; 2008.

28. Golanó P, Vega J, de Leeuw PAJ, et al. Anatomy of the ankle ligaments: a pictorial essay. Knee Surg Sports Traumatol Arthrosc 2016;24(4):944–56.

29. Jayatilaka MLT, Philpott MDG, Fisher A, et al. Anatomy of the insertion of the posterior inferior tibiofibular ligament and the posterior malleolar fracture. Foot Ankle Int 2019;40(11):1319–24.

30. Golanò P, Mariani PP, Rodríguez-Niedenfuhr M, et al. Arthroscopic anatomy of the posterior ankle ligaments. Arthroscopy 2002;18(4):353–8.

31. Martins CF, Miranda M, Cortegana IM, et al. Posteroinferior tibiofibular ligament – A cadaveric study. Foot Ankle Surg 2021;27(3):296–300.

32. Martin Oliva X, Méndez López JM, Monzo Planella M, et al. Anatomical relations of anterior and posterior ankle arthroscopy portals: a cadaveric study. Eur J Orthop Surg Traumatol 2015;25(3):577–81.

33. Paturet G. Traité d'anatomie humaine [A treatise on human anatomy], Masson, París (1951)

34. van Dijk C. On diagnostic strategies in patient with severe ankle sprain. Rodopi 1994;140–60.

35. Golano P, Vega J, de Leeuw P, et al. Anatomy of the ankle ligaments: a pictorial essay. Knee Surg Sports Traumatol Arthrosc 2010;18:557–69.

36. Sarrafian S. Anatomy of the foot and ankle. Descriptive, topographic, functional. 2nd edition. Philadelphia: Lippincott; 1993.

37. Renstrom F, Lynch S. Acute injuries of the ankle. Foot Ankle Clin 1999;4:697–711.

38. Matsui K, Oliva XM, Takao M, et al. Bony landmarks available for minimally invasive lateral ankle stabilization surgery: a cadaveric anatomical study. Knee Surg Sports Traumatol Arthrosc 2017;25(6):1916–24.

39. Milner C, Soames R. Anatomical variations of the anterior talofibular ligament of the human ankle joint. J Anat 1997;191:457–8.

40. Guerra-Pinto F, Côrte-Real N, Gomes TM, et al. Varus talar tilt combined with an internal rotation pivot stress assesses the supination instability vector in lateral ankle ligaments' injury — cadaver study. Foot Ankle Surg 2020;26(3):258–64.

41. Guerra-Pinto F, Côrte-Real N, Mota Gomes T, et al. Rotational instability after anterior talofibular and calcaneofibular ligament section: the experimental basis for the ankle pivot test. J Foot Ankle Surg 2018;57(6):1087–91.

42. van den Bekerom M, Oostra R, Golano P. The anatomy in relation to injury of the lateral collateral ligaments of the ankle: a current concepts review. Clin Anat 2008;21:619–26.

43. Kristen K-H, Seilern und Aspang J, Wiedemann J, et al. Reliability of ultrasonography measurement of the anterior talofibular ligament (ATFL) length in healthy subjects (in vivo), based on examiner experience and patient positioning. J Exp Orthop 2019;6(1):30.

44. Yang H, Su M, Chen Z, et al. Anatomic measurement and variability analysis of the anterior talofibular ligament and calcaneofibular ligament of the ankle. Orthop J Sport Med 2021;9(11):1–8.

45. Pereira BS, Andrade R, Espregueira-Mendes J, et al. Current concepts on subtalar instability. Orthop J Sport Med 2021;9(8). 232596712110213.

46. Wiersma PH, Griffioen FMM. Variations of three lateral ligaments of the ankle. A descriptive anatomical study. Foot Ankle Int 1992;2(4):218–24.

47. Mota Gomes T, Guerra-Pinto F, Soares S, et al. The vascularization of the peroneal tendons: an anatomic study. Foot Ankle Surg 2021;27(4):450–6.

48. Gould N, Seligson D, Gassman J. Early and late repair of lateral ligament of the ankle. Foot Ankle 1980;1(2):84–9.
49. Kobayashi T, Suzuki D, Kondo Y, et al. Morphological characteristics of the lateral ankle ligament complex. Surg Radiol Anat 2020;42(10):1153–9.
50. Peters JW, Trevino SG, Renstrom PA. Chronic lateral ankle instability. Foot Ankle 1991;12(3). https://doi.org/10.1177/107110079101200310.
51. Michels F, Clockaerts S, Van Der Bauwhede J, et al. Does subtalar instability really exist? A systematic review. Foot Ankle Surg 2020;26(2):119–27.
52. Poonja AJ, Hirano M, Khakimov D, et al. Anatomical study of the cervical and interosseous talocalcaneal ligaments of the foot with surgical relevance. Cureus 2017;9(6):e1382.
53. Bartoníček J, Rammelt S, Naňka O. Anatomy of the subtalar joint. Foot Ankle Clin 2018;23(3):315–40.
54. Li S-Y, Hou Z-D, Zhang P, et al. Ligament structures in the tarsal sinus and canal. Foot Ankle Int 2013;34(12):1729–36.
55. Pankovich AM, Shivaram MS. Anatomical basis of variability in injuries of the medial malleolus and the deltoid ligament: II. clinical studies. Acta Orthop Scand 1979;50(2):225–36.
56. Milner CE, Soames RW. The medial collateral ligaments of the human ankle joint: anatomical variations. Foot Ankle Int 1998;19(5):289–92.
57. Boss AP, Hintermann B. Anatomical study of the medial ankle ligament complex. Foot Ankle Int 2002;23(6):547–53.
58. Panchani S, Reading J, Mehta J. Inter and intra-observer reliability in assessment of the position of the lateral sesamoid in determining the severity of hallux valgus. Foot (Edinb) 2016;27:59–61.
59. Savage-Elliott I, Murawski CD, Smyth NA, et al. The deltoid ligament: an in-depth review of anatomy, function, and treatment strategies. Knee Surg Sports Traumatol Arthrosc 2013;21(6):1316–27.
60. Guerra-Pinto F, Fabian A, Mota T, et al. The tibiocalcaneal bundle of the deltoid ligament – Prevalence and variations. Foot Ankle Surg 2021;27(2):138–42.
61. Cain JD, Dalmau-Pastor M. Anatomy of the deltoid-spring ligament complex. Foot Ankle Clin 2021;26(2):237–47.
62. Stufkens SAS, van den Bekerom MPJ, Knupp M, et al. The diagnosis and treatment of deltoid ligament lesions in supination–external rotation ankle fractures: a review. Strategies Trauma Limb Reconstr 2012;7(2):73–85.
63. Mengiardi B, Pfirrmann CWA, Vienne P, et al. Medial collateral ligament complex of the ankle: MR appearance in asymptomatic subjects. Radiology 2007;242(3):817–24.
64. Yammine K. Evidence-based anatomy. Clin Anat 2014;27(6):847–52.
65. Jeong MS, Choi YS, Kim YJ, et al. Deltoid ligament in acute ankle injury: MR imaging analysis. Skeletal Radiol 2014;43(5):655–63.

Physical Examination of Ankle Sprain and Ankle Instability

Can We Really Divide It into Low and High Ankle Sprains?

Theodorakys Marín Fermín, MD[a],*,
Panagiotis D. Symeonidis, MD, PhD[b]

KEYWORDS

- Ankle sprain • Syndesmosis injury • Ankle instability • Clinical test
- Physical examination • Anterior drawer test • Squeeze test • Football soccer

KEY POINTS

- A comprehensive clinical examination and an early and accurate diagnosis are crucial for the successful management of low and high ankle sprains but have a limited value in the differential diagnosis between them.
- It is essential to examine both ankles for comparison. Significant variations of joint laxity exist among individuals, depending on genetics, age, and gender.
- The combination of tenderness on palpation over the anterior syndesmosis and positive Cotton and fibular translation tests are highly suggestive of a syndesmotic ankle injury.
- Based on the mechanism of injury, clinical examination plays an essential role in guiding further imaging and early diagnosis of low/high ankle instability.

INTRODUCTION

Ankle sprains are among the most frequent injuries between the normal population and athletes, accounting for 40% of them, especially in football, basketball, dancing, and running. Its incidence has been reported to range from 2 to 7 per 1000 person-years.[1,2] Similarly, syndesmotic or "high ankle" sprains are reported in 1 of every 5 athletes undergoing MRI evaluation after an acute ankle sprain and correlate with prolonged pain, dysfunction, and return to sports.[3–7] Syndesmotic injuries can be present as isolated lesions or concomitantly with ankle sprains and fractures. Associated

[a] Aspetar Orthopaedic and Sports Medicine Hospital, Inside Aspire Zone, Sports City Street, Al Buwairda St, 29222, Doha, Qatar; [b] St. Luke's Hospital, Panorama 55236, Thessaloniki, Greece
* Corresponding author.
E-mail address: theodorakysmarin@yahoo.com

Foot Ankle Clin N Am 28 (2023) 217–229
https://doi.org/10.1016/j.fcl.2022.12.004
1083-7515/23/© 2022 Elsevier Inc. All rights reserved.

foot.theclinics.com

syndesmosis compromise is encountered in almost one-quarter of ankle fractures and is linked with lateral and/or posterior malleoli fracture patterns and should always be evaluated in the presence of proximal fibular fractures.[8]

Conservative and surgical treatment options for acute lateral ankle ligament sprain and acute syndesmosis injury yield satisfactory outcomes.[9,10] However, despite its frequency, delayed diagnosis and chronicity result in poor prognosis, inferior outcomes, and a longer recovery.[11–13] Thus, a comprehensive clinical examination and an early and accurate diagnosis are crucial for a successful management.

PATHOMECHANICS

The most common mechanism of injury in an ankle sprain is supination/inversion with the ankle in plantar flexion and adduction. The anterior talofibular ligament (ATFL) is the most vulnerable among the ankle lateral ligament complex because it has the lowest load to failure. Its rupture compromises the stability of the ankle in anterior translation, internal rotation, and plantar flexion.[14] A combined injury to the calcaneofibular ligament (CFL) can further contribute to inversion instability.[15] More than two-thirds of the patients who sustained an acute ankle sprain develop chronic ankle instability due to mechanical ligament insufficiency.[16] Mechanical insufficiency can lead to episodes of recurrent sprains, pain, sensory and motor deficits, fear of reinjury, and ligament attenuation.[17]

However, in the absence of fracture, there are 2 main mechanisms associated with a syndesmotic injury: (1) forceful external rotation and pronation of the foot during ankle dorsiflexion[6] and (2) hyperdorsiflexion of the ankle.[6] The former mechanism is now recognized as a "pivot-shift mechanism" due to the similarities shared with an anterior cruciate ligament injury pattern in pivoting or cutting sports with the forefoot fixed on the ground.[18] The talar rotation in the syndesmotic mortise forces the fibula to extreme external rotation and posterior translation, detaching it from the tibial notch.

This mechanism triggers consecutive disruption of the following ligamentous complex or osseous structures: the anteroinferior tibiofibular ligament (AITFL), deep deltoid ligament or medial malleolus, interosseous ligament, and posteroinferior tibiofibular ligament.[6] In contrast, hyper-dorsiflexion injuries lead to separation of the mortise because the wider anterior talar dome surface acts as a wedge.[19] The combination with a deltoid ligament disruption represents the most unstable variant among syndesmotic injury patterns.[6]

CLINICAL PRESENTATION

The presenting symptoms of lateral ankle ligament sprains are pain, edema, and ecchymosis, with or without the inability to bear weight fully. Although physical examination in the acute setting may cause additional discomfort, its performance is essential to rule out concomitant fractures of the malleoli and the base of the fifth metatarsal. The range of motion is often limited, and palpation over the involved ligaments can elicit tenderness. A second-look examination after the pain, edema, and safeguarding mechanisms subside is particularly valuable after the initial assessment, yielding a higher sensitivity.[20,21] A relevant world consensus conference identified delayed physical examination as the method of choice for combining high sensitivity and specificity in diagnosing ankle instability.[22]

The clinical presentation of an acute syndesmotic injury may be more complex. Similarly, patients with a syndesmotic injury present with ankle pain, effusion, limited dorsiflexion, ecchymoses, and inability to bear weight.[6,23–25] Typically, tenderness is located at the level of the distal tibiofibular syndesmosis. However, pain over the

ATFL can also be present in up to 40% of patients. Less frequently, concomitant medial pain during dorsiflexion or push-off during gait can coexist in these injuries.[6,23,24,26]

Conversely, symptoms of chronic ankle instability can persist beyond 6 months.[27] Patients present a "giving way" sensation of the ankle, recurrent sprains, permanent ankle pain, edema, locking, mechanical symptoms, and loss of range of motion.[28,29] Chronic ankle instability can develop after (1) a single sprain episode with persistent pain, (2) recurrent sprains with pain-free intervals, or (3) recurrent sprains with pain between intervals. In the latter, pain and perceived instability symptoms usually build up after each episode forcing the patient to seek medical advice.[29]

CLINICAL EXAMINATION

A battery of stress tests can aid in evaluating instability in the event of a lateral collateral ligament and/or syndesmotic complex injury (**Table 1**). Interestingly, it is difficult to find in the literature a detailed original description for most of the commonly used clinical tests for assessing posttraumatic ankle instability. As a result, clinicians worldwide may perform the same tests in a considerably variable manner, as depicted even in clinical photographs of relevant publications.[37,38] Regardless of these differences, physicians must adhere to the following general principles to optimize their clinical examination efficacy.[39]

1. Most tests are ambidextrous. As a rule, the examiner stabilizes parts of the hindfoot with one hand while applying force or performing a maneuver with the other.
2. Patient positioning is crucial. Unless the patients are examined and reviewed in the same position(s), no reliable clinical conclusions can be drawn. For the purposes of the current study, the descriptions of patient positioning represent the senior author's preference.
3. It is essential to examine both ankles for comparison. Significant variations of joint laxity exist among individuals, depending on genetics, age, and gender. Because this affects both limbs equally, a comparison to the contralateral side will give the clinician a better feel of an underlying instability compared with agreed cutoff values of normal upper limits.

Table 1		
Sensitivity and specificity of low and high ankle instability clinical diagnostic tests		
Diagnostic Test	**Sensitivity**	**Specificity**
Low ankle sprain-specific		
Anterior drawer test[30–32]	36–96	43–97
High ankle sprain-specific		
Syndesmosis palpation[33]	92%	-
Dorsiflexion[30]	50	57
Dorsiflexion lunge test[33]	75	-
Squeeze test[30,34,35]	30–100	14–93.5
Cotton test[30]	29	71
Fibula translation test[30]	64	57
External rotation stress test[23,34,36]	24–71	84.4
Crossed-legged test[33]	-	83
External rotation test[30]	50	0

4. Some clinical tests can be supplemented by simultaneous imaging studies, such as ultrasonography or fluoroscopy, which can improve their efficacy.[40] Each clinician needs to utilize all available modalities in their setting in order to improve their diagnostic accuracy.

Low/Supination Ankle Sprain-Specific Clinical Tests

- Anterior drawer test: The examination is best performed with the patient seated in an elevated position, the knee flexed, and the foot hanging free. This positioning allows for the gastrocnemius complex to relax (**Fig. 1**). This is particularly important as a taut gastrocnemius can dynamically stabilize the ankle and produce a false-negative test, especially in patients with equinism. The increased anterior translation is noted after stabilizing the tibial plafond and exerting an anterior force on the hindfoot from the calcaneus. A talar translation of more than 5 mm renders a test positive. In some cases, a visible sulcus is created at the level of the torn ATFL. The test's specificity can be improved with an additional internal rotation force, minimizing the contribution of a lax deltoid ligament to the anterior translation.[41]

Rather than a mere anterior translation of the talus, the drawer test represents a rotatory movement because the intact deltoid ligament prevents the talus from moving forward on the medial side. Therefore, the ideal anterior drawer test should combine a straightforward translation and an internal rotation movement.[42]

- Talar tilt test: A hindfoot inversion force is applied with the same patient positioning, eliciting lateral opening and pain (**Fig. 2**). In theory, the test can assess the integrity of both ATFL and CFL by positioning the foot in plantar flexion or dorsiflexion, respectively.[43,44] However, concerns exist regarding the contribution of the subtalar joint in the perceived displacement.[41] Angulation of greater than 23°

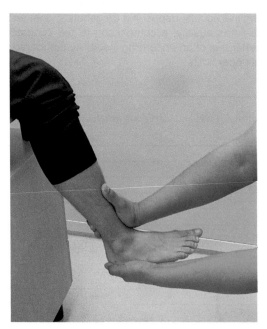

Fig. 1. Anterior drawer test.

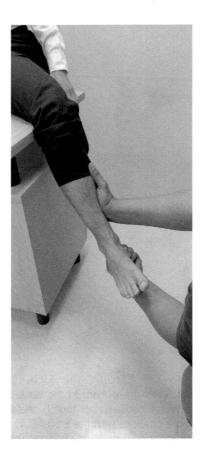

Fig. 2. Talar tilt test.

or a tilt of more than 10° as compared with the healthy side indicates insufficiency of both ligaments.[39]

High Ankle Sprain-Specific Clinical Tests

Clinical examination of syndesmotic injuries is challenging due to the lack of a gold-standard maneuver.[6,25,33] Specific tests can be harder to interpret in the acute phase and lack predictive value. However, they are essential in raising suspicion and guiding further imaging assessment in combination with a positive clinical history. The most commonly used tests are as follows:

- Tenderness on palpation over the anterior or posterior syndesmosis. Pain elicited on palpation is the test with the highest sensitivity.[33]
- Squeeze test: It consists of compression of the tibia and fibula in the mid-leg to evoke distal tibiofibular pain (**Fig. 3**). Patients with a positive squeeze test are as 9.5 times more likely to be unstable.[25,26,33]
- Cotton test[45]: The examiner stabilizes the hindfoot by locking the subtalar joint in a neutral position with the hand contralateral to the injury site. With the other hand, he applies a lateral translation of the talus within the tibiotalar fork. In a positive test, pain is elicited, and increased translation as compared with the healthy ankle is observed. Notably, the test can also be positive in deltoid ligament injuries.

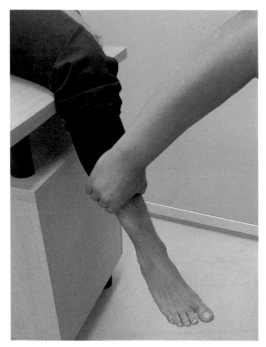

Fig. 3. Squeeze test.

- Fibular translation test: With the patient in the seated position, the physician grasps the lateral malleolus between his thumb and index and middle fingers and, while stabilizing the hindfoot with the ipsilateral hand, mobilizes the fibula in an anteroposterior translation (**Fig. 4**). In a normal syndesmosis, the movement

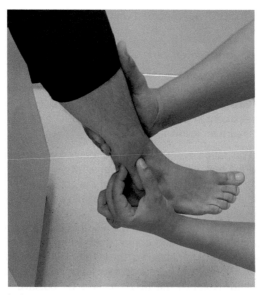

Fig. 4. Fibular translation test.

is limited with a firm endpoint. Increased movement with no firm endpoint, as compared with the contralateral side, suggests a ligamentous injury.

- Syndesmosis tenderness length: It entails the measurement of the distance from the distal tip of the fibula to the most proximal painful area on palpation between the tibia and fibula. The length of the tenderness relates to injury severity and a prolonged return to sports period.[6,23]

- Cross-legged test: The examiner asks the patient to cross the injured leg across the contralateral side resting the distal fibula on the opposite knee. Then, a gentle downward force is applied to the knee (**Fig. 5**). Pain elicited over the syndesmosis signifies a positive test.

- External rotation stress test: The physician exerts forced ankle dorsiflexion and external foot rotation for pain evaluation with the knee in 90° of flexion (**Fig. 6**). Pain in the syndesmosis joint area results in a positive test. It is the test with the most balanced sensitivity/specificity, and therefore, it has become a standard procedure to assess syndesmotic instability.[33]

- Single-leg jump test: The patient is asked to perform single-leg jumping with and without adhesive taping (stabilizing the syndesmotic complex). The test is considered positive if the patient can jump without pain when taped but painful without stabilization.

- Dorsiflexion lunge: The patient performs a lunge on the injured side, reaching as far as possible, and then it is repeated with the physician applying compression on the ankle syndesmosis. An increased range of motion or less pain is considered a positive test result.[25]

Currently, the combination of tenderness on palpation over the anterior syndesmosis and positive Cotton and fibular translation tests are highly suggestive of a

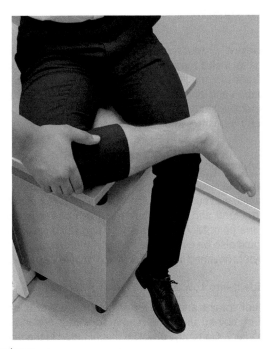

Fig. 5. Cross-legged test.

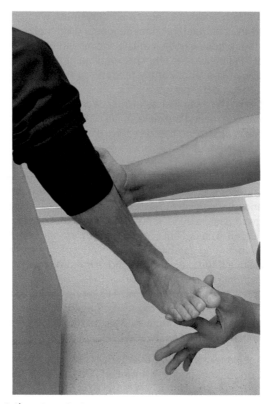

Fig. 6. External rotation stress test.

syndesmotic ankle injury.[6,46] As a result of a recent consensus, a diagnostic algorithm has been proposed that yields the highest clinical likelihood of syndesmotic injury and warrants further diagnostic imaging or arthroscopy.[33] It combines 2 highly sensitive tests (pain on palpation and dorsiflexion lunge) followed by the squeeze test. Moreover, a recent prospective study shows a significant association between an eversion injury mechanism and a positive squeeze test with a syndesmotic injury in the acute setting.[47]

Chronic Ankle Instability Clinical Tests

In the chronic setting, the clinical examination should also focus on the range of motion, including the ankle and subtalar joints. Areas of chronic pain should be identified and correlated with lateral and medial ankle ligamentous structures, peroneal tendons, and/or joint line pain. Moreover, predisposing factors such as hindfoot varus and arch height should also be evaluated.[28] Finally, the presence of anterior or posterior impingement symptoms and physical findings should be noted.

Can We Really Divide It into Low and High Ankle Sprains?

Lateral ankle ligament sprains and syndesmotic injuries are 2 different entities. However, they may be combined under the same spectrum depending on the arch of violence during the injury. Currently, physical examination in the acute setting cannot reliably discriminate between these 2 entities, neither in their isolated nor in their concomitant presentation.[37] However, it is fundamental to perform a thorough clinical examination in each case, order to raise suspicion on combined injuries and guide the subsequent imaging accordingly.

Clinical examination is, by definition, subjective. On top of that, the lack of standardization in the performance of most of the described clinical tests makes it difficult to conduct comparative, multicenter studies and undermines the value of meta-analyses. Characteristically, in their relevant textbook, van Dijk and Valderabano[37,38] describe in detail 3 ways in how *not* to perform the anterior drawer test, one of the essential tests in everyday clinical practice.

In an effort to increase their accuracy, certain tests can be performed under imaging. In the current practice, bedside ultrasonography is becoming part of standard care, particularly in ligamentous injuries and subtle instability. Among its advantages, it is fast, low-cost, and allows dynamic evaluation of the ankle ligaments without radiation exposure.[48] Moreover, the examiner can perform some of the aforementioned clinical tests under sonography. Recent studies have demonstrated 100% of sensitivity and specificity of the method when evaluating AITFL injuries.[48] However, its disadvantages comprise the limited value in assessing associated injuries and its user-dependent nature.[24,49]

Fluoroscopy can also be used simultaneously with some of the described tests such as the external rotation test. A recent meta-analysis of 5 studies showed that widening of the clear medial space of more than 1 mm compared with the uninjured side under fluoroscopy should be considered a syndesmotic instability.[50]

Finally, there have been efforts to develop disease-specific devices as an extension to available clinical tests. The so-called Syndhoo tool[24] is such a device for syndesmotic stability assessment, especially in grade II injuries. This device assesses, under dynamometric force exertion, the stability in dorsiflexion/external rotation on a rotating board while keeping the knee fixed. Preliminary studies demonstrate the high reliability of the method compared with arthroscopic evaluation.[24]

SUMMARY

Currently, the clinical examination has a limited value in the differential diagnosis between an acute ATFL rupture and a syndesmotic high ankle sprain. However, its use is indispensable for raising a high index of suspicion for detecting these injuries. Based on the mechanism of injury, clinical examination plays an essential role in guiding further imaging and early diagnosis of low/high ankle instability.

CLINICS CARE POINTS

- The presenting symptoms of lateral ankle ligament sprains are pain, edema, and ecchymosis, with or without the inability to bear weight fully.
- Physical examination in the acute setting may cause additional discomfort but its performance is essential to rule out concomitant fractures of the malleoli and the base of the fifth metatarsal.
- A second-look examination after the pain, edema, and safeguarding mechanisms subside is particularly valuable after the initial assessment, yielding a higher sensitivity.
- A comparison to the contralateral side will give the clinician a better feel of an underlying instability compared with agreed cutoff values of normal upper limits.
- The ideal anterior drawer test should combine a straightforward translation and an internal rotation movement. In some cases, a visible sulcus is created at the level of the torn ATFL.

> • The combination of tenderness on palpation over the anterior syndesmosis and positive Cotton and fibular translation tests are highly suggestive of a syndesmotic ankle injury.

CONTRIBUTIONS

T. Marín Fermín Conceptualization, Methodology, Validation, Investigation, Resources, Writing–Original Draft, Visualization.

P.D. Symeonidis Conceptualization, Methodology, Validation, Investigation, Writing–Review and Editing, Supervision, Project administration.

All authors contributed to the conception and design of the study; acquisition, analysis, and interpretation of the data; drafting the work and revising it critically for important intellectual content; agreed to be accountable for all aspects of the work in ensuring that questions related to the accuracy or integrity of any part of the study were appropriately investigated and resolved. All authors read and approved the final article.

DECLARATIONS OF INTEREST

None.

No ethics approval was required for the presented study.

FUNDING

None.

DATA AVAILABILITY STATEMENT

The data underlying this article are available in the article and its online supplementary material.

ACKNOWLEDGMENTS

Thanks to Dr Mohamed Elamin for his kind collaboration on the photographs for the present article.

REFERENCES

1. Herzog MM, Kerr ZY, Marshall SW, et al. Epidemiology of Ankle Sprains and Chronic Ankle Instability. J Athl Train 2019;54(6):603–10.
2. Waterman BR, Owens BD, Davey S, et al. The epidemiology of ankle sprains in the United States. J Bone Joint Surg Am 2010;92(13):2279–84.
3. Roemer FW, Jomaah N, Niu J, et al. Ligamentous injuries and the risk of associated tissue damage in acute ankle sprains in athletes: a cross-sectional MRI study. Am J Sports Med 2014;42:1549–57.
4. van den Bekerom MP. Diagnosing syndesmotic instability in ankle fractures. World J Orthop 2011;2(7):51–6.
5. Waldén M, Hägglund M, Ekstrand J. Time-trends and circumstances surrounding ankle injuries in men's professional football: an 11-year follow-up of the UEFA Champions League injury study. Br J Sports Med 2013;47(12):748–53.
6. D'Hooghe P, Alkhelaifi K, Abdelatif N, et al. From "low" to "high" athletic ankle sprains: a comprehensive review. Oper Tech Orthop 2018;28(2):54–60.

7. Lubberts B, D'Hooghe P, Bengtsson H, et al. Epidemiology and return to play following isolated syndesmotic injuries of the ankle: a prospective cohort study of 3677 male professional footballers in the UEFA Elite Club Injury Study. Br J Sports Med 2019;53(15):959–64.
8. Purvis GD. Displaced, unstable ankle fractures: classification, incidence, and management of a consecutive series. Clin Orthop Relat Res 1982;165:91–8.
9. Miller TL, Skalak T. Evaluation and treatment recommendations for acute injuries to the ankle syndesmosis without associated fracture. Sports Med 2014;44(2): 179–88.
10. Altomare D, Fusco G, Bertolino E, et al. Evidence-based treatment choices for acute lateral ankle sprain: a comprehensive systematic review. Eur Rev Med Pharmacol Sci 2022;26(6):1876–84.
11. Stenquist DS, Ye MY, Kwon JY. Acute and Chronic Syndesmotic Instability: Role of Surgical Stabilization. Clin Sports Med 2020;39(4):745–71.
12. Kent S, Yeo G, Marsland D, et al. Delayed stabilisation of dynamically unstable syndesmotic injuries results in worse functional outcomes. Knee Surg Sports Traumatol Arthrosc 2020;28(10):3347–53.
13. Miklovic TM, Donovan L, Protzuk OA, et al. Acute lateral ankle sprain to chronic ankle instability: a pathway of dysfunction. Phys Sportsmed 2018;46(1):116–22.
14. Slater K. Acute lateral ankle instability. Foot Ankle Clin 2018;23(4):523–37.
15. Hunt KJ, Pereira H, Kelley J, et al. The role of calcaneofibular ligament injury in ankle instability: implications for surgical management. Am J Sports Med 2019; 47(2):431–7.
16. Doherty C, Bleakley C, Hertel J, et al. Clinical tests have limited predictive value for chronic ankle instability when conducted in the acute phase of a first-time lateral ankle sprain injury. Arch Phys Med Rehabil 2018;99(4):720–5.e1.
17. Hur ES, Bohl DD, Lee S. Lateral Ligament Instability: Review of Pathology and Diagnosis. Curr Rev Musculoskelet Med 2020;13(4):494–500.
18. Tampere T, D'Hooghe P. The ankle syndesmosis pivot shift "Are we reviving the ACL story? Knee Surg Sports Traumatol Arthrosc 2021;29(11):3508–11.
19. Williams GN, Jones MH, Amendola A. Syndesmotic ankle sprains in athletes. Am J Sports Med 2007;35(7):1197–207.
20. van Dijk CN, Lim LS, Bossuyt PM, et al. Physical examination is sufficient for the diagnosis of sprained ankles. J Bone Joint Surg Br 1996;78(6):958–62.
21. Frey C, Bell J, Teresi L, et al. A comparison of MRI and clinical examination of acute lateral ankle sprains. Foot Ankle Int 1996;17(9):533–7.
22. van Dijk CN. Diagnosis of ankle sprain: history and physical examination. In: Chan KM, Karlsson J, editors. International Society of arthroscopy, knee Surgery and orthopaedic sports medicine—international Federation of sports medicine (ISAKOS–FIMS). World consensus conference on ankle instability. 2005. p. 21–2.
23. D'Hooghe P, York PJ, Kaux JF, et al. Fixation Techniques in Lower Extremity Syndesmotic Injuries. Foot Ankle Int 2017 Nov;38(11):1278–88.
24. D'Hooghe P, Bouhdida S, Whiteley R, et al. Stable versus unstable grade 2 high ankle sprains in athletes: a noninvasive tool to predict the need for surgical fixation. Clin Res Foot Ankle 2018;6(1):252–9.
25. Sman AD, Hiller CE, Refshauge KM. Diagnostic accuracy of clinical tests for diagnosis of ankle syndesmosis injury: a systematic review. Br J Sports Med 2013;47(10):620–8.
26. Calder JD, Bamford R, Petrie A, et al. Stable versus unstable grade II high ankle sprains: a prospective study predicting the need for surgical stabilization and time to return to sports. Arthroscopy 2016;32(4):634–42.

27. Terada M, Bowker S, Hiller CE, et al. Quantifying levels of function between different subgroups of chronic ankle instability. Scand J Med Sci Sports 2017; 27(6):650–60.

28. Tourné Y, Besse JL, Mabit C, et al. Chronic ankle instability. Which tests to assess the lesions? Which therapeutic options? Orthop Traumatol Surg Res 2010;96(4): 433–46.

29. Corte-Real N, Caetano J. Ankle and syndesmosis instability: consensus and controversies. EFORT Open Rev 2021 Jun 28;6(6):420–31.

30. Beumer A, Swierstra BA, Mulder PG. Clinical diagnosis of syndesmotic ankle instability: evaluation of stress tests behind the curtains. Acta Orthop Scand 2002;73(6):667–9.

31. Gribble PA. Evaluating and Differentiating Ankle Instability. J Athl Train 2019; 54(6):617–27.

32. Polzer H, Kanz KG, Prall WC, et al. Diagnosis and treatment of acute ankle injuries: development of an evidence-based algorithm. Orthop Rev (Pavia) 2012; 4(1):e5.

33. Netterström-Wedin F, Matthews M, Bleakley C. Diagnostic Accuracy of Clinical Tests Assessing Ligamentous Injury of the Talocrural and Subtalar Joints: A Systematic Review With Meta-Analysis. Sports Health 2022;14(3):336–47.

34. de César PC, Avila EM, de Abreu MR. Comparison of magnetic resonance imaging to physical examination for syndesmotic injury after lateral ankle sprain. Foot Ankle Int 2011;32(12):1110–4.

35. Nussbaum ED, Hosea TM, Sieler SD, et al. Prospective evaluation of syndesmotic ankle sprains without diastasis. Am J Sports Med 2001;29(1):31–5.

36. Schnetzke M, Vetter SY, Beisemann N, et al. Management of syndesmotic injuries: What is the evidence? World J Orthop 2016;7(11):718–25.

37. Niek van Dijk C, editor. Ankle arthroscopy: techniques developed by the amsterdam foot and ankle school. Heidelberg: Springer Berlin; 2014. https://doi.org/10.1007/978-3-642-35989-7.

38. Valderrabano V, Easley M, editors. Foot and ankle sports orthopaedics. Cham: Springer; 2014. https://doi.org/10.1007/978-3-319-15735-1_1.

39. Mahaffey D, Hilts M, Fileds KB. Ankle and foot injuries in sports. Clin Fam Pract 1999;1:233–50.

40. Mei-Dan O, Kots E, Barchilon V, et al. A dynamic ultrasound examination for the diagnosis of ankle syndesmotic injury in professional athletes: a preliminary study. Am J Sports Med 2009;37(5):1009–16.

41. Park DH, Singh D. Ankle Instability (Ankle Sprain). In: Bentley G, editor. European surgical orthopaedics and traumatology. Heidelberg: Springer Berlin; 2014. https://doi.org/10.1007/978-3-642-34746-7_221.

42. Kerkhoffs GM, Blankevoort L, Sierevelt IN, et al. Two ankle joint laxity testers: reliability and validity. Knee Surg Sports Traumatol Arthrosc 2005;13(8):699–705.

43. Frost SC, Amendola A. Is stress radiography necessary in the diagnosis of acute or chronic ankle instability? Clin J Sport Med 1999;9(1):40–5.

44. Chan KW, Ding BC, Mroczek KJ. Acute and chronic lateral ankle instability in the athlete. Bull NYU Hosp Jt Dis 2011;69(1):17–26.

45.. Cotton FJ. The ankle and foot. In: Cotton FJ, editor. *Dislocations and joint-fractures*. Philadelphia: WB Saunders Co; 1910. p. 535–88.

46. Hunt KJ, Phisitkul P, Pirolo J, et al. High Ankle Sprains and Syndesmotic Injuries in Athletes. J Am Acad Orthop Surg 2015;23(11):661–73.

47. Baltes TPA, Al Sayrafi O, Arnáiz J, et al. Acute clinical evaluation for syndesmosis injury has high diagnostic value. Knee Surg Sports Traumatol Arthrosc 2022; 30(11):3871–80.
48. Amendola A, Williams G, Foster D. Evidence-based approach to treatment of acute traumatic syndesmosis (high ankle) sprains. Sports Med Arthrosc Rev 2006;14(4):232–6.
49. Drijfhout van Hooff CC, Verhage SM, Hoogendoorn JM. Influence of fragment size and postoperative joint congruency on long-term outcome of posterior malleolar fractures. Foot Ankle Int 2015;36(6):673–8.
50. Spindler FT, Herterich V, Holzapfel BM, et al. A systematic review and meta-analysis on the value of the external rotation stress test under fluoroscopy to detect syndesmotic injuries. EFORT Open Rev 2022;7(10):671–9.

MRI in Acute Ankle Sprains

Should We Be More Aggressive with Indications?

Eun Hae Park, MD, PhD[a,b], Cesar de Cesar Netto, MD, PhD[c], Jan Fritz, MD, PD, RMSK[a,*]

KEYWORDS

- MRI • Ankle sprain • Ankle • Sprain • Ligamentous • Injuries

KEY POINTS

- Acute ankle sprains can be categorized based on the location into lateral ankle sprains, medial ankle sprains, or syndesmotic sprains.
- MRI is the most accurate test for noninvasively assessing the structural integrity and severity of deltoid, lateral collateral, and syndesmotic ligament injuries in acute ankle sprains.
- MRI adds value in confirming the absence or presence of ankle sprain–associated hindfoot and midfoot injuries, especially when subtle instability is suspected.

INTRODUCTION

An acute ankle sprain is a clinical term describing a spectrum of traumatic injuries, including stretching and partial or full-thickness tears of one or more of the capsuloligamentous structures of the ankle joint. Acute ankle sprains can be categorized based on the location into lateral ankle sprains, medial ankle sprains, or syndesmotic sprains.[1,2] Combined injuries of the different ligamentous complexes, such as combined medial and syndesmotic, as well as multidirectional and multiligamentous injuries, can also occur.

Acute ankle sprain injuries range among the most frequent sports injuries in recreational and professional athletes. Risk factors include high-velocity movements, jumps, cutting and torsion motions, abrupt accelerations and decelerations, and indoor courts with high-friction synthetic surfaces. Disciplines with higher rates of acute

[a] Division of Musculoskeletal Radiology, Department of Radiology, NYU Grossman School of Medicine, 660 1St Ave, 3rd Floor, New York, NY 10016, USA; [b] Department of Radiology, Jeonbuk National University Medical School, Jeonju, Republic of Korea; [c] Department of Orthopaedics and Rehabilitation, University of Iowa, 200 Hawkins Dr, Iowa City, IA 52242, USA
* Corresponding author.
E-mail address: jan.fritz@nyulangone.org

Foot Ankle Clin N Am 28 (2023) 231–264
https://doi.org/10.1016/j.fcl.2023.01.011
1083-7515/23/© 2023 Elsevier Inc. All rights reserved.

foot.theclinics.com

ankle sprains include basketball, volleyball, soccer, American football, and European handball.[3,4]

Acute ankle sprains typically involve the lateral collateral ligaments (LCL), with or without additional deltoid ligament injuries. High ankle sprains, by definition, include injuries to the syndesmotic ligaments. MRI is the most accurate imaging test for visualizing collateral and syndesmotic ligaments, assessing their integrity, and characterizing the number of ligaments involved and the severity of fiber disruption. However, conventional MRI in recumbent non–weight-bearing position represents a static test and may not detect the degree of ankle and syndesmotic instability involved with the associated ligamentous injuries. In addition, many ankle sprain injuries are treated conservatively,[5,6] questioning the added value of MRI assessment in acute ankle sprains.

In our practice, MRI adds value in confirming the absence or presence of associated hindfoot and midfoot injuries, especially when clinical examinations are challenging, radiographs are inconclusive, and subtle instability is suspected. MRI accurately detects and characterizes a spectrum of ankle sprain–associated injuries, including radiographically occult nondisplaced fractures; bone bruises; osteochondral lesions (OCLs); subtalar, spring ligament, sinus tarsi, and peritalar injuries; as well as tendon, nerve, and Lisfranc injuries.[7–9]

In this article, we review and illustrate the MRI appearances of the spectrum of ankle sprains and associated hindfoot and midfoot injuries.

MRI Technique

High-quality ankle MRI may be obtained with 1.5 and 3.0 Tesla (T) MRI scanners. Compared with 1.5 T scans, 3.0 T MRI scanners yield approximately twice the signal, which can be translated into higher spatial resolution for improved visibility of fine detail and faster MRI scans.[10,11] Dedicated boot-shaped surface coils improve the MRI signal further and are explicitly well-suited for clinical high spatial resolution MRI of the ankle, allowing visualization of submillimeter anatomic structures and detection of subtle tendinous and ligamentous injuries, as well as small OCLs.[12]

MRI protocols for evaluating acute ankle sprains typically consist of 5 pulse sequences with varying nonfat-suppressed and fat-suppressed contrast weightings to highlight anatomy versus signal abnormalities (**Fig. 1**) differentially. The inclusion of nonfat-suppressed and fat-suppressed pulse sequences is pivotal. Proton density and T2 contrasts display fluid as bright signal and hence are most powerful for visualizing a broad spectrum of injuries of cancellous bone and bone marrow, cortical bone, articular cartilage, synovium, ligaments, tendons, nerves, and vessels, as well as joint fluid.[10] Fat suppression is commonly applied to improve the conspicuity of bone marrow edema, soft tissue edema, small collections, and hematomas but comes at the expense of obscuring intrinsically dark structures, such as intact ligaments, for which nonfat-suppressed proton density– and T2-weighted pulse sequences are needed. T1-weighted MR images are fat-specific, displaying fat as bright and fluid as dark MRI signals. In acute ankle sprains, T1-weighted MR images are useful, but not required, for visualizing bone contusions and subtle nondisplaced fractures. However, the combination of nonfat-suppressed proton density–weighted pulse and fat-suppressed T2-weighted pulse MR images is equally powerful, and thus T1-weighted MR images can be omitted in ankle sprain protocols. However, T1-weighted pulse sequences are essential and irreplaceable components of osteomyelitis and tumor MRI protocols.[13,14]

Clinical MRI protocols for ankle sprain injuries typically include standard axial, coronal, and sagittal image plane orientations. Specialized, nonorthogonal image plane

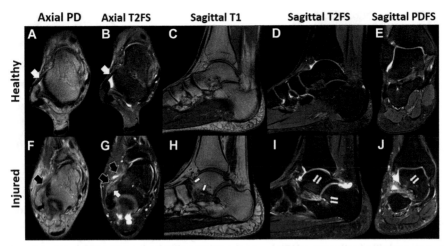

Fig. 1. Ankle sprain MRI protocol using 5 pulse sequences with different nonfat-suppressed and fat-suppressed contrasts to highlight healthy (*A–E*) and injured (*F–J*) anatomic structures and signal abnormalities differentially. Nonfat-suppressed proton density–weighted MR images (*A* and *F*) are best for assessing the structural integrity of ligaments, such as the anterior talofibular ligament (*arrows* in *A* and *F*), whereas corresponding fat-suppressed T2-weighted MR images (*white arrows B* and *G*) are best for assessing ligamentous and periligamentous edema (*black arrow* in *G*) indicating the acuity of healthy versus injured ligament. Similarly, fat-suppressed proton density and T2-weighted MR images are best for demonstrating normal (*D* and *E*) versus bone marrow edema (*I* and *J*) in bone contusions and non-displaced fractures, for example, around the sinus tarsi (*arrows* in *I* and *J*). T1-weighted MR images highlight bone marrow fat, corroborating bone contusions and non-displaced fractures, and visualize small marginal osteophytes, such as in the calcaneus (*arrows* in *H*). FS, fat suppression; PD, proton density weighting.

orientations, such as oblique axial, oblique coronal, and double oblique image plane orientations along the course of oblique ligaments, such as the anterior talofibular ligament (ATFL), calcaneofibular ligament (CFL), and anterior inferior tibiofibular ligaments (AiTFL), have been described to improve visibility (**Fig. 2**).[15–17]

In the superior-inferior dimension, acute ankle sprain MRI protocols should extend from the plantar surface to approximately 10 cm above the syndesmosis to include all ligaments and periarticular tendons, allowing the detection of high ankle sprain injuries. In the anterior-posterior dimension, the images should extend from the posterior skin surface to the base of the metatarsal bones to include the midfoot to detect Chopart joint line, sinus tarsi, Lisfranc injuries, and metatarsal base fractures.

New clinically available MRI techniques have substantially shortened the acquisition time of acute ankle sprain protocols.[18,19] Commonly applied acceleration techniques include parallel imaging, simultaneous multislice acquisition, compressed sensing, and artificial intelligence–based image reconstruction.[20,21] The combination of acceleration techniques and artificial intelligence–based image reconstruction results in scan times of 5 to 10 minutes for high-quality, high-spatial resolution 3T MRI protocols (**Table 1**).[22,23]

Clinical MRI protocols commonly use 2-dimensional (2D) MRI techniques, which enable high in-plane spatial resolution but are limited to 2- to 3-mm slice thicknesses. However, the thick slices result in volume-averaging effects, which may obscure small details, such as individual bands of the LCL complex. In comparison, 3D MRI

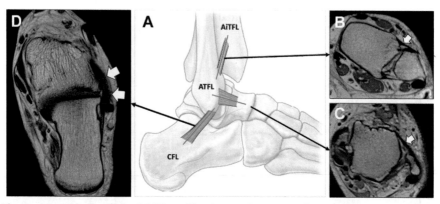

Fig. 2. Anatomically aligned MRI profile views using non-orthogonal plane orientations along the long axis of syndesmotic and lateral collateral ligaments. The anatomic illustration (A) demonstrates the anterior inferior talofibular ligament (AiTFL) of the syndesmosis, the anterior talofibular ligament (ATFL), and the calcaneofibular ligament (CFL). Anatomically aligned MRI image planes along the long axis of the ligaments (*blue lines* in A) result in profile views of the AiTFL (*arrow* in B), ATFL (*arrow* in C), and CFL (*arrows* in D), which avoids ligaments coursing obliquely through multiple images slices.

techniques can acquire much higher spatial resolution and thinner slice thickness without slice gaps, offering several advantages for MRI of acute ankle injury (**Fig. 3**).[24–27] Similar to computed tomography (CT), 3D MRI data can be acquired with isotropic voxel resolution, which means that each image voxel has the same length in all 3 dimensions, rendering them capable of reformation in virtually any spatial orientation, for example, along oblique ligaments.[12] In addition, such isotopic multiaxial 3D MRI data sets can trace and unfold curved tendons around the ankle (**Fig. 4**).

For MRI of acute ankle sprains, contrast-enhanced MR with intravenous gadolinium-based contrast injection or MR arthrography with intraarticular gadolinium-based contrast injection are typically not required.[28] In the chronic phase, MR arthrography may aid in visualizing synovial scarring and adhesions.

MRI of Acute Ankle Sprains

The clinical spectrum of ankle sprains ranges from low-grade capsular and ligamentous interstitial injuries to full-thickness disruptions of the collateral and syndesmotic ligaments. MRI is the most accurate imaging modality for visualizing collateral and syndesmotic ligaments and their integrity. MRI may be useful for evaluating the number of ligaments involved, differentiating LCL from syndesmotic ligament injuries, and characterizing the tears of individual ligaments.

The MRI appearance of intact ligaments is a well-demarcated tout linear band with low signal on all MR images. Homogeneous fat layers often surround intact ligaments. Similar to the anterior cruciate ligament of the knee, some ankle ligaments are composed of macroscopic fiber strands with interposed fat. This composition forms a striated pattern on MR images of alternating ligament fibers and high-signal interposed fat, which should not be mistaken for tears. Ankle ligaments commonly demonstrating a striated pattern include the anterior (AiTFL) and posterior (posterior inferior tibiofibular ligament [PiTFL]) syndesmotic inferior tibiofibular ligaments, the posterior tibiotalar ligament, medioplantar oblique bundle of the spring ligament, interosseous

Table 1
3.0 Tesla MRI protocol for evaluating ankle sprains

Parameters	Axial T2FS	Axial PD	Sagittal T2FS	Sagittal T1	Coronal PDFS
Repetition time [ms]	3800	3480	3700	546	3510
Echo time [ms]	60	23	56	7.1	35
Echo train length	11	11	11	4	11
Bandwidth (Hz/px)	296	354	299	355	301
Field-of-view [mm]	140 × 140	140 × 140	140 × 140	140 × 140	140 × 140
Matrix size	272 × 204	336 × 252	304 × 228	256 × 179	272 × 204
Slice thickness [mm]	3	3	3	3.5	3
Number of slices	38	38	38	28	36
Parallel imaging acceleration factor	3	3	2	3	3
Simultaneous multislice acceleration factor	2	2	2	2	2
Acquisition time [mm:ss]	0:42	0:55	1:03	0:32	1:15

Abbreviations: FS, fat suppression; PD, proton density weighting.

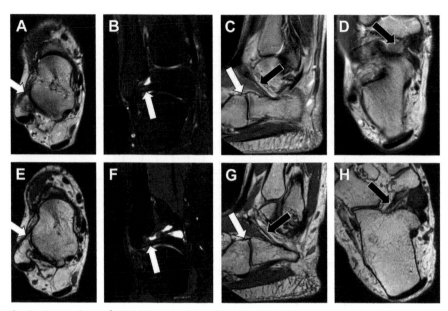

Fig. 3. Comparison of 2D MRI versus 3D ankle MRI. 2D MR images are inherently prone to partial volume defects due to comparably thicker slices (eg, 3 mm), which may an obscure fine detail of ankle ligaments (*arrows* in *A–D*). 3D MR images minimize such partial volume effects due to thinner slices (eg, 0.5 mm), resulting in sharply delineated ligaments with higher spatial resolution (*arrows* in *E–H*). From left to right, anterior talofibular ligament (*arrows* in *A* and *E*), posterior talofibular ligament (*arrows* in *B* and *F*), calcaneonavicular bifurcate ligament (*white arrows* in *C* and *G*), extensor retinaculum (*black arrows* in *C* and *G*), and medioplantar oblique plantar spring ligament (*arrows* in *D* and *H*).

talocalcaneal ligament, cervical ligament, and the deep layer of the deltoid ligament complex (**Fig. 5**).[29–31]

The spectrum of acute ligament injuries MRI can detect and characterize, in ascending severity of tissue injury, extends from low-grade interstitial injuries to partial-thickness and full-thickness tears (**Table 2**). The MRI appearance of low-grade interstitial ligament injuries shows increased internal proton density and T2 signal as a surrogate marker for interstitial edema and no visualized fiber disruption. In partial-thickness tears, MRI demonstrates disruption of some, but not all, ligament fibers in cross-sectional, longitudinal, or both planes. MRI demonstrates disruption of all ligament fibers in full-thickness or complete ligament tears, which can further characterize the proximal attachment, midsubstance, distal attachment, or combinations thereof (**Fig. 6**). These may combine with periligamentous edema, bone avulsion, and hematomas.[31,32] Clinical grading of ankle ligamentous injuries may not always match the degree of ligamentous fiber disruption seen on MRI.[33] Hence, the clinical term "sprain" should not be used in MRI reports. Descriptors characterizing the structural fiber integrity or lack thereof should be used instead, as shown in **Table 2**.

Lateral Ankle Sprains

LCL injuries occur in more than 85% of all ankle sprains.[32] The LCL complex comprises the ATFL, CFL, and posterior talofibular ligament (PTFL). The classic cascade

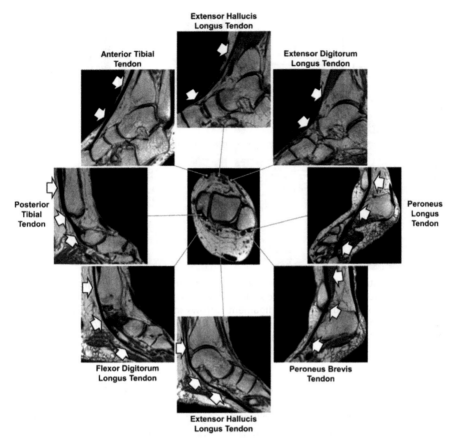

Fig. 4. 3D MRI unfolding of ankle tendons using curved planar reformation. Using a single multiaxial isotropic high-resolution 3D MRI volume dataset (center image), dedicated curved multiplanar reformation images can be created for any curved tendon about the ankle. The unfolding reformation results in a planar long-axis display of double- and triple-angulated tendons (*arrows*), thereby avoiding partial volume effects for better display and evaluation.

of injury is ATFL injury followed by CFL and PTLF[30,32]; however, patterns vary depending on the mechanisms of injury.

Anterior talofibular ligament

ATFL injuries occur in more than 75% to 80% of ankle sprains.[9] MRI has 83% to 100% sensitivity and 100% specificity for detecting and characterizing ATFL tears.[34,35] The taut cordlike low-signal ATFL is best seen in the axial plane at the level of the distal fibula, where it forms a cross-sectional commalike shape (see **Fig. 6**). The normal ligament thickness is 2 to 4 mm in anterior-to-posterior dimension and thus, appropriately visualized using 3-mm thick axial slices.[29]

The ATFL comprises 1 to 3 bundles.[16,36] Two bundles are the most common type (50%–82%). The superior bundle is thicker than the inferior bundle. Superior and inferior bundles have been assigned different functions depending on the ankle position. In a cadaveric study, the superior bundle was taut during plantar flexion, whereas the inferior bundle was relaxed and vice versa, which may be analogous to the functions of

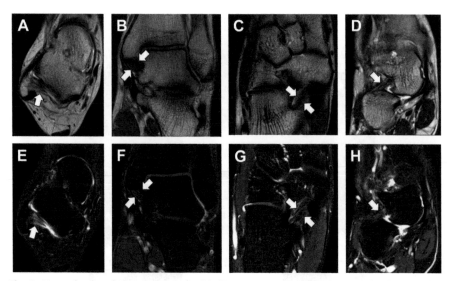

Fig. 5. Normal striated MRI pattern of ankle ligaments. Proton density–weighted MR images (*A–D*) and fat-suppressed T2-weighted MR images (*E–H*) of the posterior talofibular ligament (*arrows* in *A* and *E*), deltoid ligament (*arrows* in *B* and *F*), medioplantar oblique plantar spring ligament (*arrows* in *C* and *G*), and cervical ligament (*arrows* in *D* and *H*) show multiple strands of alternating ligament fibers and interposed fat, which should not be mistaken for tears.

anteromedial and posterolateral anterior cruciate ligament bundles in flexion and extension of the knee.[37,38] Later, the 3-bundle ATFL type was considered weaker than types 1 and 2.[36] Individually aligned imaging planes to the axial oblique ATFL course reformatted from isotropic 3D MRI datasets aid in delineating superior and inferior ATFL bundles.[16] The significance of the number of ATFL bundles for the treatment of choice is unclear. However, characterizing the bundle anatomy may aid anatomic suture anchor placement.[37] In addition, knowledge of the anatomic ATFL bundle spectrum aids in avoiding misinterpretation of tears.

Calcaneofibular ligament
The CFL is the second most commonly injured LCL, whereas approximately 20% of ankle sprains involve CFL and ATFL injuries.[39] MRI has 87% to 97% sensitivity and 75% to 98% specificity for detecting and characterizing CFL tears.[15,40] The CFL is a cordlike ligament that runs from the fibular tip to the lateral calcaneus cortex in a 10

Table 2	
MRI terminology and MRI findings of ligamentous injuries	
Ligamentous Integrity and MRI Terminology	**MRI Findings**
Interstitial injury	Increased proton density and T2 signal inside the ligament without visualized fiber disruption
Partial-thickness tear	Disrupted and intact ligament fibers
Full-thickness tear	Disruption of all ligament fibers with optional fiber retraction and displacement of torn ligament ends

Healthy   Interstitial Injury   Partial-thickness Tear   Full-thickness Tear

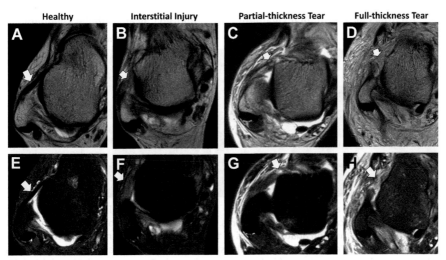

Fig. 6. MRI appearances of normal and torn anterior talofibular ligaments. Axial T2-weighted MR images (*A–D*) and axial fat-suppressed T2-weighted MR images (*E–H*) show the spectrum from normal to completely torn anterior talofibular ligament, best seen in the axial plane. Normal MRI appearance of the anterior talofibular ligament (*arrows in A and E*) showing a taut, dark cordlike, and sharply demarcated healthy ligament. Interstitial anterior talofibular ligament tear showing thickening of the ligament with increased internal edemalike protein density or T2 signal (*arrows in B and F*) but no visible fiber disruption. Partial-thickness tear of the anterior talofibular ligament showing mixed discontinuous and continuous ligament fibers (*arrows in C and G*). Full-thickness anterior talofibular ligament tear showing disruption of all ligament fibers (*arrows in D and H*).

to 45 degree anterosuperior to a posteroinferior oblique coronal plane.[29,36] The CFL courses deep to the peroneus brevis tendon and is contiguous with the tendon sheath.

Because of its curved orientation, the whole length of CFL is typically not demonstrated in standard orthogonal axial, sagittal, or coronal imaging plane, which may explain low MRI sensitivity (87%) for detecting tears.[29,30] Anatomically angulated imaging planes along the CFL long axis increases the sensitivity to 94% (see **Fig. 2** and **Fig. 7**).[15] Higher-grade CFL tears are associated with subtalar and sinus tarsi injuries (**Table 3**).[32]

Posterior talofibular ligament
Higher-grade PTFL injuries are the least common.[31,32] The MRI sensitivity and specificity for detecting and characterizing PTFL tears are less well defined but fall within the range of the diagnostic performances of ATFL and CFL tears. On conventional axial MR images, the PTFL and ATFL are visible in the same plane, where the fibula assumes a commalike shape. The normal PTFL has a multistriated MRI appearance with a fan-shaped attachment to the inner cortex of the fibular (see **Fig. 5**). Following injury and remodeling, its MRI appearance often lacks the striated pattern.

Medial ankle sprains
The deltoid ligament complex, also known as the medial collateral ligament complex, is injured in 15% or more of all ankle sprains.[41] MRI has 84% to 100% sensitivity and 93% to 100% specificity for detecting and characterizing deltoid ligament complex injuries.[40,42]

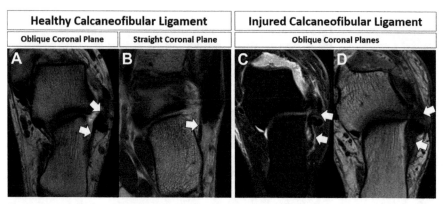

Healthy Calcaneofibular Ligament		Injured Calcaneofibular Ligament
Oblique Coronal Plane	Straight Coronal Plane	Oblique Coronal Planes

Fig. 7. Anatomically aligned coronal oblique versus straight coronal plane for visualizing healthy and injured calcaneofibular ligaments. The coronal oblique plane T2-weighted MR image aligned with the long anatomical axis of the calcaneofibular ligament (*A*) demonstrates the ligament in profile (*arrows*), whereas the standard straight coronal MR image (*B*) shows only part of the intact calcaneofibular ligament (*arrow*). Fat-suppressed T2-weighted (*C*) and proton density–weighted (*D*) coronal oblique MR images aligned with the long anatomical axis of the calcaneofibular ligament demonstrate partial ligament tears (*arrows*).

The deltoid ligament complex is a group of ligaments that restrain valgus tilt and rotational forces on the talus. A common subdivision of ligamentous fibers describes this ligamentous complex in superficial (tibionavicular, tibiocalcaneal, tibiospring, posterior superficial tibiotalar ligaments) and deep (anterior tibiotalar, posterior deep tibiotalar ligaments) layers that act synergistically (**Fig. 8**).[43] On MRI, the healthy deltoid ligament complex also demonstrates the striated pattern formed by the different ligament components, bundles, strands, and interspersed fatty tissue (see **Fig. 5**).[43,44] The striated pattern may not be apparent in older individuals and scar-remodeled

Table 3
Ligament injuries and associated injuries in acute ankle sprain injuries

Acute Ankle Sprain and Associated Lesions	
Ligament injury	Articular injury
Anterior talofibular ligament	Osteochondral lesion
Calcaneofibular ligament	Chondral lesion
Posterior talofibular ligament	Subtalar injury
Syndesmosis	Sinus tarsi injury
Deltoid ligament complex	Peritalar translation
Spring ligament	Tendon injury
Bifurcate ligament	Peroneus tendon
Bone marrow edema	Tibialis posterior
Fracture	Nerve injury
Both malleoli	Posterior tibial nerve
Talar head or dome	peroneal nerve
Navicular bone	—
Anterior articular process of calcaneus	Midfoot injury
Cuboid	Lisfranc ligament injury
Fifth metatarsal bone	Avulsion fracture

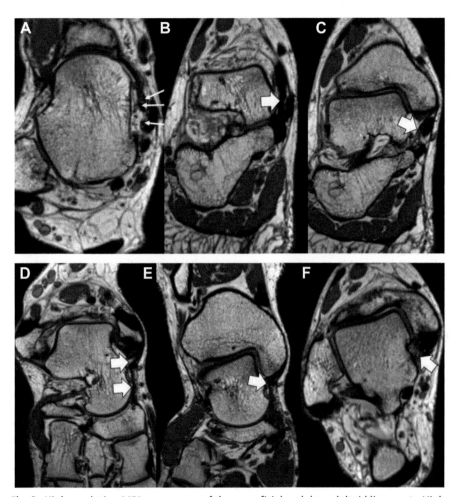

Fig. 8. High-resolution MRI appearance of the superficial and deep deltoid ligaments. High-resolution axial oblique 3D MR image (*A*) demonstrates the short axis of 3 superficial deltoid ligaments, including the tibionavicular ligament (*top arrow*), tibiospring ligament (*middle arrow*), and tibiocalcaneal ligament (*bottom arrow*). Coronal oblique MR images demonstrate the 3 superficial deltoid ligament components, including the tibiospring ligament (*arrow* in *B*), tibiocalcaneal ligament (*arrow* in *C*), and tibionavicular ligament (*arrows* in *D*). 3D MR reformation images demonstrate the deep deltoid ligament layer, including the anterior tibiotalar ligament (*arrow* in *E*) and posterior tibiotalar ligament (*arrow* in *F*).

deltoid ligaments.[43] On 3-mm coronal and axial MR images, the superficial and deep layers can be identified confidently,[43,44] whereas the 5-individual subligament portions may require high-resolution thin section 3D MRI for reliable visualization (see **Fig. 8**). The fan-shaped posterior deep tibiotalar ligament is the thickest ligament component measuring 6 to 11 mm in cross-sectional diameter.[41]

Deltoid ligament injuries are frequently associated with syndesmotic injuries, LCL injuries, malleoli fractures, flexor tendon injuries, and saphenous nerve injuries, which are less common in isolated lateral ankle sprains.[5] In a retrospective study, 72% of surgically treated chronic lateral ligament injuries had concomitant deltoid ligament complex injuries.[40] Patients with chronic lateral ankle instability requiring surgery were found to have MRI findings of deltoid ligament complex injuries in 36% and syndesmotic injuries in 42%.[42]

Syndesmotic ankle sprains

Syndesmotic injuries, or high ankle sprains, occur with a 10% to 17% incidence.[45,46] The convex shape of the distal fibula cortex and the receiving concave fibular notch of the distal tibia provide static stability. However, the syndesmotic ligaments are the major stabilizers, including the AiTFL, PiTFL, and the interosseous tibiofibular ligament (ITFL), also known as the syndesmotic plate.[5,47] The PiTFL contributes 40% to 45%, the AiTFL 35%, and the ITLF 22% to syndesmotic stability, whereas injury of 2 out of 3 syndesmotic ligaments carries a high risk for ankle instability.[48]

The AiTFL course from superomedial to inferolateral with a 30° to 45° obliquity. As such, the AiTFL are typically only partially imaged on axial images. Individually aligned axial oblique MR images, obtained with separately acquired 2D pulse sequences or individually reformatted from isotropic 3D data, can improve its visibility and assessment (**Fig. 9**).[26]

Bassett ligament is an accessory ligament just inferior and parallel to the inferior AiTFL margin that occurs with 83% to 92% prevalence.[49] An anatomic gap between the 2 ligaments should not be mistaken as an AiTFL tear. Similarly, thickening of the Bassett ligament should not be considered as injured AiTFL.

Stable versus unstable syndesmotic injuries may be diagnosed by physical examination by skilled orthopedic surgeons and radiographs. However, syndesmotic injuries have been reported as an underestimated source of chronic ankle pain and arthrosis,[5] with up to 20% being missed in the emergency room.[50] A study reported a 7.9% miss rate of syndesmotic injuries in acute ankle sprains with normal radiographs.[8] The addition of radiographic stress results in only small increases in diagnostic performance.[8,51]

MRI has a 92% to 100% sensitivity and 87% to 93% specificity for detecting and characterizing syndesmotic injuries (**Fig. 10**),[51,52] which is substantially higher than the diagnostic performance of ultrasonography.[5,50]

Clinical grade I high ankle sprains are usually limited to the AiTFL, whereas, in clinical grade IIa sprains, the interosseous ligament, and in clinical grade IIb sprains, the

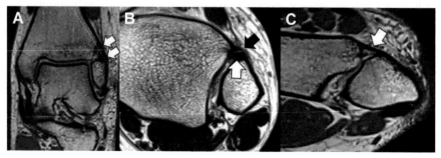

Fig. 9. Comparison of axial view versus oblique axial views of the syndesmotic anterior inferior tibiofibular ligament (AiTFL). Coronal MR image (*A*) shows the axial (*solid line*) versus axial oblique (*dashed line*) plane alignments along AiTFL (*arrows*). The straight axial MR image (*B*) cuts through the syndesmotic AiTFL bands (*white arrow*) obliquely, creating partial volume and pseudotear (*black arrow*) effects. The axial oblique MR image (*C*) is aligned along the anatomic long-axis course of the syndesmotic anterior inferior talofibular ligament (*arrow*), displaying the ligament bands in profile without partial volume and pseudotear effects.

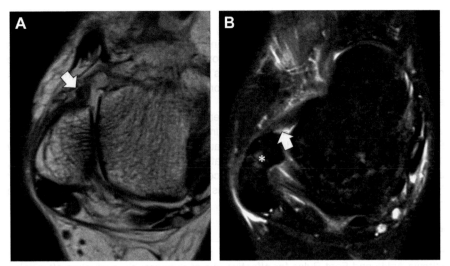

Fig. 10. A 33-year-old woman with an acute ankle sprain. Axial proton density–weighted MR image with axial oblique plane orientation along the long axis of the syndesmotic anterior inferior talofibular ligament (*A*) demonstrates a full-thickness anterior inferior talofibular ligament tear (*arrow*) with fiber detachment off the tibial attachment. Axial fat-suppressed T2-weighted MR image (*B*) at the level of the distal fibula where the fibula resembles a commalike shape (*asterisk*) shows a concomitant partial-thickness anterior talofibular ligament tear (*arrow*).

PiTFL are torn as well. Clinical grade III sprains are rare and typically also include fibular fractures.

Stable high ankle sprains may be treated conservatively with little risk for chronic instability, whereas unstable high ankle injuries typically require surgery.[53] MRI may be helpful in acute clinical grade 2 high ankle sprains presenting with subtle instability on physical examination. In clinical grade 2 syndesmotic injuries, surgically treated athletes had a high rate of return to play to their previous level, whereas untreated grade 2 injuries with microstability carry a risk of developing chronic instability and accelerated degeneration.[54]

Accurate detection and grading of deltoid ligament injuries are important, as the deltoid ligament complex supports syndesmotic stability. In a cadaveric study, dividing 2 or more syndesmotic and deltoid ligaments resulted in syndesmotic instability.[55]

ASSOCIATED INJURIES
Bone Marrow Edema

Areas of bone marrow edema are a common finding on MRI after ankle sprains. Previous reports found areas of bone marrow edema in 25% of recurrent ankle sprains[56] and 76% of ankle sprains with LCL injury.[57] Areas of marrow edema typically normalized within 2 to 12 months after trauma and have a good prognosis. However, the MRI visualization of bone marrow edema patterns is useful for recreating the injury mechanism, detecting occult nondisplaced fractures, and predicting injury patterns and recovery time. Bone marrow edema of the plantar talar head is suspicious for a peritalar subluxation event and is associated with deltoid ligament complex, LCL, talonavicular, and spring ligament injuries.[58,59]

MRI is the imaging test of choice to diagnose and monitor bone marrow edema with a virtual 100% accuracy. On MRI, bone marrow edema presents as linear subcortical or geographic proton density– and T2-weighted signal hyperintensity, best seen with fat suppression (see **Fig. 1**). T1-weighted MR images may demonstrate optional T1 hyperintensity. In acute ankle sprains, bone marrow edema areas typically indicate impact-associated bone contusion after trauma. Although there are no visible cortical or trabecular deformities or fractures, the bone marrow edema signal is thought to represent a combination of trabecular microcontusive injuries, edema, and hemorrhage.[56,58,59]

Nontraumatic causes of bone marrow edema include stress reaction, red marrow, weight-bearing–induced increased bone turnover, disuse, and degeneration.[5,58,60] Pattern or location may help differentiate traumatic from nontraumatic bone marrow edema. Traumatic bone marrow edema patterns tend to be geographic, reticular, and nonlinear and may show associated cortex deformation and disruptions.[56,60] Nontraumatic bone marrow edema patterns are often subchondral or cortical with diffuse and multifocal distribution.[58,60]

Fractures

Fractures occur with an incidence of 26% percent in acute ankle sprains.[8,61] The Ottawa Ankle and Foot Rules for effective use of radiographic evaluation after ankle sprains have a high sensitivity of 92% to 100% but low sensitivity of 11% to 79%[39,62] (**Fig. 11**). However, foot and ankle fractures are among the most common unrecognized fractures in the lower extremity.[63]

Conventional radiography is the first-line imaging test for fracture evaluation in acute ankle sprains, yet the sensitivity is low (**Fig. 12**). Weight-bearing can increase the accuracy of detecting nondisplaced fractures. However, the complex 3D foot and ankle anatomy and the 2D projections nature of radiography result in summation artifacts and potential obscuration of subtle fractures.[63,64]

In acute ankle sprains, common fracture locations include medial and lateral malleoli, talar head, talar dome, navicular bone, the anterior articular process of calcaneus, cuboid bone, and fifth metatarsal bone.[64] Subtle, minimally displaced

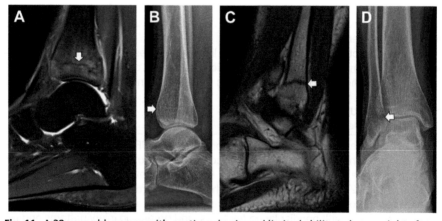

Fig. 11. A 28-year-old woman with continued pain and limited ability to bear weight after a lateral ankle sprain 3 weeks before. Sagittal fat-suppressed T2-weighted MR image (*A*) demonstrates a subacute nondisplaced distal tibia fracture (*arrow* in *A*) that is not visible on the same-day lateral radiograph (*arrow* in *B*). Sagittal proton density–weighted MR image (*C*) demonstrates a subacute nondisplaced distal tibia fracture (*arrow* in *C*) that is faintly visible on the same-day anteroposterior radiograph (*arrow* in *D*).

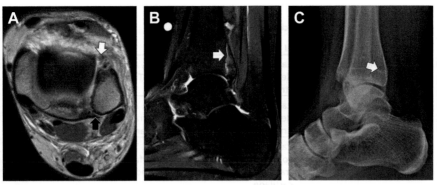

Fig. 12. A 33-year-old woman with a lateral ankle sprain. Axial proton density–weighted MR image (*A*) demonstrates a clinically unexpected syndesmotic injury, including full-thickness anterior (*white arrow*) and posterior (*black arrow*) inferior tibiofibular ligament tears. Sagittal fat-suppressed T2-weighted MR image (*B*) demonstrates a radiographically occult nondisplaced posterior malleolus fracture (*arrow* in B), which is not seen on the lateral radiograph (*arrow*) (*C*).

avulsion fractures of the lateral malleolus occur in up to 26% of lateral ankle sprains.[61] Deltoid and ATiFL ligament injuries have a higher incidence of combined medial malleolar, tibial, and fibular avulsion fractures.[65]

Radiographically occult, nondisplaced fractures can also be diagnosed with CT; however, MRI has similar or better diagnostic performance, specifically for diagnosing stress and osteochondral fractures without clearly CT-delineated fracture lines.[66] Similar to CT, 3D MRI enables the generation of 3D rendered images to display complex fractures.[28]

Small cortical and nonacute minimally displaced fractures may not be visible on conventional MRI scans,[67,68] as cortical fragments are dark in all pulse sequences and may not be associated with bone marrow edema. Opposed-phase Dixon MR images increase the sensitivity of detecting such fractures by creating dark bands around

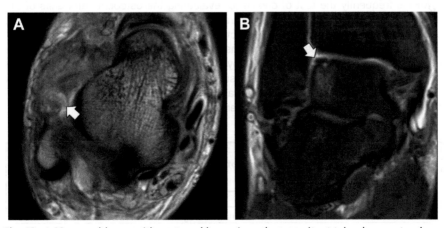

Fig. 13. A 23-year-old man with acute ankle sprain and concomitant talar dome osteochondral lesion. Axial proton density–weighted MR image (*A*) shows a full-thickness tear (*arrow*) of the anterior talofibular ligament. Coronal fat-suppressed proton density–weighted MR image (*B*) shows a concomitant lateral talar dome osteochondral lesion (*arrow*).

Table 4
Types of acute traumatic osteochondral injury

Type	MRI Appearance
Bone contusion	Focal bone marrow edema pattern. Absent cortical contour deformity. Absent fracture lines. The overlying cartilage is structurally intact.
Subchondral fracture	Focal bone marrow edema pattern. Absent cortical contour deformity. Subcortically located fracture line that parallels the articular surface. The overlying cartilage is structurally intact.
Osteochondral fracture	Focal bone marrow edema pattern. Typically presents with contour deformities, articular surface step-off, or displaced fragments. The fracture line extends through bone and articular cartilage.
Chondral fracture	Focal bone marrow edema pattern. Presents with articular cartilage contour irregularities. The separation typically occurs at the calcified-noncalcified cartilage interface near the tidemark layer. Chondral fragments may remain in situ or float in the joint cavity.

fracture margins.[67] New, clinically available MRI techniques that create CT images synthetically from MRI data may also increase the detectability of cortical fractures.[12]

Osteochondral Injuries

Ankle sprains may be associated with acute traumatic osteochondral injuries, representing a spectrum of bone contusions, subchondral, and osteochondral fractures (**Fig. 13**) (**Table 4**).

OCLs of the talus involve injury to the articular cartilage and subjacent subchondral bone of the talar dome or distal tibia articular surface. OCL can cause persistent ankle pain, stiffness, reduced range of motion, and locking. Seventy-five percent of OCLs arise from ankle sprains,[32,69] whereas 6% to 8% of patients with ankle sprains have an OCL.[8,70] Although lateral talar dome lesions are less common (25%–40%) than medial talar dome lesions, they are usually traumatic, smaller, shallower, and shearlike.[32]

MRI is frequently the test of choice for evaluating the osteochondral units of the ankle and hindfoot.[71] Proton density– and intermediate-weighted MR images most accurately detect articular cartilage defects, including fissuring, fracture, and shear injuries.[32,72,73] Fat-suppressed proton density– and T2-weighted MR images increase the detectability of subchondral injuries by isolating bone marrow edema signal, which improves the visibility of deformities and subchondral fractures. Additional information derived from MRI includes the presence and degree of subsidence, collapse, separation, cyst formation, cortication, and sclerosis of margins.

Table 5
MRI classification of osteochondral lesions of the talus

Grade	Description
1	Normal
2	Partial-thickness articular cartilage defect
3	Coapted full-thickness articular cartilage defect or exposed bone
4	Unstable but nondisplaced in-situ chondral or osteochondral fragment
5	Displaced chondral or osteochondral fragment

A grading system with a high correlation between MRI and arthroscopy differentiates 5 grades for OCL (grade 1, normal; grade 2, partial-thickness articular cartilage defect; grade 3, coapted full-thickness articular cartilage defect or exposed bone; grade 4, unstable but nondisplaced in-situ chondral or osteochondral fragment; grade 5, displaced chondral or osteochondral fragment) (**Table 5**).[72]

Spring Ligament Injuries

Spring ligament injuries occur with a reported incidence of 4% in acute ankle sprains, but the true incidence is likely higher, as spring ligament tears are challenging to diagnose. The spring ligament complex comprises the superomedial calcaneonavicular ligament and the medioplantar oblique and inferoplantar longitudinal calcaneonavicular ligaments.[74,75] Extending from the calcaneus to the tarsal navicular bone, the spring ligament complex stabilizes the talus (or talar head) and medial longitudinal arch.

The superomedial calcaneonavicular ligament is best seen on coronal and axial images, as it wraps around the talar head in a hammocklike fashion (**Fig. 14**). The medioplantar oblique calcaneonavicular (**Fig. 15**) and inferoplantar longitudinal (**Fig. 16**) ligaments are best seen on axial and sagittal MR images. The medioplantar oblique ligament (see **Fig. 15**) has a striated pattern, whereas the normal superomedial (see **Fig. 14**) and inferoplantar longitudinal calcaneonavicular (see **Fig. 16**) ligaments have low signal intensity. The normal superomedial calcaneonavicular ligament width ranges between 2 and 5 mm.[76]

Lower or higher superomedial calcaneonavicular ligament widths, edema signal within the ligament, and partial or complete fiber discontinuity indicate tears (**Fig. 17**). Spring ligament insufficiency may occur with other structures that maintain

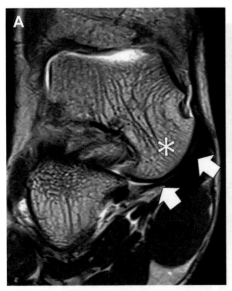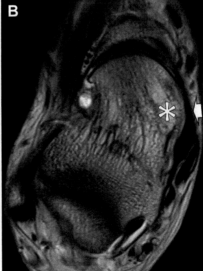

Fig. 14. MRI appearance of the normal superomedial calcaneonavicular ligament of spring ligament complex. Coronal T2-weighted MR image (*A*) shows the superomedial spring ligament (*arrows*) wrapping around the head of the talus (*asterisk*) in a hammocklike fashion. Axial T2-weighted MR image (*B*) shows the superomedial spring ligament (*arrow*) coursing medial to the talar head (*asterisk*).

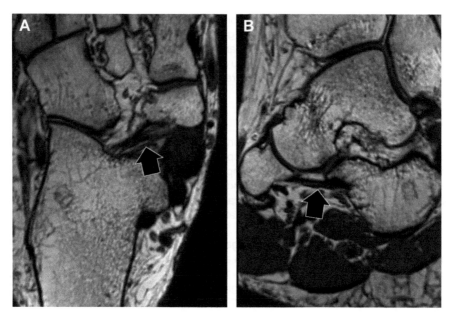

Fig. 15. MRI appearance of the normal medioplantar oblique calcaneonavicular ligament of spring ligament complex. Axial (*A*) and sagittal (*B*) proton density–weighted high-resolution 3D MR images show the striated plantar medioplantar oblique ligament (*arrows*).

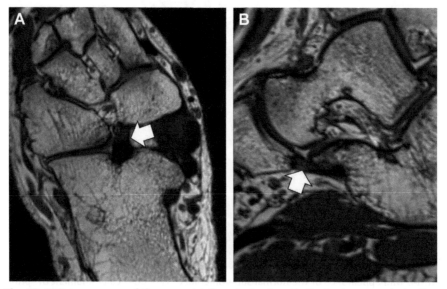

Fig. 16. MRI appearance of the normal inferoplantar longitudinal calcaneonavicular ligament of spring ligament complex. Axial (*A*) and sagittal (*B*) proton density–weighted high-resolution 3D MR images show the cordlike plantar inferomedial calcaneonavicular ligament (*arrows*).

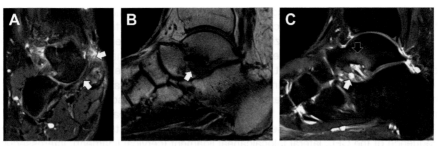

Fig. 17. A 42-year-old man with subacute ankle sprain and concomitant sinus tarsi syndrome. Coronal fat-suppressed proton density–weighted MR image (*A*) shows a superomedial calcaneonavicular spring ligament (*arrows*) partial thickness tear near the junction to the tibiospring deltoid ligament. Sagittal T1-weighted (*B*) and fat-suppressed proton density–weighted (*C*) MR images show concomitant signs of sinus tarsi syndrome, including obliteration of the sinus tarsi fat (*arrow* in *B*), ganglion cyst formation (*white arrow* in *C*), and adjacent bone marrow edema (*black arrow* in *C*).

the medial longitudinal arch (posted tibial tendon, sinus tarsi, plantar fascia), with the risk of progressive collapsing foot deformity.[76–80]

Full-thickness spring ligament tears are rare, whereas the MRI appearance of most spring ligament injuries is characterized by lengthening and loss of tensile strength of the superomedial calcaneonavicular ligament, which is difficult to detect on MR images. As such, the diagnostic performance data for MRI vary depending on the used criteria. In our experience, MRI findings of spring ligament injuries are specific but not sensitive, with the potential for a high false-negative rate of lower-grade injuries that lack substantial fiber disruption.

Sinus Tarsi Injuries

Sinus tarsi–associated symptoms may occur in up to 70% of patients after ankle sprains (see **Fig. 17**).[32,81,82] The sinus tarsi is a funnel-shaped space anterior to the posterior facet of the subtalar joint, bounded superiorly by the talus and inferiorly by

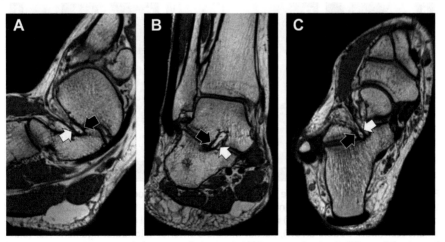

Fig. 18. MRI appearance of the normal sinus tarsi ligaments. Sagittal oblique (*A*), coronal oblique (*B*), and axial oblique (*C*) proton density–weighted 3D MR images aligned to the long anatomical axis of each ligament show the cervical (*white arrows*) and interosseous talocalcaneal (*black arrows*) ligaments.

the calcaneus. A complex arrangement of the medial, intermediate, and lateral roots of the extensor retinaculum, cervical ligament, and interosseous talocalcaneal restraints the talus and calcaneus, stabilizing the hindfoot to prevent inversion primarily through the cervical ligament and preventing excessive eversion primarily through the interosseous talocalcaneal ligament.[81,82] On standard 2D MRI, the cervical ligament and interosseous talocalcaneal ligaments are best seen on sagittal and coronal images; however, the sinus tarsi ligaments are best seen on high-resolution 3D MR images that are individually aligned to the long anatomical axis of each ligament (**Fig. 18**). Ankle sprain–associated ligament injuries around the sinus tarsi may occur in the sequence of the CFL, lateral talocalcaneal ligament (cervical ligament), interosseous ligament, and subtalar joint injury.[32]

MRI is the test of choice for evaluating the integrity of the sinus tarsi ligaments. In the acute phase, sinus tarsi edema, small collections, and ligamentous fiber disruption are the prototypical findings (**Fig. 19**). In the subacute and chronic phases, obliteration of the sinus tarsi, diffuse synovitis, and scarring dominate. Sinus tarsi injuries are associated with posterior tibial tendon tears and subtalar joint subluxation/dislocation.[81,82] Bone cysts and edemalike signal near the angle of Gissane can be nonpathologic findings from vascular remnants[60] or related to progressive collapsing foot deformity and sinus tarsi impingement.[83]

Peritalar Subluxation/Dislocation

Traumatic peritalar subluxation and dislocation include subluxation or dislocation of the talocalcaneal and talonavicular joints, whereas the calcaneocuboidal or tibiotalar joints remain preserved. Although persistent peritalar dislocation associated with high-energy trauma is rare, transient peritalar subluxation events occur in up to 19% of sports-related ankle sprains (**Fig. 20**).[84,85] Following ankle sprains with transient peritalar subluxation, radiographs may be normal, showing anatomically aligned talocalcaneal and talonavicular joints and no overt deformities or fractures. On physical examination, detecting subtle instability may be challenging in the acute phase of ankle sprains due to pain.

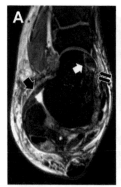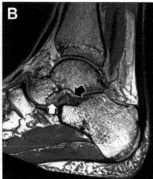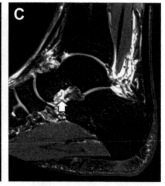

Fig. 19. MRI appearance of acute cervical and interosseous talocalcaneal ligament injury after ankle sprain with talocalcaneal translation injury. Axial fat-suppressed T2-weighted high-resolution 3D MR image (*A*) demonstrates a superomedial calcaneonavicular spring ligament tear (*black double arrow*), partial-thickness anterior talofibular ligament tear (*black arrow*), and nondisplaced anteromedial talar head fracture (*white arrow*). Sagittal proton density–weighted (*B*) and fat-suppressed T2-weighted (*C*) high-resolution 3D MR images show full-thickness cervical (*white arrows* in *B* and *C*) and interosseous talocalcaneal (*black arrows*) ligament tears.

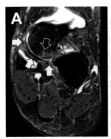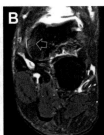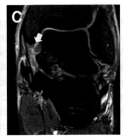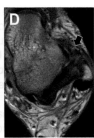

Fig. 20. A 48-year-old man with ankle sprain and concomitant peritalar translation. Coronal fat-suppressed proton density–weighted MR images (*A* and *B*) show a partial tear of the superomedial calcaneonavicular spring ligament (*white arrows* in *A*) and plantar (*black arrow* in *A*) and medial (*arrow* in *B*) talar head bone marrow contusions, indicative of a recent medioplantar peritalar subluxation or transient dislocation. Coronal fat-suppressed proton density–weighted MR image (*C*) shows a concomitant full-thickness deep deltoid ligament tear (*arrow*). Axial proton density–weighted MR image (*D*) shows a concomitant anterior talofibular ligament tear (*arrow*).

Peritalar subluxations/dislocations may occur in medial or lateral directions. Medial peritalar subluxation injuries, or "basketball foot, " occur with forced inversion to a dorsiflexed foot, with the sustentaculum tali acting as a fulcrum.[86] Lateral peritalar subluxation injuries, also known as "acquired clubfoot," occur with forced eversion to a plantarflexed foot, with the anterior calcaneal process serving as the fulcrum.[85,87] Medial peritalar translation injuries are approximately 4 times more common than lateral peritalar translation injuries.

MRI findings after peritalar translation may be subtle but characteristic. Subtle medial or lateral talar shift relative to the navicular bone may persist. Focal subcortical bone marrow edema at the medioplantar and lateroplantar talar head without or with associated cortical flattening and subcortical nondisplaced fracture risk are high suspicion for peritalar translation components in acute ankle sprains (see **Fig. 20**). Talonavicular ligament tears are frequently associated,[58] followed by less frequent calcaneofibular and deltoid ligament complex tears.[85,88] Nondisplaced talus, calcaneus, cuboid, cuneiform, navicular, medial and lateral malleolus, metatarsal, and osteochondral fractures occur in 12% to 38% (see **Fig. 19**).[88] Osseous injuries, including intraarticular osteochondral fractures, occur more commonly with lateral peritalar translation.[85] The MRI diagnosis of posterior tibial tendon, flexor hallucis longus tendon, and joint capsule entrapments aid surgical planning.[88]

Chopart Injury

Midtarsal sprains occur in up to 73% of ankle sprains.[89,90] The calcaneocuboid and talocalcaneonavicular or talonavicular joint form the midtarsal (Chopart) joint, which connects the midfoot with the hindfoot.[91,92] Both joints are stabilized with multiple ligaments, including dorsal calcaneocuboid ligament, dorsal talonavicular ligaments, bifurcate ligament, plantar calcaneocuboid ligaments, and spring ligament complex. The 2 principal Chopart joints interact with the subtalar joint forming a triple joint complex. Dysfunction of either joint affects the other 2 joints.[93] Untreated Chopart joint injuries may result in persistent pain and cuboid instability.[94]

Chopart joint injuries have 2 distinct type patterns.[95] Higher energy injuries result in Chopart joint fracture-dislocation, whereas lower energy injuries (up to 73% during inversion injury) typically result in midtarsal sprains.[89,90] The incidence of midtarsal sprain varies from 5.5% to 33%; however, the incidence may be higher because of overlapping clinical symptoms with lateral ankle sprains.[89,94,95] Up to 41% of cases may go undetected during clinical examination and radiographic evaluation.[92]

MRI is more accurate in detecting midtarsal sprains than radiography. In a comparative investigation, MRI found Chopart injuries in 76% of cases, whereas only 14% were detected with radiography.[92] MRI can delineate each stabilizing midtarsal joint ligament, including the dorsal calcaneocuboid ligament, dorsal talonavicular ligaments, bifurcate ligament, plantar calcaneocuboid ligaments, and spring ligament complex.

The dorsal talonavicular ligament is a major stabilizer of the medial Chopart joint. Radiographs can accurately detect osseous avulsion fractures of the dorsal talonavicular ligament attachments; however, the diagnostic accuracy is higher with MRI for sole ligamentous injuries (**Fig. 21**).

The bifurcate ligament complex supports calcaneocuboid joint stability and includes the calcaneocuboid and calcaneonavicular ligaments, which form a Y-shape comprised of calcaneonavicular and calcaneocuboid limbs. Both ligaments are seen in the sagittal image planes, whereas the calcaneocuboid limb of the bifurcate ligament is usually best seen (**Fig. 22**). Individually aligned image planes along the long anatomical axis of each length are best for MRI visualization.[26] Opposing bone marrow edema at the anterior process of the calcaneus and proximal dorsal cuboid is characteristic of calcaneocuboid limb tears (see **Fig. 22**).[90]

Most cases of concomitant ankle and midtarsal sprains are treated conservatively. However, concomitant ankle and midtarsal sprains may be treated with longer and more aggressive immobilization than sole lateral ligament sprains. Surgical indications include instability and early return to weight-bearing.[90,94]

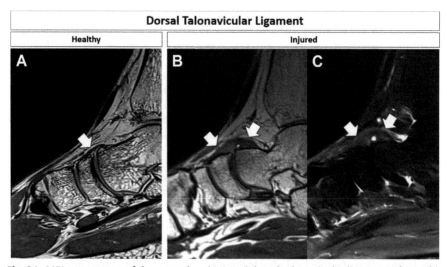

Fig. 21. MRI appearance of the normal and injured dorsal talonavicular ligament after ankle sprain with concomitant midtarsal Chopart injury. Sagittal proton density–weighted 3D MR image (A) shows the normal talonavicular ligament as a thin, taut low-signal band (arrow) extending from the talar neck to the navicular bone. Sagittal proton density–weighted (B) and fat-suppressed T2-weighted MR images (C) show a dorsal talonavicular injury with thickened, edematous, and ill-marginated ligament (arrows in B and C).

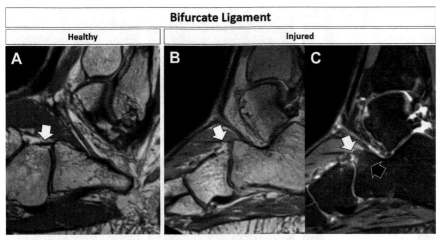

Fig. 22. MRI appearance of the normal and injured bifurcate ligament after ankle sprain with concomitant midtarsal Chopart injury. Sagittal proton density–weighted 3D MR image (*A*) shows the normal calcaneocuboid ligament as a thin, taut low-signal band (*arrow*) extending from the interprocess of the calcaneus to the cuboid bone. Sagittal proton density–weighted (*B*) and fat-suppressed T2-weighted MR images (*C*) show a bifurcate ligament injury with full-thickness calcaneocuboid ligament tear (*arrows* in *B* and *C*).

Lisfranc Injury

One-third to one-half of Lisfranc injuries and other midfoot sprains occur with low-impact trauma, including ankle sprains.[96] The oblique Lisfranc ligament courses from the medial cuneiform to the base of the second metatarsal bone. It comprises the weakest dorsal, interosseous, and strongest plantar bands. Because there is no transverse metatarsal ligament connecting the first and second metatarsal bone, the Lisfranc ligament is the primary static stabilizer of the second metatarsal base and transverse arch.[32,97]

Undertreated midfoot sprain and Lisfranc injuries may progress to midfoot instability, planovalgus deformity, substantial midfoot arthrosis, pain, decreased function, and loss of quality of life.[32,97,98] However, 30% of cases are unrecognized during the initial workup.[96,97,99] Lower-grade injuries often show intact radiographic alignment, emphasizing the need for MRI to visualize the ligament tears.[99]

The Nunley-Vertullo classification differentiates stage 1 as a low-grade sprain of the Lisfranc ligament complex and a dorsal capsular tear without diastasis, stage 2 as elongation or disruption of the Lisfranc ligament complex with 2 to 5 mm diastasis, and stage 3 as plantar Lisfranc ligament disruption with more than 5 mm diastasis and loss of arch height.[97]

The long axis of the Lisfranc ligament is best seen on axial and short axis on coronal MR images (**Fig. 23**).[32] In addition to Lisfranc ligament fiber disruption, Lisfranc interval edema and capsular tears indicate Lisfranc injuries. MRI has 94% sensitivity and 75% to 100% specificity for detecting and characterizing Lisfranc ligament tears.[100]

Tendon Injuries

Partial- and full-thickness tendon tears occur with a 1.5% to 2.5% incidence in acute ankle sprains.[9,101] MRI has 83% sensitivity and 75% specificity for detecting and characterizing tendon injuries.[102] The peroneal longus and brevis muscle-tendon units are lateral ankle stabilizers and primary investors of the foot. Although less common than

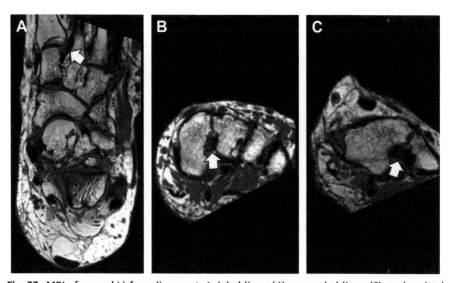

Fig. 23. MRI of normal Lisfranc ligament. Axial oblique (*A*), coronal oblique (*B*), and sagittal oblique (*C*) proton density–weighted 3D MR images of the Lisfranc ligament using dedicated planes aligned to the long and short anatomic axes of the ligament. The MRI appearance of the healthy Lisfranc ligament shows a dark signal band (*arrows*) coursing obliquely from the medial cuneiform to the base of the second metatarsal bone.

ligament tears, high-grade ankle sprains may be associated with peroneal tendon tears (**Fig. 24**), resulting in tendon displacement, pain, and dysfunction.[32,103] The close location to the LCL and peroneal tendons at the inframalleolar area may result in an underestimation of concomitant peroneal tendon injuries and prolonged lateral ankle

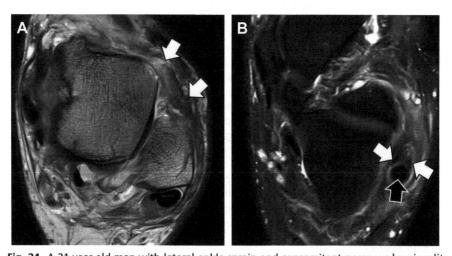

Fig. 24. A 31-year-old man with lateral ankle sprain and concomitant peroneus brevis split tear. Axial proton density–weighted MR image (*A*) shows an anterior talofibular ligament tear (*arrows*). Axial fat-suppressed T2-weighted MR image (*B*) shows a concomitant subfibular peroneus brevis tendon split tear (*white arrows*) and an intact peroneus longus tendon (*black arrow*).

Table 6
Seddon and Sunderland nerve injury classification with structural correlation

Seddon Classification	Sunderland Classification	Axonal Disruption	Endoneurium Disruption	Perineurium Disruption	Epineurium Disruption	Wallerian Degeneration
Neurapraxia	Class I	−[a]	−	−	−	−
Axonotmesis	Class II	+	−	−	−	+
	Class III	+	+	−	−	+
	Class IV	+	+	+	−	+
Neurotmesis	Class V[b]	+	+	+	+	+

[a] Axonal injury without disruption.
[b] Nerve transection.

Table 7
MRI findings in nerve injuries

	Neurapraxia	Axonotmesis	Neurotmesis
Nerve conduction study	Slowing or focal conduction block	Initial conduction block followed by recovery	Persistent conduction block
Electromyography	No or minimal denervation	Denervation occurs after 2–3 wk	Persistent denervation
MRI of injured nerve	Abnormal T2 signal hyperintensity	Nerve enlargement and abnormal T2 signal hyperintensity distal to injury followed by normalization with nerve regeneration	Nerve discontinuity with abnormal T2 signal hyperintensity distal to injury followed by delayed normalization
MRI muscle denervation effects	None	Muscle edema pattern, followed by normalization with nerve regeneration	Muscle edema pattern, followed by progressive atrophy and fatty infiltration

pain. Diagnosis of peroneal tendon injuries may also be important for planning surgical reconstruction and choice of graft, such as the peroneus brevis tendon.[104] MRI findings of traumatic peroneus tears include partial-thickness and full-thickness cross-sectional and longitudinal tears and tendon subluxation and dislocation.[32]

Inversion-type lateral ankle sprains are associated with superior peroneal retinaculum tears, representing a fibro-osseous tunnel that encloses and stabilizes the peroneal tendon in the retromalleolar groove. Superior peroneal retinaculum tears may result in peroneal tendon micro- and macroinstability and progression to tendon fissuring and rupture.[32,105] Superior peroneal retinaculum tears may be partial or complete. However, in both instances, peroneal tendon subluxation and dislocation may occur dynamically, meaning the peroneal tendons may be located anatomically during MRI in recumbent non–weight-bearing position.[105] In such cases, dynamic ultrasound examination is the test of choice to visualize peroneal tendon subluxation and dislocation.

Nerve Injuries

Ankle sprains can also be associated with posterior tibial nerve, medial and lateral plantar nerve, peroneal nerve, and sural nerve injuries.[106–109] Posterior tibial nerve injuries have been reported in 17% of clinical grade 2 and 86% of clinical grade 3 ankle sprains, whereas peroneal nerve injuries have been reported in 10% of clinical grade 2 and 83% of clinical grade 3 ankle sprains.[106]

Depending on the injury grade, ankle sprain–associated nerve injury symptoms range from sensory loss to motor weakness with eventual muscle atrophy. The evaluation of nerve injuries is based on neurologic examination and invasive electrodiagnostic studies, including electromyography (EMG) and nerve conduction studies. MRI can aid in the early noninvasive diagnosis of nerve injuries, differentiate low-grade from high-grade nerve injuries, and define the side of injury, including external compression. EMG change can often occur late, and in this case, muscle edema associated with denervation effects is seen earlier with MRI.[110]

The Seddon classification of nerve injuries differentiates neurapraxia, axonotmesis, and neurotmesis (Table 6). In neurapraxia and axonotmesis, the injured nerves remain microscopically continuous. Neurapraxia indicates axonal disruption, whereas axonotmesis indicates axonal disruption with a preserved myelin sheath. In neurotmesis, the nerve is transected. The more diversified Sunderland classification includes classes I to V (see Table 6). Sunderland class I corresponds to neurapraxia. Classes II to IV correspond to axonotmesis with axonal disruption (class II), endoneurial disruption (class III), and additional fascicular disruption (class IV). Class V represents neurotmesis.

Sunderland class I nerve injuries are low severity and characterized by transient clinical symptoms. MRI shows nerve edema (increased T2 signal) at the injury site. Muscle denervation effects are typically absent. Injured nerves typically recover fully.

Motor function occurs with increasing frequency in Sunderland class II to IV nerve injuries. MRI shows nerve swelling and accompanying muscle edema in the nerve distribution area in the acute phase. The muscle edema may be mild in class II and more pronounced in class III and IV. Nerve and muscle edema may normalize with axonal regeneration. Lack of regeneration may indicate a Sunderland IV, further corroborated by the MRI demonstration of internal nerve scarring, manifesting as neuroma in continuity with fusiform nerve enlargement and heterogeneous internal fascicular pattern (Table 7).[111] MRI differentiates low-grade Sunderland class I to III from high-grade Sunderland IV to V injuries with 75% sensitivity and 83% specificity. MR neurography findings of architectural nerve distortion, fusiform enlargement, perineural fibrosis, nerve discontinuity, and skeletal muscle denervation effects were most useful for differentiation.[112]

SUMMARY

MRI is the most accurate noninvasive test for assessing the structural integrity and severity of deltoid, lateral collateral, and syndesmotic ligament injuries in acute ankle sprains. Lateral collateral ligament injuries may be treated conservatively; however, high-grade deltoid ligament and syndesmotic injuries may require surgical reconstruction. MRI adds value in confirming the absence or presence of ankle sprain–associated hindfoot and midfoot injuries, especially when clinical examinations are challenging and radiographs are normal. The threshold for ankle MRI investigation following ankle sprains should be low, particularly in the setting of clinically more severe and recurrent injuries. Misdiagnosing associated injuries and minor residual instability following recurrent or multiligamentous injuries may contribute to 30% of the end-stage ankle arthritis cases with a clinical history of a prior sprain.[113] A more consistent MRI investigation of acute ankle sprains could lead to a better and more complete assessment of these injuries, allowing more accurate diagnoses and adequate treatment of the more severe, multiligament and potentially more unstable ankles with associated injuries.

CLINICS CARE POINTS

- Advances in ankle MRI resulted in increased image quality and decreased acquisition time.
- MRI provides high-resolution visualization of ankle ligaments for accurate diagnosis and grading.
- MRI adds value in confirming the absence or presence of ankle sprain–associated hindfoot and midfoot injuries, especially when clinical examinations are challenging and radiographs are normal.

REFERENCES

1. Southerland JT, Boberg JS, Downey MS, et al. McGlamry's comprehensive textbook of foot and ankle surgery. 4th edition. Philadelphia: Lippincott Williams & Wilkins; 2012.
2. Maughan KL, Jackson J. Ankle sprain in adults: evaluation and diagnosis. In: UpToDate, Post TW(Ed), UpToDate, Walham, MA. (Accessed on January 13, 2023). Available at: https://www.uptodate.com/contents/ankle-sprain-in-adults-evaluation-and-diagnosis?search=acute%20ankle%20sprain&source=search_result&selectedTitle=1~150&usage_type=default&display_rank=1.
3. Fritz B, Parkar AP, Cerezal L, et al. Sports imaging of team handball injuries. Semin Muscoskel Radiol 2020;24(3):227–45.
4. Waterman BR, Owens BD, Davey S, et al. The epidemiology of ankle sprains in the United States. J Bone Joint Surg Am 2010;92(13):2279–84.
5. Coughlin MJ, Saltzman CL, Mann RA. Mann's surgery of the foot and ankle: expert consult-online. 9th edition. Philadelphia: Elsevier Health Sciences; 2013.
6. Pihlajamäki H, Hietaniemi K, Paavola M, et al. Surgical versus functional treatment for acute ruptures of the lateral ligament complex of the ankle in young men: a randomized controlled trial. J Bone Joint Surg Am 2010;92(14):2367–74.
7. Hintermann B, Boss A, Schäfer D. Arthroscopic findings in patients with chronic ankle instability. Am J Sports Med 2002;30(3):402–9.

8. Langner I, Frank M, Kuehn JP, et al. Acute inversion injury of the ankle without radiological abnormalities: assessment with high-field MR imaging and correlation of findings with clinical outcome. Skeletal Radiol 2011;40(4):423–30.

9. Roemer FW, Jomaah N, Niu J, et al. Ligamentous injuries and the risk of associated tissue damage in acute ankle sprains in athletes: a cross-sectional MRI study. Am J Sports Med 2014;42(7):1549–57.

10. Khodarahmi I, Fritz J. The value of 3 Tesla field strength for musculoskeletal magnetic resonance imaging. Invest Radiol 2021;56(11):749–63.

11. Chhabra A, Soldatos T, Chalian M, et al. 3-Tesla magnetic resonance imaging evaluation of posterior tibial tendon dysfunction with relevance to clinical staging. J Foot Ankle Surg 2011;50(3):320–8.

12. Kijowski R, Fritz J. Emerging technology in musculoskeletal MRI and CT. Radiology 2023;306(1):6–19.

13. Alaia EF, Chhabra A, Simpfendorfer CS, et al. MRI nomenclature for musculoskeletal infection. Skeletal Radiol 2021;50(12):2319–47.

14. Walter SS, Fritz J. MRI of muscular neoplasms and tumor-like lesions: a 2020 World Health Organization classification-based systematic review. Semin Roentgenol 2022;57(3):252–74.

15. Park HJ, Lee SY, Park NH, et al. Usefulness of the oblique coronal plane in ankle MRI of the calcaneofibular ligament. Clin Radiol 2015;70(4):416–23.

16. Choo HJ, Lee SJ, Kim DW, et al. Multibanded anterior talofibular ligaments in normal ankles and sprained ankles using 3D isotropic proton density-weighted fast spin-echo MRI sequence. AJR Am J Roentgenol 2014;202(1): W87–94.

17. Hermans JJ, Ginai AZ, Wentink N, et al. The additional value of an oblique image plane for MRI of the anterior and posterior distal tibiofibular syndesmosis. Skeletal Radiol 2011;40(1):75–83.

18. Del Grande F, Guggenberger R, Fritz J. Rapid musculoskeletal MRI in 2021: value and optimized use of widely accessible techniques. AJR Am J Roentgenol 2021;216(3):704–17.

19. Fritz J, Guggenberger R, Del Grande F. Rapid musculoskeletal MRI in 2021: clinical application of advanced accelerated techniques. AJR Am J Roentgenol 2021;216(3):718–33.

20. Fritz J, Fritz B, Zhang J, et al. Simultaneous multislice accelerated turbo spin echo magnetic resonance imaging: comparison and combination with in-plane parallel imaging acceleration for high-resolution magnetic resonance imaging of the knee. Invest Radiol 2017;52(9):529–37.

21. Fritz J, Raithel E, Thawait GK, et al. Six-fold acceleration of high-spatial resolution 3D SPACE MRI of the knee through incoherent k-space undersampling and iterative reconstruction-first experience. Invest Radiol 2016;51(6):400–9.

22. Lin DJ, Walter SS, Fritz J. Artificial intelligence-driven ultra-fast superresolution MRI: 10-Fold accelerated musculoskeletal turbo spin echo MRI within reach. Invest Radiol 2023;58(1):28–42.

23. Del Grande F, Rashidi A, Luna R, et al. Five-minute five-sequence knee MRI using combined simultaneous multislice and parallel imaging acceleration: comparison with 10-minute parallel imaging knee MRI. Radiology 2021;299(3): 635–46.

24. Fritz J, Fritz B, Thawait GG, et al. Three-dimensional CAIPIRINHA SPACE TSE for 5-minute high-resolution MRI of the knee. Invest Radiol 2016;51(10):609–17.

25. Fritz B, Bensler S, Thawait GK, et al. CAIPIRINHA-accelerated 10-min 3D TSE MRI of the ankle for the diagnosis of painful ankle conditions: Performance evaluation in 70 patients. Eur Radiol 2019;29(2):609–19.

26. Fritz B, Fritz J, Sutter R. 3D MRI of the ankle: a concise state-of-the-art review. Semin Muscoskel Radiol 2021;25(3):514–26.

27. Kalia V, Fritz B, Johnson R, et al. CAIPIRINHA accelerated SPACE enables 10-min isotropic 3D TSE MRI of the ankle for optimized visualization of curved and oblique ligaments and tendons. Eur Radiol 2017;27(9):3652–61.

28. Siriwanarangsun P, Bae WC, Statum S, et al. Advanced MRI techniques for the ankle. AJR Am J Roentgenol 2017;209(3):511–24.

29. Rosenberg ZS, Beltran J, Bencardino JT. From the RSNa refresher courses. radiological society of North America. MR imaging of the ankle and foot. Radiographics 2000;20 Spec No:S153–79.

30. Perrich KD, Goodwin DW, Hecht PJ, et al. Ankle ligaments on MRI: appearance of normal and injured ligaments. AJR Am J Roentgenol 2009;193(3):687–95.

31. Salat P, Le V, Veljkovic A, et al. Imaging in foot and ankle instability. Foot Ankle Clin 2018;23(4):499–522.e28.

32. Stoller DW, Tirman PF, Miriam AB, et al. Magnetic Resonance Imaging in Orthopaedics and Sports Medicine. 3rd edition. Philadelphia: Lippincott Williams & Wilkins; 2007.

33. de César PC, Avila EM, de Abreu MR. Comparison of magnetic resonance imaging to physical examination for syndesmotic injury after lateral ankle sprain. Foot Ankle Int 2011;32(12):1110–4.

34. Joshy S, Abdulkadir U, Chaganti S, et al. Accuracy of MRI scan in the diagnosis of ligamentous and chondral pathology in the ankle. Foot Ankle Surg 2010; 16(2):78–80.

35. Oae K, Takao M, Uchio Y, et al. Evaluation of anterior talofibular ligament injury with stress radiography, ultrasonography and MR imaging. Skeletal Radiol 2010; 39(1):41–7.

36. Edama M, Takabayashi T, Inai T, et al. Relationships between differences in the number of fiber bundles of the anterior talofibular ligament and differences in the angle of the calcaneofibular ligament and their effects on ankle-braking function. Surg Radiol Anat 2019;41(6):675–9.

37. van den Bekerom MP, Oostra RJ, Golanó P, et al. The anatomy in relation to injury of the lateral collateral ligaments of the ankle: a current concepts review. Clin Anat 2008;21(7):619–26.

38. Amis AA, Dawkins GP. Functional anatomy of the anterior cruciate ligament. Fibre bundle actions related to ligament replacements and injuries. J Bone Joint Surg Br 1991;73(2):260–7.

39. Halabchi F, Hassabi M. Acute ankle sprain in athletes: clinical aspects and algorithmic approach. World J Orthop 2020;11(12):534–58.

40. Crim JR, Beals TC, Nickisch F, et al. Deltoid ligament abnormalities in chronic lateral ankle instability. Foot Ankle Int 2011;32(9):873–8.

41. Mengiardi B, Pfirrmann CW, Vienne P, et al. Medial collateral ligament complex of the ankle: MR appearance in asymptomatic subjects. Radiology 2007;242(3): 817–24.

42. Chun KY, Choi YS, Lee SH, et al. Deltoid ligament and tibiofibular syndesmosis injury in chronic lateral ankle instability: magnetic resonance imaging evaluation at 3T and comparison with arthroscopy. Korean J Radiol 2015;16(5):1096–103.

43. Chhabra A, Subhawong TK, Carrino JA. MR imaging of deltoid ligament patho-logic findings and associated impingement syndromes. Radiographics 2010; 30(3):751–61.

44. Muhle C, Frank LR, Rand T, et al. Collateral ligaments of the ankle: high-resolution MR imaging with a local gradient coil and anatomic correlation in ca-davers. Radiographics 1999;19(3):673–83.

45. Bencardino J, Rosenberg ZS, Delfaut E. MR imaging in sports injuries of the foot and ankle. Magn Reson Imaging Clin N Am 1999;7(1):131–49, ix.

46. Espinosa N, Smerek JP, Myerson MS. Acute and chronic syndesmosis injuries: pathomechanisms, diagnosis and management. Foot Ankle Clin 2006;11(3): 639–57.

47. Rammelt S, Zwipp H, Grass R. Injuries to the distal tibiofibular syndesmosis: an evidence-based approach to acute and chronic lesions. Foot Ankle Clin 2008; 13(4):611–33, vii-viii.

48. Ogilvie-Harris DJ, Reed SC, Hedman TP. Disruption of the ankle syndesmosis: biomechanical study of the ligamentous restraints. Arthroscopy 1994;10(5): 558–60.

49. Bassett FH 3rd, Gates HS 3rd, Billys JB, et al. Talar impingement by the ante-roinferior tibiofibular ligament. A cause of chronic pain in the ankle after inver-sion sprain. J Bone Joint Surg Am 1990;72(1):55–9.

50. Tourné Y, Molinier F, Andrieu M, et al. Diagnosis and treatment of tibiofibular syn-desmosis lesions. Orthop Traumatol Surg Res 2019;105(8s):S275–86.

51. Chun DI, Cho JH, Min TH, et al. Diagnostic accuracy of radiologic methods for ankle syndesmosis injury: a systematic review and meta-analysis. J Clin Med 2019;8(7):968.

52. Oae K, Takao M, Naito K, et al. Injury of the tibiofibular syndesmosis: value of MR imaging for diagnosis. Radiology 2003;227(1):155–61.

53. van Dijk CN, Longo UG, Loppini M, et al. Classification and diagnosis of acute isolated syndesmotic injuries: ESSKA-AFAS consensus and guidelines. Knee Surg Sports Traumatol Arthrosc 2016;24(4):1200–16.

54. Calder JD, Bamford R, Petrie A, et al. Stable versus unstable grade II high ankle sprains: a prospective study predicting the need for surgical stabilization and time to return to sports. Arthroscopy 2016;32(4):634–42.

55. Massri-Pugin J, Lubberts B, Vopat BG, et al. Role of the deltoid ligament in syn-desmotic instability. Foot Ankle Int 2018;39(5):598–603.

56. Pinar H, Akseki D, Kovanlikaya I, et al. Bone bruises detected by magnetic reso-nance imaging following lateral ankle sprains. Knee Surg Sports Traumatol Ar-throsc 1997;5(2):113–7.

57. Khor YP, Tan KJ. The anatomic pattern of injuries in acute inversion ankle sprains: a magnetic resonance imaging study. Orthop J Sports Med 2013; 1(7). 2325967113517078.

58. Passon T, Germann C, Fritz B, et al. Bone marrow edema of the medioplantar talar head is associated with severe ligamentous injury in ankle sprain. Skeletal Radiol 2022;51(10):1937–46.

59. Gorbachova T, Wang PS, Hu B, et al. Plantar talar head contusions and osteo-chondral fractures: associated findings on ankle MRI and proposed mechanism of injury. Skeletal Radiol 2016;45(6):795–803.

60. Szaro P, Geijer M, Solidakis N. Traumatic and non-traumatic bone marrow edema in ankle MRI: a pictorial essay. Insights Imaging 2020;11(1):97.

61. Haraguchi N, Toga H, Shiba N, et al. Avulsion fracture of the lateral ankle ligament complex in severe inversion injury: incidence and clinical outcome. Am J Sports Med 2007;35(7):1144–52.
62. Jonckheer P, Willems T, De Ridder R, et al. Evaluating fracture risk in acute ankle sprains: any news since the ottawa ankle rules? A systematic review. Eur J Gen Pract 2016;22(1):31–41.
63. Wei CJ, Tsai WC, Tiu CM, et al. Systematic analysis of missed extremity fractures in emergency radiology. Acta Radiol 2006;47(7):710–7.
64. Kou JX, Fortin PT. Commonly missed peritalar injuries. J Am Acad Orthop Surg 2009;17(12):775–86.
65. Hermans JJ, Beumer A, Hop WC, et al. Tibiofibular syndesmosis in acute ankle fractures: additional value of an oblique MR image plane. Skeletal Radiol 2012;41(2):193–202.
66. Collin D, Geijer M, Göthlin JH. Computed tomography compared to magnetic resonance imaging in occult or suspect hip fractures. A retrospective study in 44 patients. Eur Radiol 2016;26(11):3932–8.
67. You JH, Kim IH, Hwang J, et al. Fracture of ankle: MRI using opposed-phase imaging obtained from turbo spin echo modified Dixon image shows improved sensitivity. Br J Radiol 2018;91(1088):20170779.
68. Lohman M, Kivisaari A, Kallio P, et al. Acute paediatric ankle trauma: MRI versus plain radiography. Skeletal Radiol 2001;30(9):504–11.
69. Rikken QGH, Kerkhoffs G. Osteochondral lesions of the talus: an individualized treatment paradigm from the amsterdam perspective. Foot Ankle Clin 2021;26(1):121–36.
70. Liu SH, Jason WJ. Lateral ankle sprains and instability problems. Clin Sports Med 1994;13(4):793–809.
71. Gold GE, Chen CA, Koo S, et al. Recent advances in MRI of articular cartilage. AJR Am J Roentgenol 2009;193(3):628–38.
72. Mintz DN, Tashjian GS, Connell DA, et al. Osteochondral lesions of the talus: a new magnetic resonance grading system with arthroscopic correlation. Arthroscopy 2003;19(4):353–9.
73. Griffith JF, Lau DT, Yeung DK, et al. High-resolution MR imaging of talar osteochondral lesions with new classification. Skeletal Radiol 2012;41(4):387–99.
74. Cain JD, Dalmau-Pastor M. Anatomy of the deltoid-spring ligament complex. Foot Ankle Clin 2021;26(2):237–47.
75. Taniguchi A, Tanaka Y, Takakura Y, et al. Anatomy of the spring ligament. J Bone Joint Surg Am 2003;85(11):2174–8.
76. Williams G, Widnall J, Evans P, et al. MRI features most often associated with surgically proven tears of the spring ligament complex. Skeletal Radiol 2013;42(7):969–73.
77. Balen PF, Helms CA. Association of posterior tibial tendon injury with spring ligament injury, sinus tarsi abnormality, and plantar fasciitis on MR imaging. AJR Am J Roentgenol 2001;176(5):1137–43.
78. Toye LR, Helms CA, Hoffman BD, et al. MRI of spring ligament tears. AJR Am J Roentgenol 2005;184(5):1475–80.
79. Myerson MS, Thordarson DB, Johnson JE, et al. Classification and nomenclature: progressive collapsing foot deformity. Foot Ankle Int 2020;41(10):1271–6.
80. de Cesar Netto C, Deland JT, Ellis SJ. Guest editorial: expert consensus on adult-acquired flatfoot deformity. Foot Ankle Int 2020;41(10):1269–71.
81. Arshad Z, Bhatia M. Current concepts in sinus tarsi syndrome: a scoping review. Foot Ankle Surg 2021;27(6):615–21.

82. Beltran J. Sinus tarsi syndrome. Magn Reson Imaging Clin N Am 1994;2(1): 59–65.

83. de Cesar Netto C, Saito GH, Roney A, et al. Combined weightbearing CT and MRI assessment of flexible progressive collapsing foot deformity. Foot Ankle Surg 2021;27(8):884–91.

84. DeLee JC, Curtis R. Subtalar dislocation of the foot. J Bone Joint Surg Am 1982; 64(3):433–7.

85. Hoexum F, Heetveld MJ. Subtalar dislocation: two cases requiring surgery and a literature review of the last 25 years. Arch Orthop Trauma Surg 2014;134(9): 1237–49.

86. Perugia D, Basile A, Massoni C, et al. Conservative treatment of subtalar dislocations. Int Orthop 2002;26(1):56–60.

87. Heck BE, Ebraheim NA, Jackson WT. Anatomical considerations of irreducible medial subtalar dislocation. Foot Ankle Int 1996;17(2):103–6.

88. Melenevsky Y, Mackey RA, Abrahams RB, et al. Talar fractures and dislocations: a radiologist's guide to timely diagnosis and classification. Radiographics 2015; 35(3):765–79.

89. Walter WR, Hirschmann A, Alaia EF, et al. Normal anatomy and traumatic injury of the midtarsal (chopart) joint complex: an imaging primer. Radiographics 2019;39(1):136–52.

90. Walter WR, Hirschmann A, Alaia EF, et al. JOURNAL CLUB: MRI evaluation of midtarsal (Chopart) Sprain in the setting of acute ankle injury. AJR Am J Roentgenol 2018;210(2):386–95.

91. Keener BJ, Sizensky JA. The anatomy of the calcaneus and surrounding structures. Foot Ankle Clin 2005;10(3):413–24.

92. Hirschmann A, Walter WR, Alaia EF, et al. Acute fracture of the anterior process of calcaneus: does it herald a more advanced injury to chopart joint? AJR Am J Roentgenol 2018;210(5):1123–30.

93. Benirschke SK, Meinberg EG, Anderson SA, et al. Fractures and dislocations of the midfoot: Lisfranc and Chopart injuries. Instr Course Lect 2013;62:79–91.

94. Rammelt S, Schepers T. Chopart injuries: when to fix and when to fuse? Foot Ankle Clin 2017;22(1):163–80.

95. Walter WR, Hirschmann A, Tafur M, et al. Imaging of chopart (Midtarsal) joint complex: normal anatomy and posttraumatic findings. AJR Am J Roentgenol 2018;211(2):416–25.

96. Renninger CH, Cochran G, Tompane T, et al. Injury characteristics of low-energy lisfranc injuries compared with high-energy injuries. Foot Ankle Int 2017;38(9): 964–9.

97. Siddiqui NA, Galizia MS, Almusa E, et al. Evaluation of the tarsometatarsal joint using conventional radiography, CT, and MR imaging. Radiographics 2014; 34(2):514–31.

98. Philbin T, Rosenberg G, Sferra JJ. Complications of missed or untreated Lisfranc injuries. Foot Ankle Clin 2003;8(1):61–71.

99. Haapamaki VV, Kiuru MJ, Koskinen SK. Ankle and foot injuries: analysis of MDCT findings. AJR Am J Roentgenol 2004;183(3):615–22.

100. Sripanich Y, Weinberg MW, Krähenbühl N, et al. Imaging in Lisfranc injury: a systematic literature review. Skeletal Radiol 2020;49(1):31–53.

101. Fallat L, Grimm DJ, Saracco JA. Sprained ankle syndrome: prevalence and analysis of 639 acute injuries. J Foot Ankle Surg 1998;37(4):280–5.

102. Lamm BM, Myers DT, Dombek M, et al. Magnetic resonance imaging and surgical correlation of peroneus brevis tears. J Foot Ankle Surg 2004;43(1):30–6.

103. Philbin TM, Landis GS, Smith B. Peroneal tendon injuries. J Am Acad Orthop Surg 2009;17(5):306–17.
104. Umans H, Cerezal L, Linklater J, et al. Postoperative MRI of the ankle and foot. Magn Reson Imaging Clin N Am 2022;30(4):733–55.
105. Rosenberg ZS, Bencardino J, Astion D, et al. MRI features of chronic injuries of the superior peroneal retinaculum. AJR Am J Roentgenol 2003;181(6):1551–7.
106. Nitz AJ, Dobner JJ, Kersey D. Nerve injury and grades II and III ankle sprains. Am J Sports Med 1985;13(3):177–82.
107. Nobel W. Peroneal palsy due to hematoma in the common peroneal nerve sheath after distal torsional fractures and inversion ankle sprains. J Bone Joint Surg Am 1966;48(8):1484–95.
108. O'Neill PJ, Parks BG, Walsh R, et al. Excursion and strain of the superficial peroneal nerve during inversion ankle sprain. J Bone Joint Surg Am 2007;89(5): 979–86.
109. Fabre T, Montero C, Gaujard E, et al. Chronic calf pain in athletes due to sural nerve entrapment. A report of 18 cases. Am J Sports Med 2000;28(5):679–82.
110. Kamath S, Venkatanarasimha N, Walsh MA, et al. MRI appearance of muscle denervation. Skeletal Radiol 2008;37(5):397–404.
111. Chhabra A, Ahlawat S, Belzberg A, et al. Peripheral nerve injury grading simplified on MR neurography: as referenced to Seddon and Sunderland classifications. Indian J Radiol Imaging 2014;24(3):217–24.
112. Ahlawat S, Belzberg AJ, Fayad LM. Utility of magnetic resonance imaging for predicting severity of sciatic nerve injury. J Comput Assist Tomogr 2018;42(4): 580–7.
113. Saltzman CL, Salamon ML, Blanchard GM, et al. Epidemiology of ankle arthritis: report of a consecutive series of 639 patients from a tertiary orthopaedic center. Iowa Orthop J 2005;25:44–6.

Advanced Imaging in the Chronic Lateral Ankle Instability: An Algorithmic Approach

Adham do Amaral e Castro, MD, PhD[a,b],
Alexandre Leme Godoy-Santos, MD, PhD[a,c],
Atul K. Taneja, MD, PhD[a,d,*]

KEYWORDS

• Ankle • Instability • Lateral ligament • MRI • Imaging

KEY POINTS

• Imaging studies are fundamental in chronic lateral ankle instability (CLAI), especially when physical examination tests are negative in patients with symptoms.

• Plain radiographs are used as the initial investigative imaging test, and stress radiographs have a high specificity in actively detecting CLAI.

• Ultrasound has the advantage of being widely available, with low cost and absence of ionizing radiation. It allows the dynamic assessment of superficial structures, such as tendons and ligaments, with high sensitivity and specificity depending on the examiner.

• Magnetic Resonance Imaging brings additional information and detailed images of intra-articular and periarticular structures with high accuracy in the setting of CLAI, which is beneficial in preoperative planning. However, a negative MRI study should be interpreted cautiously and not replace arthroscopy, especially in cases with clinical-radiological dissociation.

INTRODUCTION

Ankle sprain is one of the most common musculoskeletal injuries, and its occurrence is extremely frequent among athletes at various levels, with most of the cases being treated in emergencies.[1,2] Such sprains have significant cost impact on health systems[3] being associated with high risk of reinjury, and the development of chronic ankle instability (CLAI). There is much overlap between these conditions, which can trigger

[a] Hospital Israelita Albert Einstein, Av. Albert Einstein, 627 - Jardim Leonor, São Paulo - SP, 05652-900, Brasil; [b] Universidade Federal de São Paulo, Rua Napoleão de Barros, 800 - Vila Clementino - CEP 04024-002 - São Paulo, SP, Brasil; [c] Faculdade de Medicina, USP, R. Dr. Ovídio Pires de Campos, 333 - Cerqueira César, São Paulo - SP, 05403-010, Brasil; [d] Department of Radiology, UT Southwestern Medical Center, 5323 Harry Hines Boulevard, Dallas, Texas 75390-9316, USA
* Corresponding author. Department of Radiology, UT Southwestern Medical Center, 5323 Harry Hines Boulevard, Dallas, Texas 75390-9316.
E-mail address: atul.taneja@utsouthwestern.edu

Foot Ankle Clin N Am 28 (2023) 265–282
https://doi.org/10.1016/j.fcl.2022.12.005
1083-7515/23/© 2022 Elsevier Inc. All rights reserved.
foot.theclinics.com

the development of ankle osteoarthritis.[1] CLAI is defined by the International *Ankle Consortium*[4] as the presence of residual symptoms after a significant ankle torsion, and due to the great subjectivity involved, few tools for evaluation have been developed and applied primarily in research settings.[4,5]

In 2017, the *Ankle Instability Group of European Society of Sports, Traumatology, Knee Surgery and Arthroscopy–Ankle and Foot Associates*[6] administered questionnaires to an international group of 30 orthopedic surgeons with clinical and scientific experience in CLAI, addressing several questions about the topic. In this study, regarding preoperative imaging evaluation, 40% of the orthopedic surgeons answered that they usually request stress radiographs, 87% of them request Magnetic Resonance Imaging (MRI), and 10% recommend ultrasonography (US).[6] This article discusses the role of imaging in evaluating CLAI, including the main methods used in this setting and proposes an evaluation algorithm based on the current literature.

ANATOMY AND IMAGING METHODS

The ligaments around the ankle can be divided into three main groups according to their location: lateral ligament complex, medial (deltoid), and ligaments of the distal tibiofibular syndesmosis.[7] In this article, the authors focus on the lateral complex that includes the anterior talofibular ligament (ATFL), calcaneofibular ligament (CFL), and posterior talofibular ligament (PTFL) (**Fig. 1**).

All mentioned ligamentous structures can be adequately evaluated either by US or MRI, which are considered the gold standard in imaging evaluation.[8–11] On the other hand, computed tomography (CT) scanning is not usually used for ligament evaluation, but it may add relevant information about the effects of ligament injuries on biomechanics and joint instability.[11–13]

The typical appearance of these ligaments on MRI is to present with a low signal intensity on all sequences (**Fig. 2**), whereas on US, they present as hyperechogenic structures with a fibrillar appearance[8–10] (**Fig. 3**). On MRI, T1-weighted and proton density-weighted images are ideal for the evaluation of anatomical structures, whereas fluid-sensitive images such as T2-weighted with fat suppression are used to detect pathological processes.[8] Standard 2-dimensional (2D) images are generally used in institutional protocols with good quality images (high signal-to-noise ratio [SNR] and contrast-to-noise ratio) but with a potential disadvantage of partial volume

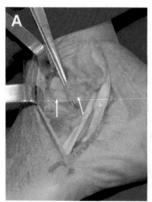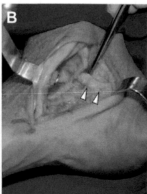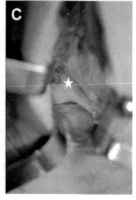

Fig. 1. Cadaveric dissection showing the lateral ligament complex, formed by anterior talofibular (straight *arrows* in (*A*), calcaneofibular (*arrowheads* in *B*), and posterior talofibular (star in *C*) ligaments.

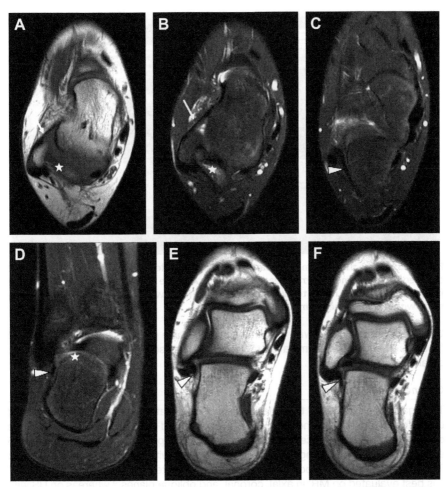

Fig. 2. MR images in axial T1 (*A*), axial T2 fat sat (*B* and *C*), coronal T2 fat sat (*D*), and oblique coronal proton-density (PD) (*E* and *F*) show normal appearance of lateral ankle ligaments: anterior talofibular (straight *arrow*), calcaneofibular (*arrowheads*), and posterior talofibular (star).

effect due to the high slice thickness. MR aquisition with 3-dimensional (3D) volumetric sequences (**Fig. 4**) have reduced slice thickness and allow multiplanar reformatting, avoiding partial volume effect. With the advent of image acceleration protocols using artificial intelligence, these sequences can potentially replace some of the 2D sequences and optimize study protocol time.[14,15] **Fig. 5** shows the positioning to evaluate lateral complex ligaments under MRI and US studies.

Anterior Talofibular Ligament

Generally composed of two bands, this ligament originates at the anterior margin of the lateral malleolus about 10 mm from its distal end and inserts into the talus body, close to the talofibular joint, having a close relationship with its capsule. With a horizontal orientation with the ankle in the neutral position, its average width ranges from 6 to 10 mm,[7] being about 10–16 mm long and with an average thickness of 2.19 mm.[16–18] The best plane for its MRI evaluation is the axial plane,[8] whereas at

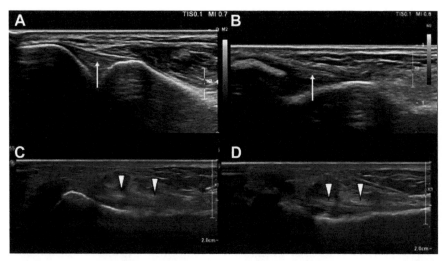

Fig. 3. US images show normal appearance of anterior talofibular (*arrow* in *A* and *B*) and calcaneofibular ligaments (*arrowheads* in *C* and *D*). As these ligaments present in an oblique fashion, the operator needs to avoid anisotropy artifacts, which may decrease the echogenicity within the ligament simulating tear.

US, it is better evaluated with the patient in the supine position, knee flexed with the foot placed flat on the examination table, and the transducer positioned horizontally, parallel to the table.[9,10]

Calcaneofibular Ligament

This ligament originates in the anterior aspect of the lateral malleolus and is located below the inferior band of the ATFL. With an oblique and posterior orientation, it inserts distally on the lateral surface of the calcaneus. Usually, presents a diameter between 6 and 8 mm and length ranging from 12 to 23 mm, with average thickness around 2.13 mm.[16–18] The CFL is located deep to the peroneal tendons, as if it was their floor.[7] It is best evaluated on MRI in axial, coronal, and oblique planes,[8] whereas on US with

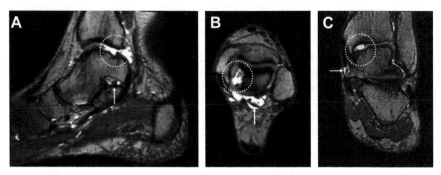

Fig. 4. MRI with volumetric acquisition allows multiplanar reformats (*A*, sagittal; *B*, Axial; and *C*, Coronal), with higher resolution and optimized protocols. In this case of chronic lateral ankle instability, 3D turbo-spin echo (TSE) MRI was acquired with 0.7 mm of slice thickness and shows a large osteochondral lesion at the medial talar dome (*circles*), with displaced loose bodies (*arrows*) and joint effusion. Case courtesy of Dr. Avneesh Chhabra (UT Southwestern Medical Center, Dallas, TX, USA).

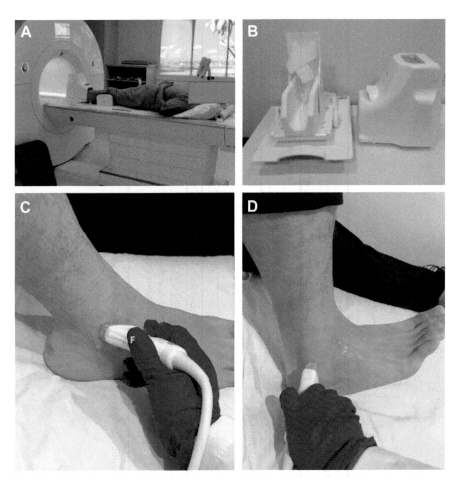

Fig. 5. *Imaging techniques.* In (*A*), the usual positioning of the patient for ankle MR scanning is demonstrated, and in (*B*), the corresponding ankle coil. In (*C*), a standard approach in ultrasound to evaluate the anterior talofibular ligament, with the foot placed flat and the probe positioned parallel to the table. In (*D*), the calcaneofibular ligament is evaluated with the US probe positioned in the long axis of the ligament, whereas the ankle is dorsiflexed.

the patient in the supine position, foot in dorsiflexion, and the transducer positioned obliquely in the long axis of the ligament.[9,10]

Posterior Talofibular Ligament

It represents the strongest, thickest, and deepest ligament of the lateral complex and originates in the lateral malleolar fossa. It has a posterior and horizontal orientation, inserted into the talus posterolateral aspect.[7] Studies show average values for length between 22.0 and 29.6 mm and mean thickness of 3.3 mm.[19,20] On MRI, it is best evaluated in the axial and coronal planes,[8] whereas on US, although it is not routinely assessed, it can be seen posteriorly with the transducer positioned lateral to the calcaneal tendon in a transverse fashion.[9,10]

Table 1 summarizes the anatomical information of the lateral ligaments, their orientation, best evaluation planes on MRI, and transducer positioning on US.

Table 1
Summary of anatomic features and imaging techniques to assess lateral ligament complex in chronic ankle instability

Ligament Features	ATFL	CFL	PTFL
Origin	Anterior margin of lateral malleolus	Anterior aspect of lateral malleolus, below inferior band of ATFL	Lateral malleolar fossa
Insertion	Talus body, adjacent to talofibular joint	Lateral surface of calcaneus	Posterolateral aspect of the talus
Thickness	2.19 mm	2.13 mm	3.3 mm
Length	10–16 mm	12–23 mm	22–29.6 mm
Orientation	Horizontal	Oblique and posterior	Posterior and horizontal
MRI plane for best assessment	Axial	Axial, coronal, and oblique	Axial and coronal
US approach technique	Transducer parallel to the table	Foot in dorsiflexion and transducer positioned obliquely	Lateral to calcaneal tendon in transverse fashion (not routinely assessed)

Abbreviations: ATFL, anterior talofibular ligament; CFL, calcaneofibular ligament; PTFL, posterior talofibular ligament.

IMAGING EVALUATION

Evaluating lateral ankle instability can be optimized through multimodality imaging studies, according to the assessment, clinical need, and physician expertise in choosing the best method.[21] A systematic review study with meta-analysis found that, when clinical tests to assess ankle ligament injury are negative, the presence of ligament injury cannot be excluded and further imaging evaluation becomes necessary.[22] This is also in line with the opinion of experts.

As mentioned in the section above, the diagnostic methods available to evaluate CLAI include plain and stress radiographs, CT, US, and MRI, each presenting its respective role and accuracy.[21] CT and MRI arthrograms are also used, but since they are invasive, they are targeted mostly to cases with suspected osteochondral injury.[23]

Weight-Bearing X-rays and Stress Views

Plain radiographs should be used to start the investigation, yet it does not provide much information on the lateral ligament complex unless there is an evident instability, such as articular widening or lateral avulsion bone fragments in ligaments attachment sites.[21,24] A standard radiographic evaluation in CLAI should comprise the following views: standing anteroposterior, lateral, mortise, and comparative *Saltzman* or *Méary* views, the latter being useful to assess hindfoot alignment.[23] Radiographs also provide information about the morphology of the hindfoot, associated osteochondral lesions of the talar dome, or signs of osteoarthritis[25] (**Fig. 6**).

Comparative stress radiographs with anterior drawer test and varus tilt have high specificity but low sensitivity for CLAI, being of clinical value only if they show positive

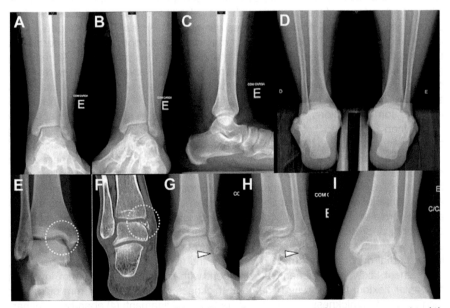

Fig. 6. Weight-bearing normal ankle radiographs are presented in anteroposterior (*A*), mortise (*B*), lateral (*C*), and comparative Saltzman (*D*) views. A case of medial talar dome osteochondral lesion is presented in (*E* and *F*), seen in AP radiograph and coronal CT reformat (*circles*). Images *G* and *H* demonstrate ankle radiographs in oblique (*G*) and mortise (*H*) presenting a sequelae of avulsion fracture at the tip of lateral malleolus (*arrowhead*). In (*I*), advanced tibiotalar arthrosis is seen in AP view radiograph.

findings.[23] As for accuracy , studies indicate low sensitivity, reaching about 57%, but high specificity, up to 100%.[25] In a more recent systematic review with meta-analysis considering arthroscopy as gold standard of diagnosis, the sensitivity and specificity values of this imaging modality were 81% and 92%, respectively.[26] Regarding some experts, once they feel confident with the findings of the physical examination, they often do not request stress radiographs.[6]

In radiographic studies with stress, the tibiotalar joint can be dynamically accessed, whereas a clinical laxity test is performed simultaneously by the orthopedic surgeon manually, by the patient himself with active control, or with the aid of stress devices.[25,27] These different methodologies make radiographic stress testing results variable and heterogeneous. Thus, many authors advocate that one should evaluate the findings compared with the healthy contralateral limb rather than sticking to predetermined reference values.[28]

The *anterior drawer test* aims to assess the anterior talar displacement in the lateral view and is considered diagnostic of ankle instability if greater than 10 mm (or 5 mm compared with the contralateral).[27,29] On the other hand, the *talar tilt stress test* measures the angle between the talar dome and tibial plafond in the anteroposterior view, being considered positive if greater than 10 mm or degrees (or 5 mm or degrees compared with contralateral)[21,25,27,29,30] (**Fig. 7**). However, such measurements are subject to criticism due to varied methodologies and references in the orthopedic literature, including studies suggesting lower reference values than those usually considered diagnostic for CLAI.[31]

Ultrasound

Using US to evaluate patients with CLAI has been more common, in part due to the inherent advantages of the method, such as availability, low cost, and absence of radiation. Moreover, high-resolution probes can accurately assess the integrity of the lateral ankle ligaments.[10] Conveniently, it may even be an option to be performed at the bedside, with the potential for earlier intervention in the context of CLAI, reducing the total costs of treatment.[32] One of the method's main advantages is the real-time dynamic evaluation, allowing comparison to the contralateral side and evaluation of superficial soft tissue structures, especially tendons.[21,23,33] On the other hand, US also has some limitations, such as being operator-dependent, with higher accuracy rates when performed by skilled professionals, and the restriction to evaluating deep structures, such as chondral lesions, occult fractures, and bone contusions.[10,33]

Tear of a ligament on US can be evidenced by the absence of its fibers at the respective anatomical site, and findings suggestive of chronic changes usually include thickening, loss of the fibrillar pattern, and calcifications.[10] Parameters used to verify ankle ligament integrity specifically in the context of CLAI at US vary among studies and comprise scales based on scores, presence of hypoechoic lesions, ligamentous disruption, and/or laxity[34] (**Fig. 8**). Arthroscopic-confirmed lesions of ATFL in CLAI setting were described in the study by Hua and colleagues[35] as follow: (1) ligament injury: partial or total interruption of fibers at the fibular, talar, or medial fibers site; (2) ligament laxity: the ligament remains bent with the ankle in maximum inversion or plantar flexion; (3) thickened ligament: thickness greater than 2.4 mm or greater than 20% of the thickness of the normal contralateral ligament; (4) absorbed: uncharacterized ligament fibers; and (5) nonunion or avulsion fracture of the lateral malleolus.

Regarding the diagnostic value of US in the context of CLAI, a systematic review by Radwan and colleagues[34] found that sensitivity and specificity values of the method ranged from 84.6 to 100% and 87 to 90.9%, respectively. In line with this, another systematic review with meta-analysis by Cao and colleagues[26] demonstrated sensitivity

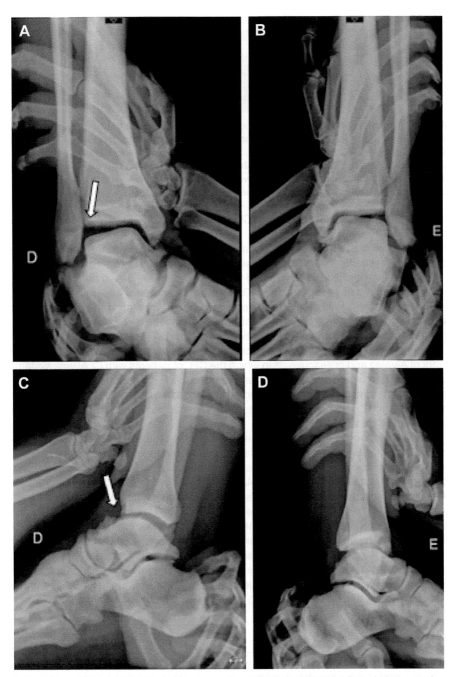

Fig. 7. Comparative ankle radiographs in mortise (*A* and *B*) and lateral (*C* and *D*) views taken under stress maneuvers applied by the orthopedic surgeon. Widening of the tibiotalar joint space (*arrow* in *A*) and a positive anterior drawer (*arrow* in *C*) are seen on the right ankle when compared to the left (*B* and *D*).

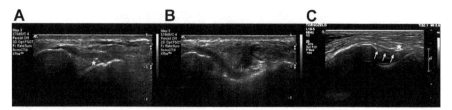

Fig. 8. US images in (*A* and *B*) show scarring changes of the anterior talofibular (*arrows* in *A*) and calcaneofibular (*arrows* in *B*) ligaments, with thickening, hypoechogenicity and loss of the fibrillar pattern. In (*A*), a small, distal, hyperechoic fragment representing a bone avulsion is also observed (*star*). The sonographic image on (*C*) shows a chronic thinning of the anterior talofibular ligament (*arrows*), with loss of the fibrillar pattern and an avulsed bone fragment at the distal end of its fibers (*star*).

and specificity of US in the context of CLAI of 99% and 91% for ATFL injury and 94% and 91% for CFL injury, respectively.

On dynamic maneuvers by US, Mizrahi and colleagues[36] compared the evaluation of the ATFL in healthy volunteers with patients with clinical diagnosis of CLAI and verified the presence of laxity. They found differences between stress and neutral positions in healthy volunteers being of 0.44 mm for men and 0.43 mm for women, whereas in patients with CLAI, this difference was 1.26 mm (mean).[36] These findings are similar to the results from another study[37] which found a positive relationship between stress US and physical examination (anterior drawer test) of patients with CLAI.

There are few studies focused on specifically evaluating CFL. One example is the work of Alvarez and colleagues, [38] in which the CFL of patients with CLAI was systematically evaluated with dorsiflexion stress, and the following parameters were considered consistent with a lesion: thickening, thinning, loss of tension during a dynamic maneuver, and hypoechogenicity due to the difficulty in visualizing its fibers near the fibular insertion site.

In addition, a technique that has been increasingly studied for US in multiple scenarios, including in the evaluation of lateral ankle ligaments, is the *shear wave elastography*, which can measure the elastic properties of tissues.[39–41] Gimber and colleagues[39] studied the shear wave elastography values for ATFL and CFL in 23 ankles of healthy male volunteers and observed a significant difference in ankle stiffness in stress maneuvers compared with the neutral position. Hotfiel and colleagues[40] also evaluated the technique for ATFL in healthy volunteers of both genders and established normality values for this ligament. Furthermore, Chen and colleagues[41] assessed elastography for ATFL and showed altered values for acute and subacute injuries, but not for chronic cases. The investigators attribute these latter findings to a gradual recovery of the ligament tissue to its original state or due to the small sample size, suggesting that before concluding in this context, studies with larger samples are needed.[41]

MRI

In cases of CLAI, MRI can not only confirm the presence of chronic ligament injuries but also detect the associated lesions, such as osteochondral lesions, concurrent tendon injuries, anterolateral impingement, bone spurs, or loose bodies[23,42–45] (**Fig. 9**). Michels and colleagues evaluated the opinions of several experts and showed that most of them routinely request MRI to detect associated intra-articular findings as they can be the cause of recurrent symptoms if not adequately addressed, even after a successful surgical approach to the ligament reconstruction itself.[6,43]

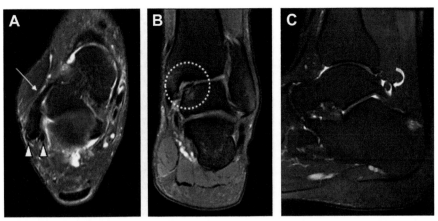

Fig. 9. MR images in axial T2 fat sat (*A*), coronal T2fat sat, and (*B*) sagittal T2 fat sat (*C*) show associated lesions that can be seen in the setting of chronic instability. In (*A*), thickening of the anterior talofibular ligament (*arrow*) and a longitudinal split-type tear of the peroneal brevis tendon (*arrowheads*). In (*B*), an osteochondral lesion of the medial talar dome (*circle*), with low-signal intensity in situ bone fragment, along with subchondral edema and cysts. In (*C*), small posterior tibiotalar joint effusion with an intra-articular loose body (*curved arrow*).

Direct findings of subacute or chronic injury to the lateral ligaments under MRI include fiber signal heterogeneity, wavy contours, lengthening, and even ligament attenuation or noncharacterization, whereas indirect findings include reduced adjacent fat signal (indicating healing or synovial proliferation); thickening and low signal intensity can be seen in scar tissue and chronic fibrosis[21] (**Fig. 10**).

A systematic review with meta-analysis by Cao and colleagues[26] demonstrated sensitivity and specificity values for MRI in chronic ATFL lesions of 83% and 88% and values of 56% and 79% for chronic CFL lesions. Although the information provided by MRI is of utmost importance, it can sometimes underestimate some additional findings, such as anterolateral impingement, bone spurs, loose bodies, and peroneal tendinopathy; therefore, arthroscopy remains the gold standard to evaluate associated lesions, as stated by Staats and colleagues.[42] As MRI presents lower sensitivity for some findings such as loose bodies, a negative result should be interpreted with caution, especially in cases with clinical-radiological discrepancy, where MRI should not replace an arthroscopic evaluation.[6,23,42]

Recent studies have tested if MRI under stress could potentially increase the diagnostic value of MRI by assessing the ankle's biomechanical function.[46] In a pilot study by Wenning and colleagues, the investigators performed stress MRI on 10 patients (seven with mechanical ankle instability vs. three controls). They observed a reduction in lateral bone constriction and in the weight-bearing surface of patients relative to controls while in the plantarflexion-supination position.[47] This same study group cross-sectionally evaluated 25 patients with mechanical ankle instability vs. controls using clinical testing, stress US, and stress MRI and found a potential cutoff point of 43% for loss in fibulotalar joint surface contact area at MRI, with a sensitivity of 71% and specificity of 80% for mechanical instability within subjects with CLAI.[48]

Some studies have evaluated ATFL signal intensity among other parameters under MRI for patients with CLAI in the preoperative setting.[49–51] Liu and colleagues[50] observed that such patients had ATFL with greater length, width, and signal intensity

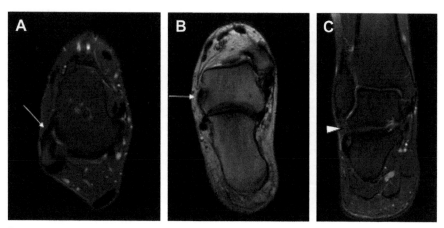

Fig. 10. MR images in axial T2 fat sat (*A*), coronal oblique PD, and (*B*) coronal T2 fat sat (*C*) show scarring and thickening of the anterior talofibular ligament (*arrows* in *A* and *B*) and chronic thinning of the calcaneofibular ligament (*arrowhead* in *C*).

than controls. Ahn and colleagues[51] assessed ATFL features and compared them with arthroscopy, finding that SNR correlates to ligament quality, presence of tear, and degree of tension; a SNR of 11.2 was found as a cutoff for differentiating normal from an abnormal but repairable ATFL, and 32.3 for determining repairable from non-repairable ATFL.[51]

Although conventional MRI can directly visualize osteoarthritis-related findings such as osteophytes, cysts, and subchondral bone edema, there are MRI techniques capable of characterizing and quantifying the biochemical composition of cartilage, with the potential for early detection of chondral changes, such as T2-mapping.[52] For example, Kim and colleagues[53] presented significant differences between T2 relaxation values of the subtalar cartilage patients who underwent surgical intervention compared with controls, with an increased value in patients with CLAI. In a study by Tao and colleagues,[54] T2-mapping of the cartilage and American Orthopaedic Foot and Ankle Society (AOFAS) scoring were evaluated in patients with CLAI with isolated ATFL or combined ATFL + CFL injury and demonstrated (a) higher T2-mapping values in patients compared with controls, (b) higher values in cases with combined ATFL + CFL injuries compared with isolated ATFL injury, and (c) negative correlation of T2-mapping values of anterior medial aspect of the talar cartilage with the AOFAS scoring.[54] The same study group analyzed T2-mapping of the cartilage in patients with CLAI before and 3 years after ligament repair surgery[55] and showed higher values compared with controls and improvement only of the anteromedial talar dome cartilage after 3 years, despite improvement of AOFAS scores.[55]

POSTOPERATIVE EVALUATION

The postsurgical appearance of ATFL on MRI includes decreased signal intensity of ligament fibers, indicating the presence of scar tissue and tightness and sometimes accompanied by changes in the ligament thickness and/or length.[50]

Surgical treatment of CLAI can be performed using either anatomical or nonanatomical techniques.[56,57] A deeper discussion on surgical indications and techniques is beyond the scope of this article; thus, for purposes of illustration we present the modified *Broström* technique, one of the most common techniques, consisting in anatomic shortening and reinsertion of the ATFL and CFL ligaments[56–59] (**Fig. 11**).

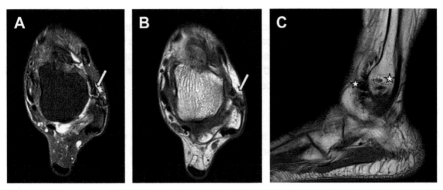

Fig. 11. MR images in axial T2 fat sat (*A*), axial T1 (*B*), and sagittal T1 (*C*) show post-operative status from anterior talofibular ligament reconstruction (18 months prior). The repaired ligament appears thickened and irregular, with low signal intensity (*arrows* in *A* and *B*). Foci of magnetic susceptibility artifacts are observed within the fibers and surgical insertion site in lateral malleolus (*stars* in *C*).

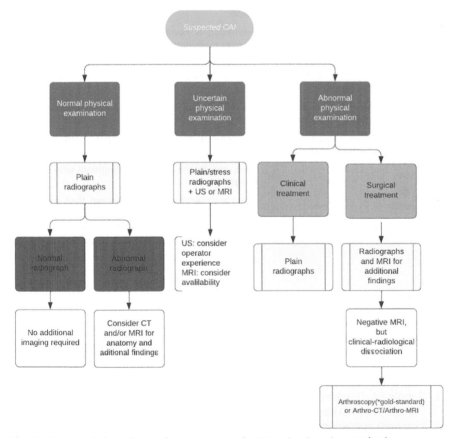

Fig. 12. Proposed algorithm on how to approach CLAI using imaging methods.

In order to assess postoperative results, [57] stress radiographs and Clinical Outcome Measurement Scales should stand as reference tools. Regarding postsurgical ankle biomechanics, Wainright and colleagues[60] evaluated patients with CLAI before and after surgery using MRI and fluoroscopy: they presented improvement in ankle kinematics and joint motion illustrated by a reduction in anterior translation and internal rotation of the talus after the procedure.

SUMMARY

A flowchart summarizing the best imaging methods to use in each clinical scenario of CLAI is presented in **Fig. 12**, based on the most recent literature and authors' experience.

DISCLOSURES

The authors declare that there are no commercial or financial conflicts of interest.

CLINICS CARE POINTS

- Is imaging indicated in the context of chronic lateral ankle instability (CLAI)? Based on the recent literature and the authors' experience, the answer is yes and the physical examination plays a key role regarding which test to order.
- If CLAI is suspected but physical examination is normal, imaging study of choice is radiograph, with no need for further imaging examination if normal.
- If changes are detected on radiography in the context of normal physical examination, one should proceed with CT and/or MRI studies in order to better access the anatomy to search for additional information.
- If physical examination is uncertain, stress radiographs can be used, and its association with ultrasonography or MRI is recommended.
- In the case of an altered physical examination and a conservative therapeutic decision, imaging examination of choice is radiographic study.
- However, in the case of surgical treatment, one should associate radiographs with MRI to investigate preoperative additional findings.
- If additional findings are clinically suspected but preoperative MRI is normal, then arthro-CT or arthro-MRI investigation plays a role, but it is crucial to keep in mind that arthroscopy is the gold standard method for the investigation of intra-articular pathologies.

REFERENCES

1. Herzog MM, Kerr ZY, Marshall SW, et al. Epidemiology of Ankle Sprains and Chronic Ankle Instability. J Athletic Train 2019;54(6):603–10.
2. Doherty C, Delahunt E, Caulfield B, et al. The incidence and prevalence of ankle sprain injury: a systematic review and meta-analysis of prospective epidemiological studies. Sports Med 2014;44(1):123–40.
3. Gribble PA, Bleakley CM, Caulfield BM, et al. Evidence review for the 2016 International Ankle Consortium consensus statement on the prevalence, impact and long-term consequences of lateral ankle sprains. Br J Sports Med 2016;50(24):1496–505.

4. Gribble PA, Delahunt E, Bleakley C, et al. Selection criteria for patients with chronic ankle instability in controlled research: a position statement of the International Ankle Consortium: Table 1. Br J Sports Med 2014;48(13):1014–8.
5. Lin CI, Houtenbos S, Lu YH, et al. The epidemiology of chronic ankle instability with perceived ankle instability- a systematic review. J Foot Ankle Res 2021; 14(1):41.
6. The ESSKA-AFAS Ankle Instability Group, Michels F, Pereira H, Calder J, et al. Searching for consensus in the approach to patients with chronic lateral ankle instability: ask the expert. Knee Surg Sports Traumatol Arthrosc 2018;26(7): 2095–102.
7. Golanó P, Vega J, de Leeuw PAJ, et al. Anatomy of the ankle ligaments: a pictorial essay. Knee Surg Sports Traumatol Arthrosc 2010;18(5):557–69.
8. Pezeshk P, Rehwald C, Khodarahmi I, et al. 3-T MRI of the ankle tendons and ligaments. Clin Sports Med 2021;40(4):731–54.
9. Döring S, Provyn S, Marcelis S, et al. Ankle and midfoot ligaments: ultrasound with anatomical correlation: A review. Eur J Radiol 2018;107:216–26.
10. Sconfienza LM, Orlandi D, Lacelli F, et al. Dynamic high-resolution US of ankle and midfoot ligaments: normal anatomic structure and imaging technique. RadioGraphics 2015;35(1):164–78.
11. Sterzik A, Mueck F, Wirth S, et al. Evaluation of ankle ligaments with CT: a feasibility study. Eur J Radiol 2021;134:109446.
12. Rodrigues JC, Santos ALG, Prado MP, et al. Comparative CT with stress manoeuvres for diagnosing distal isolated tibiofibular syndesmotic injury in acute ankle sprain: a protocol for an accuracy- test prospective study. BMJ Open 2020; 10(9):e037239.
13. Godoy-Santos AL, Cesar Netto CD. Weight-bearing computed tomography of the foot and ankle: an update and future directions. Acta ortop bras 2018;26(2): 135–9.
14. Fritz B, Fritz J, Sutter R. 3D MRI of the ankle: a concise state-of-the-art review. Semin Musculoskelet Radiol 2021;25(3):514–26.
15. Park HJ, Lee SY, Park NH, et al. Three-dimensional isotropic T2-weighted fast spin-echo (VISTA) ankle MRI versus two-dimensional fast spin-echo T2-weighted sequences for the evaluation of anterior talofibular ligament injury. Clin Radiol 2016;71(4):349–55.
16. Hertel J. Functional Anatomy, Pathomechanics, and Pathophysiology of Lateral Ankle Instability. J Athl Train 2002;37(4):364–75.
17. Dimmick S, Kennedy D, Daunt N. Evaluation of thickness and appearance of anterior talofibular and calcaneofibular ligaments in normal versus abnormal ankles with MRI. J Med Imaging Radiat Oncol 2008;52(6):559–63.
18. Yıldız S, Yalcın B. The anterior talofibular and calcaneofibular ligaments: an anatomic study. Surg Radiol Anat 2013;35(6):511–6.
19. Kobayashi T, Suzuki D, Kondo Y, et al. Morphological characteristics of the lateral ankle ligament complex. Surg Radiol Anat 2020;42(10):1153–9.
20. Stella SM, Ciampi B, Del Chiaro A, et al. Sonographic visibility of the main posterior ankle ligaments and para-ligamentous structures in 15 healthy subjects. J Ultrasound 2021;24(1):23–33.
21. Salat P, Le V, Veljkovic A, et al. Imaging in Foot and Ankle Instability. Foot Ankle Clin 2018;23(4):499–522.e28.
22. Schneiders A, Karas S. The accuracy of clinical tests in diagnosing ankle ligament injury. Eur J Physiother 2016;18(4):245–53.

23. Guillo S, Bauer T, Lee JW, et al. Consensus in chronic ankle instability: Aetiology, assessment, surgical indications and place for arthroscopy. Orthopaedics Traumatol Surg Res 2013;99(8):S411–9.
24. Sy JW, Lopez AJ, Lausé GE, et al. Correlation of stress radiographs to injuries associated with lateral ankle instability. WJO 2021;12(9):710–9.
25. Tourné Y, Besse JL, Mabit C. Chronic ankle instability. Which tests to assess the lesions? Which therapeutic options? Orthopaedics Traumatol Surg Res 2010; 96(4):433–46.
26. Cao S, Wang C, Ma X, et al. Imaging diagnosis for chronic lateral ankle ligament injury: a systemic review with meta-analysis. J Orthop Surg Res 2018;13(1):122.
27. Sarcon AK, Heyrani N, Giza E, et al. Lateral ankle sprain and chronic ankle instability. Foot & Ankle Orthopaedics 2019;4(2). 247301141984693.
28. Tarczyńska M, Sekuła P, Gawęda K, et al. Stress radiography in the diagnosis and assessment of the outcomes of surgical treatment of chronic anterolateral ankle instability. Acta Radiol 2020;61(6):783–8.
29. Hoffman E, Paller D, Koruprolu S, et al. Accuracy of plain radiographs versus 3D analysis of ankle stress test. Foot Ankle Int 2011;32(10):994–9.
30. Chan KW, Ding BC, Mroczek KJ. Acute and chronic lateral ankle instability in the athlete. Bull NYU Hosp Jt Dis 2011;69(1):17–26.
31. Dowling LB, Giakoumis M, Ryan JD. Narrowing the Normal Range for Lateral Ankle Ligament Stability with Stress Radiography. J Foot Ankle Surg 2014; 53(3):269–73.
32. Lee SH, Yun SJ. The feasibility of point-of-care ankle ultrasound examination in patients with recurrent ankle sprain and chronic ankle instability: Comparison with magnetic resonance imaging. Injury 2017;48(10):2323–8.
33. Seok H, Lee SH, Yun SJ. Diagnostic performance of ankle ultrasound for diagnosing anterior talofibular and calcaneofibular ligament injuries: a meta-analysis. Acta Radiol 2020;61(5):651–61.
34. Radwan A, Bakowski J, Dew S, et al. Effectiveness of ultrasonography in diagnosing chronic lateral ankle instability:a systematic review. Int J Sports Phys Ther 2016;11(2):164–74.
35. Hua Y, Yang Y, Chen S, et al. Ultrasound examination for the diagnosis of chronic anterior talofibular ligament injury. Acta Radiol 2012;53(10):1142–5.
36. Mizrahi DJ, Nazarian LN, Parker L. Evaluation of the Anterior Talofibular Ligament via Stress Sonography in Asymptomatic and Symptomatic Populations: Stress Sonography of the Anterior Talofibular Ligament. J Ultrasound Med 2018;37(8): 1957–63.
37. Lee KT, Park YU, Jegal H, et al. New method of diagnosis for chronic ankle instability: comparison of manual anterior drawer test, stress radiography and stress ultrasound. Knee Surg Sports Traumatol Arthrosc 2014;22(7):1701–7.
38. Alvarez CAD, Hattori S, Kato Y, et al. Dynamic high-resolution ultrasound in the diagnosis of calcaneofibular ligament injury in chronic lateral ankle injury: a comparison with three-dimensional magnetic resonance imaging. J Med Ultrason 2020;47(2):313–7.
39. Department of VA – Menlo Park Campus, Uniformed Services University, National Teleradiology Program, United States, Gimber LH, Latt LD. Department of Orthopaedic Surgery, The University of Arizona College of Medicine Banner- University Medical Center, United States, Caruso C, Department of Medical Imaging, The University of Arizona College of Medicine Banner- University Medical Center, United States, et al. Ultrasound shear wave elastography of the anterior

talofibular and calcaneofibular ligaments in healthy subjects. J Ultrason 2021; 21(85):e86–94.

40. Hotfiel T, Heiss R, Janka R, et al. Acoustic radiation force impulse tissue characterization of the anterior talofibular ligament: a promising noninvasive approach in ankle imaging. Physician and Sports Med 2018;46(4):435–40.

41. Chen X, Wang L, Li X, et al. Can virtual touch tissue imaging quantification be a reliable method to detect anterior talofibular ligament type I injury at the acute, subacute, and chronic stages? Quant Imaging Med Surg 2021;11(10):4334–41.

42. Staats K, Sabeti-Aschraf M, Apprich S, et al. Preoperative MRI is helpful but not sufficient to detect associated lesions in patients with chronic ankle instability. Knee Surg Sports Traumatol Arthrosc 2018;26(7):2103–9.

43. Ahn BH, Cho BK. Persistent Pain After Operative Treatment for Chronic Lateral Ankle Instability. ORR 2021;13:47–56.

44. Taneja AK, Simeone FJ, Chang CY, et al. Peroneal tendon abnormalities in subjects with an enlarged peroneal tubercle. Skeletal Radiol 2013;42(12):1703–9.

45. Gill CM, Taneja AK, Bredella MA, et al. Osteogenic relationship between the lateral plantar process and the peroneal tubercle in the human calcaneus. J Anat 2014;224(2):173–9.

46. Ringleb SI, Udupa JK, Siegler S, et al. The effect of ankle ligament damage and surgical reconstructions on the mechanics of the ankle and subtalar joints revealed by three-dimensional stress MRI. J Orthop Res 2005;23(4):743–9.

47. Wenning M, Lange T, Paul J, et al. Assessing mechanical ankle instability via functional 3D stress-MRI – A pilot study. Clin Biomech 2019;70:107–14.

48. Wenning M, Gehring D, Lange T, et al. Clinical evaluation of manual stress testing, stress ultrasound and 3D stress MRI in chronic mechanical ankle instability. BMC Musculoskelet Disord 2021;22(1):198.

49. Li H, Hua Y, Li H, et al. Activity Level and Function 2 Years After Anterior Talofibular Ligament Repair: A Comparison Between Arthroscopic Repair and Open Repair Procedures. Am J Sports Med 2017;45(9):2044–51.

50. Liu W, Li H, Hua Y. Quantitative magnetic resonance imaging (MRI) analysis of anterior talofibular ligament in lateral chronic ankle instability ankles pre- and postoperatively. BMC Musculoskelet Disord 2017;18(1):397.

51. Ahn J, Choi JG, Jeong BO. The signal intensity of preoperative magnetic resonance imaging has predictive value for determining the arthroscopic reparability of the anterior talofibular ligament. Knee Surg Sports Traumatol Arthrosc 2021; 29(5):1535–43.

52. Guermazi A, Alizai H, Crema MD, et al. Compositional MRI techniques for evaluation of cartilage degeneration in osteoarthritis. Osteoarthritis and Cartilage 2015; 23(10):1639–53.

53. Kim HS, Yoon YC, Sung KS, et al. Comparison of T2 Relaxation Values in Subtalar Cartilage between Patients with Lateral Instability of the Ankle Joint and Healthy Volunteers. Eur Radiol 2018;28(10):4151–62.

54. Tao H, Hu Y, Qiao Y, et al. T_2-Mapping evaluation of early cartilage alteration of talus for chronic lateral ankle instability with isolated anterior talofibular ligament tear or combined with calcaneofibular ligament tear: Early Cartilage Alteration of Talus. J Magn Reson Imaging 2018;47(1):69–77.

55. Tao H, Zhang Y, Hu Y, et al. Cartilage Matrix Changes in Hindfoot Joints in Chronic Ankle Instability Patients After Anatomic Repair Using T2 -Mapping: Initial Experience With 3-Year Follow-Up. Magn Reson Imaging 2022;55(1):234–43.

56. Hassan S, Thurston D, Sian T, et al. Clinical Outcomes of the Modified Broström Technique in the Management of Chronic Ankle Instability After Early, Intermediate, and Delayed Presentation. J Foot Ankle Surg 2018;57(4):685–8.
57. Spennacchio P, Meyer C, Karlsson J, et al. Evaluation modalities for the anatomical repair of chronic ankle instability. Knee Surg Sports Traumatol Arthrosc 2020; 28(1):163–76.
58. Buerer Y, Winkler M, Burn A, et al. Evaluation of a modified Broström–Gould procedure for treatment of chronic lateral ankle instability: A retrospective study with critical analysis of outcome scoring. Foot Ankle Surg 2013;19(1):36–41.
59. Gould N, Seligson D, Gassman J. Early and Late Repair of Lateral Ligament of the Ankle. Foot & Ankle. 1980;1(2):84–9.
60. Wainright WB, Spritzer CE, Lee JY, et al. The Effect of Modified Broström-Gould Repair for Lateral Ankle Instability on In Vivo Tibiotalar Kinematics. Am J Sports Med 2012;40(9):2099–104.

Can Weight-Bearing Computed Tomography Be a Game-Changer in the Assessment of Ankle Sprain and Ankle Instability?

François Lintz, MD, MS, FEBOT[a],*, Alessio Bernasconi, MD, PhD, FEBOT[b], Eric I. Ferkel, MD[c]

KEYWORDS

- Weight-bearing CT • Ankle instability • Ankle sprain • Distance mapping
- Dynamic imaging

KEY POINTS

- The use of cone beam weight-bearing computed tomography (WBCT) in the diagnostic pathway of ankle sprain (AS) and chronic ankle instability (CLAI) may be crucial to reduce the number of unseen associated lesions, thus reducing the number of unnecessary immobilizations in isolated AS and supporting the prescription of appropriate immobilization where necessary.
- WBCT axial loading measurements in syndesmotic injuries is sensitized by adding external torque.
- More advanced visualization tools, such as segmentation and distance mapping, are already available but not common practice yet. They enable three-dimensional volumetric measurements, which demonstrate superior sensitivity as compared with radiographic and nonweight-bearing CT measurements to diagnose subtle syndesmotic lesions.

INTRODUCTION

Ankle sprain (AS) and chronic lateral ankle instability (CLAI) are complex conditions and challenging to treat. Cone beam weight-bearing computed tomography (WBCT) is an innovative imaging modality that has gained popularity in the past several years, with a body of literature reporting reduced radiation exposure and operating time, and

[a] UCP Foot & Ankle Center, Ramsay Healthcare Clinique de L'Union, Saint-Jean, Toulouse, France; [b] Federico 2 University of Napoli, Napoli, Italy, [c] Southern California Orthopedic Institute, In Affiliation with UCLA Health, Los Angeles, CA, USA
* Corresponding author. Ramsay Sante Clinique de l'Union, Boulevard de Ratalens, Saint Jean, Occitanie 31240, France.
E-mail address: dr.f.lintz@gmail.com

Foot Ankle Clin N Am 28 (2023) 283–295
https://doi.org/10.1016/j.fcl.2023.01.003
1083-7515/23/© 2023 Elsevier Inc. All rights reserved.
foot.theclinics.com

shortened examination time and a decreased time interval between injury and diagnosis. In our opinion, this supports its use as a primary means of investigation common foot and ankle conditions and therefore applies to AS and CLAI.

To date, there is little literature available on the use of WBCT to diagnose and manage AS and CLAI themselves. Some authors have provided interesting insight into the role of WBCT and more largely cone beam CT (CBCT) in the setting of accident and emergency departments. The bulk of the literature in this field is related to the early diagnosis of associated lesions, such as osteochondral lesions of the talus, fibular, navicular, talar, calcaneal or cuboid avulsion fracture, or Lisfranc and Jones fractures. In some cases, more severe fractures have also been reported, such as talar neck or body fractures. Some authors have focused on syndesmotic instability and Lisfranc fracture-dislocations after AS detected through WBCT. In this article, we make clearer the advantages of this technology and encourage researchers to investigate the area, and clinicians to use it as a primary mode of investigation. We also present clinical cases provided by the authors to illustrate those possibilities using advanced imaging tools. We deliberately do not investigate here the role of WBCT in subtalar instability nor peritalar instability.[1–3]

WEIGHT-BEARING COMPUTED TOMOGRAPHY AND ANKLE SPRAINS (ACUTE TRAUMA)

WBCT provides three-dimensional (3D) imaging of the foot and ankle with radiation doses equivalent to a conventional two-dimensional (2D) radiographic (2DXR) setup (anteroposterior, lateral, and dorsa-plantar). Furthermore, in a conventional radiographic setup, additional views are often required, such as multiple oblique views, which are often performed to uncover hidden lesions caused by bone superimpositions. Although the term "weight-bearing" was coined in the literature because of its historical appeal to foot and ankle surgeons, most devices provide a mobile gantry with possibility of seating the patient. Thus, WBCT does not have to be weight-bearing. We refer to WBCT in the setting of secondary referral where weight-bearing is possible, and to CBCT in the setting of acute trauma, when weight-bearing is not possible or contraindicated.

Although differing slightly between epidemiologic sources, AS represents roughly around 20% to 30% of all lower limb trauma and around 60% to 70% of all ankle trauma.[4,5] AS is the most frequent cause for consultation for lower limb trauma in emergency departments around the world. Such a high incidence associated with the generally benign natural history of the condition unfortunately often leads the clinician to manage AS without sufficient attention, increasing the risk of misdiagnosis for associated lesions. In this scenario, WBCT or CBCT has a huge potential to help formulating a correct diagnosis and at the same time reducing waiting times and freeing slots in conventional CT for other health issues. In technical terms, the cone beam technology has a 0.27 to 0.35 mm spatial resolution, which is better than conventional CT (0.5 mm). However, being less powerful (cone beam requires less photons and less powerful photons for bone imaging, than conventional multidetector CT [MDCT]), it is not as good in terms of contrast and at this stage it cannot be recommended for soft tissue analysis. Therefore, its indications are clearly for suspicion of bone lesions, including fracture, osteochondral lesions, small avulsion lesions, and subtle joint dislocations. Detecting such lesions, which often go undiagnosed after AS, is where CBCT is most useful in emergency departments, on the condition that it is systematically used as a primary means of investigation.

Publications regarding the impact that 3D imaging could have in this setting are mostly recent, but some others based on conventional CT (also known as MDCT) are informative regarding the amount of missed diagnoses because of 2D conventional radiography. In a 2004 paper, Haapamaki and colleagues[6,7] reported that 24% of Lisfranc dislocation-fractures had gone unseen on initial 2DXR evaluation. In a review of the literature in 2012, Van Rijn and coworkers[8] reported one-third false-negatives. We found no specific report on AS in our literature search.

Since 2017, we found seven papers relevant to the subject, all underlining the risk of missed diagnoses on 2DXR taken in emergency rooms. Lau and colleagues[9] reported 20% missed Lisfranc injuries. De Los Santos-Real and coworkers[10] reported more generally 13% to 24% of missed or delayed Lisfranc diagnoses. Borel and colleagues[11] reported: "Because of its low radiation dose, we believe that CBCT can be used in current practice as a replacement or supplement to radiographs to detect these fractures and optimize the cost-effectiveness ratio by limiting the number of needless immobilizations." This remark is indeed justified; because of the known risk of false-negatives, many patients with AS are immobilized out of apprehension rather than medical reasons. This results in delayed onset of physiotherapy, in a situation where it is known that the earlier is the better. In 2019, Ricci and colleagues[12] reported 14% false-negatives using XR compared with CBCT, looking at Lisfranc fractures in the foot and ankle, tibial plateau fractures, wrist, and elbow fractures. When evaluating AS, 2DXR may cause false-negatives, which in practice are easily discarded as just an AS. We see these patients every day in our consultations, resulting in delayed diagnoses and avoidable sequelae. In the former paper, Ricci and colleagues[12] stated that "We can say that if compared to standard X-ray, CBCT has higher sensitivity and specificity in the proper identification and typing of these kinds of lesions with low exposition dose if compared to MDCT."[12] In 2020, Mattijssen-Horstink and coworkers[13] produced a retrospective study on 26,000 fractures at an accident and emergency department of a Dutch teaching hospital and identified 1% of missed fractures, 17% of which concerned the foot or the ankle and 9% of which required surgery. The same year, Allen and colleagues[14] published a study on the combined use of ultrasound and CBCT in the assessment of ankle injuries. They reported 20% of missed major fractures including talar neck fractures and 42% of missed avulsion fractures. They stated "Fractures in the foot and ankle are detected more precisely with CBCT compared to radiographs. CBCT delivers similar doses of radiation compared to conventional radiographs which is around 10% of that resulting from conventional CT." Finally, in 2021, Jacques and coworkers[15] published a prospective comparative study reporting on 165 emergency patients going through the classical 2DXR ± MDCT pathway versus 224 patients for which CBCT was used as primary imaging modality. They reported a 35% reduction in radiation dose and a 15% reduction in turnover time. It is noteworthy that those most recent papers were published by radiologists, mostly in radiology journals, indicating that the scope of the technology is now on a larger public health level and not just limited to the foot and ankle field where it has been soon recognized as a clinical and research asset.

In summary, the problem with AS in and of itself in the context of acute ankle trauma is not necessarily diagnosis, but the need clearly is to reduce the number of false-negatives or delayed diagnosis of other pathology, misdiagnosed as Cotton on 2DRX. Therefore, WBCT/CBCT can contribute positively to this by helping reduce radiation exposure, time to diagnosis, time spent in the emergency department, and direct and secondary costs.

WEIGHT-BEARING COMPUTED TOMOGRAPHY AND CHRONIC ANKLE INSTABILITY

In what concerns CLAI, the literature is even more scarce, but landmark WBCT papers, such as by Richter and coworkers,[16] have been published, concerning more than 11,000 general foot and ankle cases, with 10% reduction in radiation dose, 75% reduction in time spent to acquire the images, and significant cost savings.

In multiple studies, WBCT has proven reliable and accurate in measuring hindfoot alignment.[17–22] A correlation between bony alignment, in particular a varus hindfoot, and the risk to develop CLAI has been hypothesized for years. This relationship, which had been hinted and commented on in the past, has been published more recently with the help of WBCT. Previous results by Van Bergeyk and coworkers,[23] which had reported increased varus associated with CLAI patients in a prospective comparative study, were confirmed in a 2019 WBCT study.[24] The authors reported on a series of 189 patients, 34 of which had CLAI, and found using multivariable logistic regression adjusted for age and sex, a 35% increased odds ratio of CLAI per 1% increase in varus hindfoot alignment. It is the authors' view that such relationships uncovered by a broader use of WBCT will in the future enable more precise prognostication of our patient's pathologic evolution based on their anatomy and medical history. Ultimately, this will enable surgeons to provide more precise and timely surgical indications.

In terms of diagnostic benefit, this is not where patients will benefit most immediately from the systematic use of WBCT. However, it is possible to consider performing dynamic WBCT imaging to explore CLAI, less so in the context of AS because of the pain in the context of acute trauma. This would enable 3D measurement of talar tilt and rotation, which has been found in the past to be a significant component of tibiotalar instability.[25]

To best illustrate these possibilities, the first author of this paper (FL), who presents with CLAI on his left ankle, treated it conservatively, and has provided images from his own dataset (**Fig. 1**). As with traditional varus and anterior drawer dynamic imaging of the ankle, the ability to perform bilateral comparative imaging is informative when the comparative side can be considered devoid of pathology, or with at least clinical asymmetry (**Fig. 2**). Furthermore, on this dataset, semiautomatic segmentation has been performed. We remind the reader that segmentation is a computerized technique, which requires dedicated software and results in separating and naming the different bones of interest. This is done manually (bones are contoured and named by the human), semiautomatically (bones are contoured by the software, but named by the human), or fully automatically (bones are contoured and named by the software alone). Once segmentation is done, the software tools offer infinite possibilities, from automatic axes calculation to advanced features, such as fracture detection.

In **Fig. 3** we illustrate the possibility to use distance mapping, a 3D point-to-point, bone-to-bone distance analysis algorithm, to best quantify tibiotalar tilt. The colorized map is a convenient and immediate qualitative tool for the clinician, which corresponds to a precise numeric quantification of the distance between articular surfaces in a defined area. In the setting of CLAI, this is crucial to assess objectively the tibiotalar tilt, with a huge potential in the initial clinical staging of the condition, in the comparison between before and after treatment, and in the follow-up of the patient. Although these tools are already available and described in the literature, further studies are warranted to validate their use in the clinical setting. Two of the most inconvenient downsides of dynamic imaging are the generally poor reproducibility and the increased possibility of motion artifacts. The use of standardized jigs (**Fig. 4**) could be helpful to solve these, but a validated scientific consensus is necessary before their use in clinical practice.

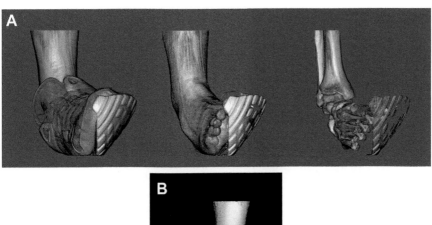

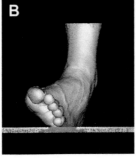

Fig. 1. (A) 3D rendering of the shod right foot. (B) 3D skin rendering of the left foot.

One other clinically impactful aspect of using WBCT to assess CLAI is the potential evolution toward ankle osteoarthritis. A recent publication by Richter and colleagues[26] has looked at the evaluation of ankle osteoarthritis using WBCT. In their paper the authors proposed a four-stage classification of OA on WBCT, combining the classical

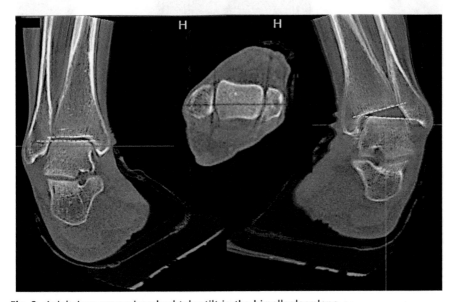

Fig. 2. Axial view comparing shod talar tilt in the bimalleolar plane.

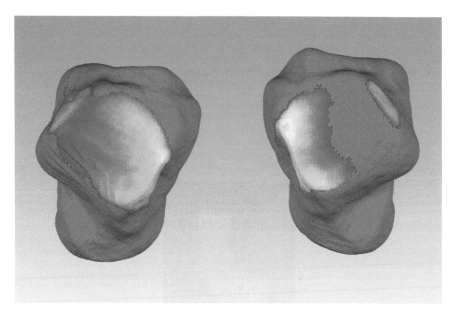

Fig. 3. Distance mapping after segmentation of the tali, showing approximation in the medial gutter and medial talar dome and distancing in the lateral aspect of the tibiotalar joint.

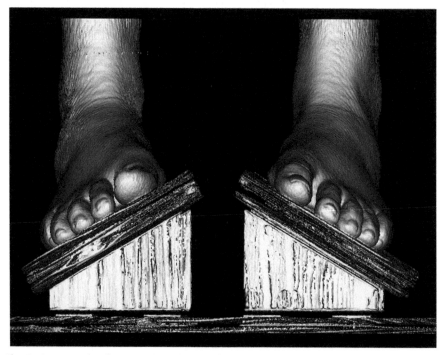

Fig. 4. An example of custom inversion jigs (Images courtesy of Curvebeamai Corp.)

signs with 3D visualization, stating the importance of alignment assessment to enable precise deformity correction using customized, patient-specific guides either to perform supramalleolar correction osteotomy[27] or total ankle replacement[28] in the varus arthritic ankle.

WEIGHT-BEARING COMPUTED TOMOGRAPHY AND ANKLE INSTABILITY ASSOCIATED LESIONS: THE IMPORTANCE OF HIGH ANKLE SPRAINS

Associated lesions are the core problem in AS and CLAI. In AS, associated fractures, most often avulsion type, of the fibula, navicular, calcaneus, or talus must not be over-looked. They account for severe sprains, fractures, or dislocations of the Chopart or Lisfranc joints, such as the Jones fracture of the fifth metatarsal base. Osteochondral lesions of the talus can also go underseen when conventional 2D radiographs are used as the primary modality of imaging. Concerning all those diagnoses, little specific literature exists. Most of what is published was described in the first section, in the context of emergency departments and looking at the clinical impact of WBCT in general.

High AS (HAS), or distal syndesmotic tibiofibular injury, is an often-overlooked lesion, not easily tackled using past modalities because of its complex 3D anatomy and the inherent limitations of conventional 2DXR.[29] Up to 10% of AS are considered HAS with associated syndesmotic injury.[30] Surprisingly, although less frequent than AS, HAS have been the most investigated subject pertaining to ankle trauma during the recent 10-year advent of WBCT in orthopedics. Because WBCT allows for immediate, loaded investigation and bilateral comparison (for some devices on the market) with a potentially uninjured contralateral side, we understand the preeminence of HAS over AS in WBCT literature as a search for a more precise diagnostic method in HAS. Using this new tool, studies have concentrated on the definition of normal values for the syndesmosis, the value of weight-bearing, of comparison with the contralateral side, and of the application of external torque.

Regarding measurements, only a few studies are available.[31–35] Lepojarvi and colleagues[34] described the normal rotational (3° external rotation) and translational (1.5 mm posterior translation) dynamics of the distal tibiofibular joint using WBCT with less than 1° and 1-mm interobserver variability. Shakoor and colleagues[36] found that WBCT provides reliable 2D linear measurements, which is not surprising because the spatial definition is even finer than MDCT (0.2–0.3 mm vs 0.5 mm). They also found that weight-bearing only seemed to increase medial clear space compared with non-weightbearing. The same team also set a standard that seemed to have stayed in the literature, to use an axial slice at 1 cm above the tibial plafond to perform the linear measurements and reported excellent intraobserver and interobserver reliability. Malhotra and colleagues[37] in a study comparing MDCT and WBCT found that weight-bearing results in lateral and posterior translation and external rotation of the fibula in relation to the incisura.

Conversely, Hamard and colleagues[38] found that anteroposterior translation is better seen on MDCT so they advocate that weight-bearing is not necessary and could even be counterproductive in identifying syndesmotic lesions, compared with MDCT. This is a fundamental misunderstanding of WDCT: it is not because the technology has been coined WBCT that the examination has to take place with a weight-bearing patient. Most devices on the market can have the patient sitting while images are acquired. In this case, WBCT still has the advantage over MDCT that it is faster, cheaper, and causes less radiation exposure. It seems that just applying axial load in unstable syndesmotic joints may not be the transformative diagnostic experience that foot and ankle surgeons hoped for. One explanation could be the impact of the extent of syndesmotic lesions, as investigated by Krähenbühl and coworkers[39] in a cadaver study, reporting that axial loading had little effect on linear measurements assessing the syndesmosis. Only complete injuries transecting the anterior inferior tibiofibular ligament, the deltoid ligament, and the interosseous membrane resulted in significant differences in axial measurements.

The effect of applying torque to sensitize the scans has been investigated as a means to increase the effect of axial loading. In a cadaveric study, Burssens and colleagues[40] proved that axial load increased lateral translation but with submillimeter differences until torque was applied with a mean 3.1-mm posterior translation and 4.7° external rotation. Similar results were reported by Krähenbühl and colleagues[41,42] in two other cadaveric studies, including that torque helps diagnose incomplete lesions.

Another important aspect of defining normal measurements was to investigate whether a contralateral, uninjured side could be used as comparison with the injured side. This was specifically reported by Patel and colleagues[32] in a retrospective study if 200 feet in 100 patients who reported no difference between left and right sides in this population of patients devoid of known syndesmotic pathology. Hagemeijer and colleagues[33] also came to the same conclusion in a series of 36 patients with bilateral WBCT scans.[43]

However, although it is important to redescribe linear measurements as a matter of comparison with existing gold standards, WBCT enables surface and volumetric measurements. Indeed, Krähenbühl and coworkers[29,44] showed that foot positioning has a distorting effect on syndesmotic linear measurements on digitally reconstructed radiographs, reconstructed from WBCT datasets, although this is not the case with axial surface measurements. For example, in a systematic review that included 11 studies, Raheman and colleagues[31] found values of 112.5 ± 7.1 mm^2 versus 157.5 ± 9.6 mm^2 combining results of 408 uninjured patients and 151 patients with syndesmotic instability, respectively. They also found that the syndesmotic area increases with weight-bearing and decreases with age. Del Rio and colleagues[35] have performed a prospective comparative study of bilateral scans and reported intraobserver and interobserver reliability measures greater than 95%, indicating that syndesmotic area increased by a mean 23 mm^2 in WBCT scans compared with 10 mm^2 when nonweight-bearing. Dynamic change caused by weight-bearing was reported to increase by +3.1% on average.

Beyond surface measurement, the future of syndesmotic lesion diagnosis lies with volumetric measurements. Moreover, the authors of this review deem this is true for all measurements, in all the foot and ankle and beyond in orthopedics. This will elevate the debate from the 2D world to the 3D world, which requires the development of efficient and validated computerized tools.[45] This means segmentation of the bones (a time-consuming procedure), which will in due course be performed via specific software based on artificial intelligence. A few publications have reported its use, enlightening its potential, but also its remaining downsides, such as limitations in the presence of metal and variability between different software and hand measurements.[22,46–49] Despite being at this early stage of development, other authors have successfully segmented the tibia and fibula to perform comparative volumetric measurements of the syndesmosis, reporting increased sensitivity to subtle syndesmotic injuries.[50,51] Segmentation can also be used to template injured sides on contralateral healthy sides in 3D, as described by Burssens and colleagues[52] in a 2018 clinical study reporting 1-mm medial diastasis and 4° and 7°, respectively, in HAS alone or associated with a fibula external rotation fracture. In a 2022 paper, Peiffer and colleagues[53] used a similar computerized technique to investigate syndesmotic "open book" lesions. This required "statistical shape modeling" of the syndesmosis and "ligament wrapping" techniques, which proved extremely precise (0.23 mm in shape modeling and 0.53 mm in the prediction of ligament insertions) and found significantly different ligament lengths between healthy control subjects and injured cases.

We did not find relevant literature reporting the use of these techniques in AS. We hypothesize that this is the case because the need for a new and better diagnostic tool in HAS is known and desired by the clinical foot and ankle community, when it is not such an acute problem in AS. However, we see no reason why these techniques could not be applied also to AS, especially when we consider that 90% of AS are isolated, which accounts for a much larger number of patients: so despite the need not being so acutely felt, it would be truly impactful for AS too.

SUMMARY

There is an immense opportunity for future research on the impact of WBCT and CBCT in diagnosing, evaluating, and treating AS, HAS, and chronic ankle instability. As we have seen from early studies the effect on future management of ankle soft tissue injuries, lower limb alignment, and foot and ankle trauma from use of WBCT and CBCT can potentially be impactful from a cost saving and clinical management perspective. WBCT and CBCT has already changed the understanding of ankle pathology and is about to revolutionize the management of ligamentous injuries and concomitant pathology.

CLINICS CARE POINTS

- The most important word in WBCT is "cone beam," meaning that WBCT does not have to be weight-bearing. It can be acquired sitting or prone. Nonweight-bearing is not a contraindication to cone beam, especially in the context of ankle trauma in accident and emergency department units.

- Cone beam is technologically closer to radiography, albeit in 3D rather than 2D, which is why it has (inaccurately) been coined "CT"; cone beam WBCT is in fact equivalent to 3D radiography. The most important advantage is immediate access to 3D images, resulting in faster and better diagnostic capabilities. Up to 40% missed diagnoses of ankle trauma associated fractures could theoretically be avoided with primary use of WBCT in accident and emergency departments.

- The most important pitfall with WBCT is its slow development because of lack of awareness. As clinicians it is our responsibility to promote education, research, and standardization of practice using WBCT. Collaboration with academic and radiology teams is essential.

DISCLOSURE

The authors discloses the following: F. Lintz: AFCP Board Member, EFAS Committee Member, Newclip Technics: Paid Consultancy, Royalties, Pragon28: Stock holder, Paid Consultancy, CurvebeamAI: Stock holder, Paid Consultancy, International Weight Bearing CT Society: President. A. Bernasconi: CurvebeamAI: Stock holder, Paid Consultancy, International Weight Bearing CT Society: Board Member, EFAS Committee Chair; E.I Ferkel: AAOS: Board or committee member, American Orthopedic Foot and Ankle Society: Board or committee member, American Orthopedic Society for Sports Medicine: Board or committee member, Arthrex, Inc: Paid consultant; Paid presenter or speaker, Arthroscopy Association of North America: Board or committee member, DJ Orthopedics: Research support, Ferring Pharmaceuticals: Paid consultant; Paid presenter or speaker, Medartis: Paid consultant, Mitek: Paid consultant; Research support, Organogenesis: Stock or stock Options, Ossio: Paid consultant, Ossur: Research support, Smith & Nephew: Paid consultant; Research support.

ACKNOWLEDGMENTS

The authors thank Sorin Siegler (Drexel University, Philadelphia, PA) for providing the figures regarding advanced visualization techniques, such as distance mapping of the first author's ankles.

REFERENCES

1. Lintz F, de Cesar Netto C. Is advanced imaging a must in the assessment of progressive collapsing foot deformity? Foot Ankle Clin 2021;26(3):427–42.
2. de Cesar Netto C, Myerson MS, Day J, et al. Consensus for the use of weight-bearing CT in the assessment of progressive collapsing foot deformity. Foot Ankle Int 2020;41(10):1277–82.
3. Burssens A, Krähenbühl N, Lenz AL, et al. Interaction of loading and ligament injuries in subtalar joint instability quantified by 3D weightbearing computed tomography. J Orthop Res 2022;40(4):933–44.
4. Lambers K, Ootes D, Ring D. Incidence of patients with lower extremity injuries presenting to US emergency departments by anatomic region, disease category, and age. Clin Orthop Relat Res 2012;470(1):284–90.
5. Hunt KJ, Hurwit D, Robell K, et al. Incidence and epidemiology of foot and ankle injuries in elite collegiate athletes. Am J Sports Med 2017;45(2):426–33.
6. Haapamaki V, Kiuru M, Koskinen S. Lisfranc fracture-dislocation in patients with multiple trauma: diagnosis with multidetector computed tomography. Foot Ankle Int 2004;25(9):614–9.
7. Haapamaki VV, Kiuru MJ, Koskinen SK. Ankle and foot injuries: analysis of MDCT findings. AJR Am J Roentgenol 2004;183(3):615–22.
8. van Rijn J, Dorleijn DMJ, Boetes B, et al. Missing the Lisfranc fracture: a case report and review of the literature. J Foot Ankle Surg 2012;51(2):270–4.
9. Lau S, Bozin M, Thillainadesan T. Lisfranc fracture dislocation: a review of a commonly missed injury of the midfoot. Emerg Med J 2017;34(1):52–6.
10. De Los Santos-Real R, Canillas F, Varas-Navas J, et al. Lisfranc joint ligament complex reconstruction: a promising solution for missed, delayed, or chronic Lisfranc injury without arthritis. J Foot Ankle Surg 2017;56(6):1350–6.
11. Borel C, Larbi A, Delclaux S, et al. Diagnostic value of cone beam computed tomography (CBCT) in occult scaphoid and wrist fractures. Eur J Radiol 2017;97:59–64.
12. Ricci PM, Boldini M, Bonfante E, et al. Cone-beam computed tomography compared to X-ray in diagnosis of extremities bone fractures: a study of 198 cases. Eur J Radiol Open 2019;6:119–21.
13. Mattijssen-Horstink L, Langeraar JJ, Mauritz GJ, et al. Radiologic discrepancies in diagnosis of fractures in a Dutch teaching emergency department: a retrospective analysis. Scand J Trauma Resusc Emerg Med 2020;28(1):38.
14. Allen GM, Wilson DJ, Bullock SA, et al. Extremity CT and ultrasound in the assessment of ankle injuries: occult fractures and ligament injuries. Br J Radiol 2020;93(1105):20180989.
15. Jacques T, Morel V, Dartus J, et al. Impact of introducing extremity cone-beam CT in an emergency radiology department: a population-based study. Orthop Traumatol Surg Res 2021;107(2):102834.

16. Richter M, Lintz F, de Cesar Netto C, et al. Results of more than 11,000 scans with weightbearing CT: impact on costs, radiation exposure, and procedure time. Foot Ankle Surg 2019;26(5):518–22.

17. Lintz F, Barton T, Millet M, et al. Ground reaction force calcaneal offset: a new measurement of hindfoot alignment. Foot Ankle Surg 2012;18(1):9–14.

18. Lintz F, Welck M, Bernasconi A, et al. 3D biometrics for hindfoot alignment using weightbearing CT. Foot Ankle Int 2017;38(6):684–9.

19. de Cesar Netto C, Bernasconi A, Roberts L, et al. Foot alignment in symptomatic National Basketball Association players using weightbearing cone beam computed tomography. Orthop J Sports Med 2019;7(2). 2325967119826081.

20. Zhang JZ, Lintz F, Bernasconi A, et al, Weight Bearing CT International Study Group. 3D biometrics for hindfoot alignment using weightbearing computed tomography. Foot Ankle Int 2019;40(6):720–6.

21. Richter M, Lintz F, Zech S, et al. Combination of PedCAT weightbearing CT with pedography assessment of the relationship between anatomy-based foot center and force/pressure-based center of gravity. Foot Ankle Int 2018;39(3):361–8.

22. de Cesar Netto C, Bang K, Mansur NS, et al. Multiplanar semiautomatic assessment of foot and ankle offset in adult acquired flatfoot deformity. Foot Ankle Int 2020;41(7):839–48.

23. Van Bergeyk AB, Younger A, Carson B. CT analysis of hindfoot alignment in chronic lateral ankle instability. Foot Ankle Int 2002;23(1):37–42.

24. Lintz F, Bernasconi A, Baschet L, et al, Weight BCT International Study Group. Relationship between chronic lateral ankle instability and hindfoot varus using weight-bearing cone beam computed tomography. Foot Ankle Int 2019;40(10): 1175–81.

25. Kobayashi T, Koshino Y, Miki T. Abnormalities of foot and ankle alignment in individuals with chronic ankle instability: a systematic review. BMC Musculoskelet Disord 2021;22(1):683.

26. Richter M, de Cesar Netto C, Lintz F, et al. The assessment of ankle osteoarthritis with weight-bearing computed tomography. Foot Ankle Clin 2022;27(1):13–36.

27. van Raaij T, van der Wel H, Beldman M, et al. Two-step 3D-guided supramalleolar osteotomy to treat varus ankle osteoarthritis. Foot Ankle Int 2022;43(7):937–41.

28. Thompson MJ, Consul D, Umbel BD, et al. Accuracy of weightbearing CT scans for patient-specific instrumentation in total ankle arthroplasty. Foot Ankle Orthop 2021;6(4). 24730114211061492.

29. Lintz F, International Weight Bearing CT Society, Barg A, et al. Comments on the paper: "Impact of the rotational position of the hindfoot on measurements assessing the integrity of the distal tibio-fibular syndesmosis. Foot Ankle Surg 2020; 26(7):833–4.

30. Bejarano-Pineda L, DiGiovanni CW, Waryasz GR, et al. Diagnosis and treatment of syndesmotic unstable injuries: where we are now and where we are headed. JAAOS - Journal of the American Academy of Orthopaedic Surgeons 2021; 29(23):905–97.

31. Raheman FJ, Rojoa DM, Hallet C, et al. Can weightbearing cone-beam CT reliably differentiate between stable and unstable syndesmotic ankle injuries? A systematic review and meta-analysis. Clin Orthop Relat Res 2022;480(8):1547–62.

32. Patel S, Malhotra K, Cullen NP, et al. Defining reference values for the normal tibiofibular syndesmosis in adults using weight-bearing CT. Bone Joint Lett J 2019; 101-B(3):348–52.

33. Hagemeijer NC, Chang SH, Abdelaziz ME, et al. Range of normal and abnormal syndesmotic measurements using weightbearing CT. Foot Ankle Int 2019;40(12): 1430–7.

34. Lepojärvi S, Niinimäki J, Pakarinen H, et al. Rotational dynamics of the normal distal tibiofibular joint with weight-bearing computed tomography. Foot Ankle Int 2016;37(6):627–35.

35. Del Rio A, Bewsher SM, Roshan-Zamir S, et al. Weightbearing cone-beam computed tomography of acute ankle syndesmosis injuries. J Foot Ankle Surg 2020;59(2):258–63.

36. Shakoor D, Osgood GM, Brehler M, et al. Cone-beam CT measurements of distal tibio-fibular syndesmosis in asymptomatic uninjured ankles: does weight-bearing matter? Skeletal Radiol 2019;48(4):583–94.

37. Malhotra K, Welck M, Cullen N, et al. The effects of weight bearing on the distal tibiofibular syndesmosis: a study comparing weight bearing-CT with conventional CT. Foot Ankle Surg 2019;25(4):511–6.

38. Hamard M, Neroladaki A, Bagetakos I, et al. Accuracy of cone-beam computed tomography for syndesmosis injury diagnosis compared to conventional computed tomography. Foot Ankle Surg 2020;26(3):265–72.

39. Krähenbühl N, Bailey TL, Weinberg MW, et al. Is load application necessary when using computed tomography scans to diagnose syndesmotic injuries? A cadaver study. Foot Ankle Surg 2020;26(2):198–204.

40. Burssens A, Krähenbühl N, Weinberg MM, et al. Comparison of external torque to axial loading in detecting 3-dimensional displacement of syndesmotic ankle injuries. Foot Ankle Int 2020;41(10):1256–68.

41. Krähenbühl N, Bailey TL, Weinberg MW, et al. Impact of torque on assessment of syndesmotic injuries using weightbearing computed tomography scans. Foot Ankle Int 2019;40(6):710–9.

42. Krähenbühl N, Bailey TL, Presson AP, et al. Torque application helps to diagnose incomplete syndesmotic injuries using weight-bearing computed tomography images. Skeletal Radiol 2019;48(9):1367–76.

43. Osgood GM, Shakoor D, Orapin J, et al. Reliability of distal tibio-fibular syndesmotic instability measurements using weightbearing and non-weightbearing cone-beam CT. Foot Ankle Surg 2019;25(6):771–81.

44. Krähenbühl N, Akkaya M, Dodd AE, et al. Impact of the rotational position of the hindfoot on measurements assessing the integrity of the distal tibio-fibular syndesmosis. Foot Ankle Surg 2020;26(7):810–7.

45. Lintz F, de Cesar Netto C, Barg A, et al, International Study Group. Weight-bearing cone beam CT scans in the foot and ankle. EFORT Open Rev 2018; 3(5):278–86.

46. Richter M, Schilke R, Duerr F, et al. Automatic software-based 3D-angular measurement for weight-bearing CT (WBCT) provides different angles than measurement by hand. Foot Ankle Surg 2021;S1268-7731(21):00235–6.

47. Bernasconi A, Cooper L, Lyle S, et al. Intraobserver and interobserver reliability of cone beam weightbearing semi-automatic three-dimensional measurements in symptomatic pes cavovarus. Foot Ankle Surg 2020;26(5):564–72.

48. Day J, de Cesar Netto C, Richter M, et al. Evaluation of a weightbearing CT artificial intelligence-based automatic measurement for the M1-M2 intermetatarsal angle in hallux valgus. Foot Ankle Int 2021;42(11):1502–9.

49. de Carvalho KAM, Walt JS, Ehret A, et al. Comparison between weightbearing-CT semiautomatic and manual measurements in hallux valgus. Foot Ankle Surg 2022;S1268-7731(22):00043–51.

50. Ashkani Esfahani S, Bhimani R, Lubberts B, et al. Volume measurements on weightbearing computed tomography can detect subtle syndesmotic instability. J Orthop Res 2022;40(2):460–7.
51. Bhimani R, Ashkani-Esfahani S, Lubberts B, et al. Utility of volumetric measurement via weight-bearing computed tomography scan to diagnose syndesmotic instability. Foot Ankle Int 2020;41(7):859–65.
52. Burssens A, Vermue H, Barg A, et al. Templating of Syndesmotic Ankle Lesions by Use of 3D Analysis in Weightbearing and Nonweightbearing CT. Foot Ankle Int 2018;39(12):1487–96.
53. Peiffer M, Burssens A, De Mits S, et al. Statistical shape model-based tibiofibular assessment of syndesmotic ankle lesions using weight-bearing CT. J Orthop Res 2022;40(12):2873–84.

Ankle Sprain and Chronic Lateral Ankle Instability
Optimizing Conservative Treatment

Mandeep S. Dhillon, MS, Sandeep Patel, MS*, Vishnu Baburaj, MS

KEYWORDS

- Ankle sprain • Chronic ankle instability • Ankle rehabilitation • Ankle bracing
- Conservative management

KEY POINTS

- Ankle sprains can frequently convert to recurrent instability if not adequately managed.
- Optimal conservative management should be individualized depending on the degree of trauma and patient requirements.
- Initial bracing should be rigid in severe injuries and could be semirigid in others.
- RICE (Rest, Ice, Compression, Elevation) protocol has been optimized to PEACE & LOVE, with initial protection and aggressive rehabilitation being included.
- Sports-related rehabilitation should be added when swelling and pain subside.

BACKGROUND

Ankle sprains are very commonly encountered in clinical practice, constituting around 15% to 30% of all musculoskeletal injuries.[1,2] Stability to the ankle laterally is given by the anterior and posterior talofibular ligaments (anterior talofibular ligament [ATFL] and posterior talofibular ligament [PTFL]), along with the calcaneofibular ligament (CFL); medially the principal restraint is the deltoid ligament.[3] The term "ankle sprain" denotes a spectrum of ligamentous injuries around the ankle, ranging from simple stretch injuries to complete ligamentous rupture. Lateral ankle sprain is most commonly caused by an inversion stress to the foot along with external rotation of the leg[4]; the common stress in a plantarflexed foot injures the ATFL, whereas the uncommon stress in a dorsiflexed ankle, if it does not cause a fracture, could injure the CFL.[5]

Many reports have documented an incidence of up to 73% of patients getting at least 1 more episode of ankle twist after 1 episode of acute ankle sprain; 30% to 70% of acute ankle sprains with inadequate treatment end up with chronic ankle

Department of Orthopedic Surgery, PGIMER Chandigarh
* Corresponding author.
E-mail address: sandeepdrpatelortho@gmail.com

Foot Ankle Clin N Am 28 (2023) 297–307
https://doi.org/10.1016/j.fcl.2022.12.006
1083-7515/23/© 2023 Elsevier Inc. All rights reserved.

instability.[6,7] Chronic ankle instability may be defined as a case of ankle sprain with a persistent feeling of the ankle "*giving way*" lasting for more than 1 year from the initial trauma, with or without pain and swelling.[8] This may be mechanical or functional; mechanical instability is due to excessively lax or torn ligaments and can be elicited during clinical examination. Functional instability is associated with frequent subjective symptoms of the ankle "*giving way*," which may have more of a sensory loss than actual frank ligament laxity. These 2 types of instability may coexist in the same patient, or maybe present independently.[9] Chronic instability is associated with functional impairment, reduced activity levels, and frequent episodes of ankle sprains and may ultimately lead to the development of ankle osteoarthritis.[10]

Optimizing athletic injury management is the aim of any sports physician or surgeon. Because ankle injuries are fairly common irrespective of sport, optimal management is a key determinant for return to sports. The treatment itself can be focused from 2 aspects: how do we treat an acute sprain and how do we manage chronic instability. Many parameters for ankle instability management are already given in the current literature[11–13]; the focus of this article is to identify and stress on parameters that can either be modified or further optimized; we present a review of the current evidences of interventions that expedite the athlete's return to sports.

DISCUSSION
Management of Acute Ankle Sprains

Currently, the conservative management protocol for acute ankle sprains involves a 3-phase rehabilitation protocol, with each phase having its own goals.[14] Phase 1 aims at limiting the degree of injury, phase 2 on bringing back the joint range of motion and strength, and phase 3 focuses on agility and endurance. In athletes, the final phase involves gradually increasing training protocols to facilitate a return to sports (**Fig. 1**).

Phase 1 in conservative treatment
Immediate management of acute ankle sprains involves a period of splinting the ligaments (protection), rest, ice application, compression bandaging, and elevation of the

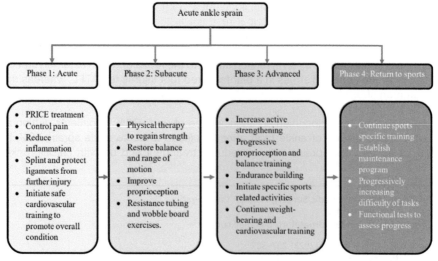

Fig. 1. Phases in the management of acute ankle sprain.

limb (traditionally called the "*RICE treatment*"), along with adequate analgesia. Over the years, many authors have advocated the use of this RICE protocol.[15–17] An extension of the standard RICE treatment, the "*PEACE & LOVE protocol*," described by Dubois and colleagues[18] is now being used to optimize acute phase management (**Fig. 2**). The main aim of management at this phase is to control pain, protect soft tissues from further injury, facilitate their healing, reduce the amount of swelling, and decrease inflammation. Although the RICE treatment has been conventionally popular among physicians, there is limited evidence in literature regarding its efficacy. Vuurberg and colleagues,[19] in a pooled analysis of 33 RCTs, reported that it was unclear if cryotherapy improves acute symptoms of ankle sprain. They also found no conclusive benefit with the use of compressive bandaging and insufficient evidence for the individual benefits of rest and elevation.[19]

The role of immobilization in acute ankle sprains is now debated. Some authors still recommend immobilization with a cast or slab,[20,21] whereas others suggest that early mobilization improves functional outcomes.[22,23] For severe cases, it seems logical that some immobilization (plaster slab, pneumatic walking boot, or an ankle-foot orthosis) is needed to provide mediolateral stability to protect the acutely injured ligaments. A pneumatic walking boot is excellent for walking because it provides stability and offloads the ligaments; however, it has certain disadvantages, such as bulky size, variable lengths, and discomfort to wear at bedtime. However, ankle-foot orthosis, which provides mediolateral stability, is lighter, can be worn with sports shoes, and is comfortable to wear at bedtime. A multicenter randomized controlled trial by Lamb and colleagues[24] compared the efficacy of 3 immobilization techniques (Below knee cast, Aircast brace, and Bledsoe boot) with that of a compression bandage. The results of the study indicated that patients who received below knee cast had the best outcomes, followed by those who received Aircast brace, with lowest quality outcomes with compression bandage. To optimize outcomes, it may be better to give a below-knee slab in noncompliant patients who tend to remove wearable orthosis.

Some therapists also use tape support to decrease edema and provide splintage. A randomized controlled trial by van Den Bekerom and colleagues[25] found that acute ankle sprains treated with tape, semirigid brace, and lace-up brace had comparable outcomes. Another option is the less frequently used lateral heel wedge, which

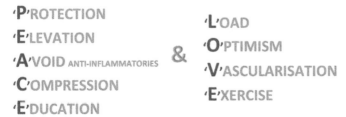

Fig. 2. Initial management of acute ankle sprains. The mnemonic stands for protection (of ligaments by avoiding activities/brief immobilization), elevation of the injured limb, avoiding analgesic drugs, compression with an elastic bandage to decrease swelling, education, and avoiding unnecessary investigations, gradually increasing load/weight-bearing as tolerated, optimism, vascularization by choosing pain-free cardiovascular workouts, and exercises to bring back strength and range of motion.

offloads the injured lateral ligaments. Patients who have antalgic gait or painful weight-bearing should take the help of crutches or walking aids.

However, Kerkhoffs and colleagues[26] reviewed some randomized studies and concluded that immobilization for a prolonged period is associated with poor functional outcomes. Functional weight-bearing should be encouraged while ensuring that the injured ligaments remain supported and are not prone to further injury. We think that the decision to immobilize an ankle sprain has to be individualized based on the extent of soft tissue injury, tenderness, and pain on walking. An inversion injury leading to an ATFL tear may lead to varied soft tissue injury on the lateral aspect of the foot. Most cases may be managed by functional bracing but some patients having more severe soft tissue injury may need cast immobilization.

Active joint mobilization is initiated early, and grade 1 and 2 sprains should be mobilized as quickly as the patient tolerates. Stretching of the Achilles tendon should be started in the first 48 to 72 hours to counteract the tendency of the muscle to contract following injury. Inversion exercises are to be avoided to prevent stretching of the already injured lateral ligaments. Bleakley and colleagues[27] conducted a randomized controlled trial in patients with acute ankle sprains wherein the intervention group was subjected to an accelerated rehab protocol with an early initiation of exercises in the first week itself. They found that the intervention group had significantly better ankle function than the standard group receiving standard care (RICE treatment) in the first week.

Electrical muscle stimulation may also be used in order to ensure that lateral compartment muscles do not undergo atrophy.

Phase 2 in conservative treatment

The next phase starts once the pain and swelling subside. This could be as soon as 4 to 5 days from injury in grade 1 sprains and 7 to 12 days for more severe sprains.

This consists of physical therapy to regain normal strength, balance, and range of motion.[28]

Resisted exercises are initially started as isometric exercises, gradually progressing to increasing resistance with weights and elastic tubing.[28] The resisted exercises should be carried out in sets, with the aim that when the prescribed set is finished, the target muscle is fully fatigued. Two to 3 such sets are carried out daily, and resistance is gradually increased. Each muscle group (anterior compartment, tibialis posterior, gastro-soleus, peroneal muscles) is targeted with a specific exercise (**Fig. 3**). For the anterior compartment musculature, the tubing is wound around the dorsum of the foot, secured to the floor, and the ankle is dorsiflexed against resistance (see **Fig. 3B**). The tibialis anterior may be targeted by the inversion of the foot when it nears terminal dorsiflexion. The gastro-soleus is targeted by reversing the tubing and plantar flexing the ankle against resistance (see **Fig. 3A**). For the tibialis posterior, the tubing is wound around the medial aspect of the head of the first metatarsal and secured laterally (see **Fig. 3C**). Inversion of the foot is carried out with the ankle in plantar flexion. Peroneal muscles prevent inversion of the foot, and strong peroneal musculature decreases the incidence of recurrent inversion sprains. Hence, peroneal strengthening is of prime importance in this phase of rehabilitation. The peronei are targeted by winding the tubing over the lateral aspect of the head of the fifth metatarsal and securing it medially (see **Fig. 3D**). The foot is everted against resistance while the ankle is kept in plantar flexion.

Proprioception is a key sense that protects against recurrent sprains. The role of proprioception training in the rehabilitation of ankle sprains has been highlighted by several authors, including Kaminski and colleagues,[29] Mattacola and Dwyer,[28] and

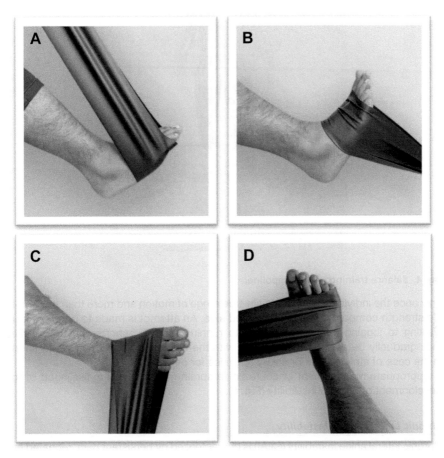

Fig. 3. (A–D) Theraband strengthening of specific muscle groups.

Lazarou and colleagues.[30] Straightforward tasks such as standing on a single leg while maintaining balance are started initially. This is advanced by adding various activities on single-leg standing, such as catching and tossing balls. Balance training is done with the help of a trampoline (**Fig. 4**).[31] A wobble board is also used to develop proprioception (**Fig. 5**). This is a flat circular platform with a hemispherical base. Patients are made to stand on the wobble board that is kept adjacent to a wall using their sprained limb. They are made to perform a fixed set of clockwise and counterclockwise rotations while keeping a finger on the wall if required. There are increasing levels for the wobble board wherein the exercise is initiated at the easiest level and progressed gradually.[32] Wright and colleagues[32] in their randomized controlled trial of 40 patients indicated that wobble board training is likely to be more effective than training using resistance tubing.

Phase 3 in conservative management
In the last phase, endurance-building and specific sports-related activities are introduced. The aim at this stage is to gradually return to preinjury activities and to prevent repeated episodes of sprain. Transition to subsequent phases should be done only once the goals of the previous phase have been achieved. This phase should begin

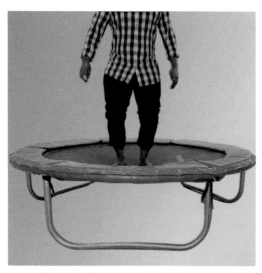

Fig. 4. Balance training with trampoline.

only once the individual regains a pain-free range of motion and more than 80% muscle strength compared with the uninjured side. An attempt is made to progress from walking to jogging and subsequently to running. Specific sports-related activities may gradually be added in this phase, with the ultimate goal of returning to sports in the case of athletes and preinjury activities for others.

Appropriate management of acute ankle sprain may reduce the likelihood of the development of chronic instability (**Fig. 6**).

Chronic Lateral Ankle Instability

Chronic lateral ankle instability (CLAI) is characterized by persistent pain, repeated episodes of ankle sprains, and multiple episodes of the ankle *"giving way."* Issues to be

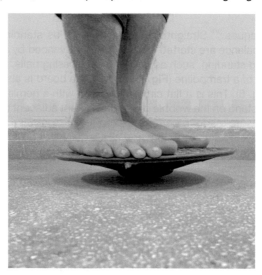

Fig. 5. Wobble board training.

addressed in CLAI include weak musculature, defects in posture control, reduced joint range of motion, and recurrent ankle sprains.[33,34] This symptom complex could prove to be a major impairment to individuals who lead an active lifestyle, and more so for athletes.

In the 1990s, conservative management played a dominant role in the management of CLAI.[35] Maffulli and colleagues,[11] in 2008, said that it still has a role and should always be offered before considering surgery. The protocol is similar to acute ankle sprain but it starts from phase 2 directly without carrying out the "RICE" treatment. Rehabilitation involves specific therapy that targets the established deficits focusing muscle strength, joint range of motion, balance, and proprioception, along with functional training and bracing (**Fig. 7**).

Strength training is carried out with the help of elastic bands, as described above. CLAI has been found to be associated with alterations in the joint range of motion, such as increased anterior laxity, decreased posterior glide of the talus, and reduced ankle dorsiflexion.[36–38] Static stretching exercises have been shown to be beneficial in improving ankle dorsiflexion.[17] Insufficiency of the ATFL is thought to lead to changes in the anterior positioning of the talus within the tibial plafond.[39] Such altered positioning may lead to a reduction in dorsiflexion by restricting the posterior glide of the talus. Joint mobilization exercises effectively enhance joint kinematics, increasing the range of motion.[40]

Balance and proprioception training is vital in preventing recurrent episodes of injury. The initial stages of this therapy involve maintaining balance on a single limb stance and are progressed by adding various challenges and complexities such as removing the visual input, altering the surface morphology, making the patient carry out trivial tasks, and so forth. Activities such as jumping are added subsequently to improve dynamic balance. CLAI patients tend to have a longer reaction time for the

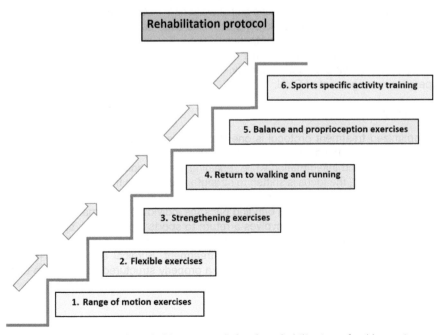

Fig. 6. Authors' suggested stepladder approach for the rehabilitation of ankle sprains.

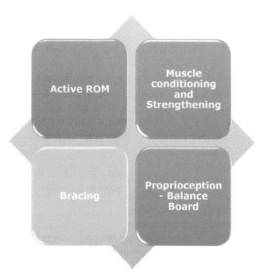

Fig. 7. Four cornerstones of effective rehabilitation.

peroneal muscles, making them prone to additional inversion injuries.[41] An ankle tilt board may be used for peroneal strengthening and proprioceptive training, facilitating ankle stabilization exercises in the entire range of motion, and developing better ankle position in the presence of external forces.[42] This improves the dynamic stability of the ankle and decreases the risk of future injuries.[41,43] Linens and colleagues[44] did a randomized controlled trial and reported that wobble board training done 3 days a week for 4 weeks significantly improved balance impairments in CLAI patients.

Patients with CLAI frequently have gait alterations.[45,46] Gait retraining and functional therapy in the form of tasks simulating activities such as jumping and landing allow these patients to establish motion tactics.

Despite strict compliance with this rehabilitation protocol, some patients tend to have persistent symptoms of instability. These patients are the ideal cases for the operative management of CLAI.

SUMMARY

An optimized treatment protocol is one that can be individualized for each case of ankle sprain. In all, the goals of acute phase treatment are to control pain and to bring down swelling and inflammation while regaining joint motion. Once the acute phase has been treated, the focus is shifted to strength and balance training. Targeted exercises are initiated to improve proprioception and neuromuscular control. The final phase of rehabilitation includes bringing back the individual to normal preinjury functional level. For athletes, this involves a return to sports, and specific sports-related tasks are added in this phase. Management of chronic ankle sprains is done in a similar manner, omitting the acute phase treatment. Surgical stabilization may be considered for cases that fail to respond to a properly structured conservative treatment protocol.

DISCLOSURE

Nothing to disclose.

CLINICS CARE POINTS

- Conservative management is always the first line of treatment in acute ankle sprains and should also be offered initially in chronic lateral instability before considering surgical intervention.
- Initial management of acute injuries is done with the PRICER protocol, which includes protection of injured ligaments, rest, ice application, compressive bandaging, limb elevation, and rehabilitation.
- Severe cases with extensive soft tissue injuries should be immobilized for a brief period to facilitate healing.
- Physical therapy is initiated as early as possible to regain normal strength, balance, proprioception, and range of motion.
- Endurance-building and sports-specific activities are in the last stage of rehabilitation, intending to bring the athlete or person to the preinjury activity level.
- Chronic lateral instability is managed with a similar protocol, excluding the initial PRICER treatment.
- Surgery may be considered in cases with persistent instability symptoms despite strictly following this rehabilitation protocol.

REFERENCES

1. Adler H. Therapy and prognosis of fresh external ankle ligament lesions (author's transl). Unfallheilkunde 1976;79(3):101.
2. Komenda GA, Ferkel RD. Arthroscopic findings associated with the unstable ankle. Foot Ankle Int 1999;20(11):708.
3. Bozkurt M, Doral MN. Anatomic factors and biomechanics in ankle instability. Foot Ankle Clin 2006;11(3):451.
4. Garrick JG. The frequency of injury, mechanism of injury, and epidemiology of ankle sprains. Am J Sports Med 1977;5(6):241.
5. Bennett W. Lateral ankle sprains. Part I: anatomy, biomechanics, diagnosis, and natural history. Orthopaedic Rev 1994;23(5):381.
6. Yeung M, Chan K-M, So C, et al. An epidemiological survey on ankle sprain. Br J Sports Med 1994;28(2):112.
7. Garrick JG, Requa RK. The epidemiology of foot and ankle injuries in sports. Clin Sports Med 1988;7(1):29.
8. Delahunt E, Coughlan GF, Caulfield B, et al. Inclusion criteria when investigating insufficiencies in chronic ankle instability. Med Sci Sports Exerc 2010;42(11):2106.
9. Ajis A, Maffulli N. Conservative management of chronic ankle instability. Foot Ankle Clin 2006;11(3):531.
10. Wikstrom EA, Hubbard-Turner T, McKeon PO. Understanding and treating lateral ankle sprains and their consequences. Sports Med 2013;43(6):385.
11. Maffulli N, Ferran NA. Management of acute and chronic ankle instability. J Am Acad Orthop Surg 2008;16(10):608.
12. Webster KA, Gribble PA. Functional rehabilitation interventions for chronic ankle instability: a systematic review. J Sport Rehabil 2010;19(1):98.
13. Chen ET, McInnis KC, Borg-Stein J. Ankle sprains: evaluation, rehabilitation, and prevention. Curr Sports Med Rep 2019;18(6):217.

14. Sammarco VJ. Principles and techniques in rehabilitation of the athlete's foot: Part III: rehabilitation of ankle sprains. Tech Foot Ankle Surg 2003;2(3):199.
15. Hing W, Lopes J, Hume PA, et al. Comparison of multimodal physiotherapy and" RICE" self-treatment for early management of ankle sprains. NZ J Physiother 2011;39(1):13.
16. Terada M, Pietrosimone BG, Gribble PA. Therapeutic interventions for increasing ankle dorsiflexion after ankle sprain: a systematic review. J Athl Train 2013;48(5): 696–709.
17. Terada M, Pietrosimone BG, Gribble PA. Therapeutic interventions for increasing ankle dorsiflexion after ankle sprain: a systematic review. J Athl Train 2013; 48(5):696.
18. Dubois B, Esculier JF. Soft-tissue injuries simply need PEACE and LOVE. Br J Sports Med 2020;54(2):72–3.
19. Vuurberg G, Hoorntje A, Wink LM, et al. Diagnosis, treatment and prevention of ankle sprains: update of an evidence-based clinical guideline. Br J Sports Med 2018;52(15):956.
20. Walker J. Assessment and management of patients with ankle injuries. Nurs Stand 2014;28(50):52–9.
21. Bhandari PS, KC G, Uprety S. Comparative study on management of acute moderate and severe lateral ankle sprain using immobilization in below knee slab versus stirrup ankle brace. J Soc Surg Nepal 2015;18(1):10.
22. Ardèvol J, Bolíbar I, Belda V, et al. Treatment of complete rupture of the lateral ligaments of the ankle: a randomized clinical trial comparing cast immobilization with functional treatment. Knee Surg Sports Traumatol Arthrosc 2002;10(6):371.
23. Mohammadi H, Ghafarian-Shiraz H, Saniee F, et al. Functional treatment comparing with immobilization after acute ankle sprain. Zahedan J Res Med Sci 2013;15(2):28–31.
24. Lamb S, Marsh J, Hutton J, et al. Mechanical supports for acute, severe ankle sprain: a pragmatic, multicentre, randomised controlled trial. Lancet 2009; 373(9663):575.
25. van Den Bekerom M, van Kimmenade R, Sierevelt I, et al. Randomized comparison of tape versus semi-rigid and versus lace-up ankle support in the treatment of acute lateral ankle ligament injury. Knee Surg Sports Traumatol Arthrosc 2016; 24(4):978.
26. Kerkhoffs GM, Rowe BH, Assendelft WJ, et al. Immobilisation for acute ankle sprain. Arch Orthop Trauma Surg 2001;121(8):462.
27. Bleakley CM, O'Connor SR, Tully MA, et al. Effect of accelerated rehabilitation on function after ankle sprain: randomised controlled trial. BMJ 2010;340.
28. Mattacola CG, Dwyer MK. Rehabilitation of the ankle after acute sprain or chronic instability. J Athl Train 2002;37(4):413.
29. Kaminski T, Buckley B, Powers M, et al. Effect of strength and proprioception training on eversion to inversion strength ratios in subjects with unilateral functional ankle instability. Br J Sports Med 2003;37(5):410.
30. Lazarou L, Kofotolis N, Pafis G, et al. Effects of two proprioceptive training programs on ankle range of motion, pain, functional and balance performance in individuals with ankle sprain. J Back Musculoskelet Rehabil 2018;31(3):437.
31. Kidgell DJ, Horvath DM, Jackson BM, et al. Effect of six weeks of dura disc and mini-trampoline balance training on postural sway in athletes with functional ankle instability. J Strength Cond Res 2007;21(2):466.
32. Wright CJ, Linens SW, Cain MS. A randomized controlled trial comparing rehabilitation efficacy in chronic ankle instability. J Sport Rehabil 2017;26(4):238.

33. Smith RW, Reischl SF. Treatment of ankle sprains in young athletes. Am J Sports Med 1986;14(6):465.
34. Hertel J. Functional anatomy, pathomechanics, and pathophysiology of lateral ankle instability. J Athletic Train 2002;37(4):364.
35. Karlsson J, Lansinger O. Chronic lateral instability of the ankle in athletes. Sports Med 1993;16(5):355.
36. Hubbard TJ, Kaminski TW, Vander Griend RA, et al. Quantitative assessment of mechanical laxity in the functionally unstable ankle. Med Sci Sports Exerc 2004;36(5):760.
37. Drewes LK, McKeon PO, Kerrigan DC, et al. Dorsiflexion deficit during jogging with chronic ankle instability. J Sci Med Sport 2009;12(6):685.
38. Denegar CR, Hertel J, Fonseca J. The effect of lateral ankle sprain on dorsiflexion range of motion, posterior talar glide, and joint laxity. J Orthop Sports Phys Ther 2002;32(4):166.
39. Wikstrom EA, Hubbard TJ. Talar positional fault in persons with chronic ankle instability. Arch Phys Med Rehabil 2010;91(8):1267.
40. Hoch MC, Andreatta RD, Mullineaux DR, et al. Two-week joint mobilization intervention improves self-reported function, range of motion, and dynamic balance in those with chronic ankle instability. J Orthop Res 2012;30(11):1798.
41. Karlsson J, Andreasson GO. The effect of external ankle support in chronic lateral ankle joint instability: an electromyographic study. Am J Sports Med 1992; 20(3):257.
42. Cooper PS. Proprioception in injury prevention and rehabilitation of ankle sprains. In: Sammarco GJ, editor. Rehabilitation of the Foot and Ankle. St Louis, MO: Mosby; 1995. p. 95.
43. Clanton TO. Instability of the subtalar joint. Orthop Clin North Am 1989;20(4):583.
44. Linens SW, Ross SE, Arnold BL. Wobble board rehabilitation for improving balance in ankles with chronic instability. Clin J Sport Med 2016;26(1):76.
45. Delahunt E, Monaghan K, Caulfield B. Changes in lower limb kinematics, kinetics, and muscle activity in subjects with functional instability of the ankle joint during a single leg drop jump. J Orthop Res 2006;24(10):1991.
46. Chinn L, Dicharry J, Hertel J. Ankle kinematics of individuals with chronic ankle instability while walking and jogging on a treadmill in shoes. Phys Ther Sport 2013;14(4):232.

Acute Ankle Sprain in Elite Athletes

How to Get Them Back to the Game?

Theodorakys Marín Fermín, MD*,
Ayyoub A. Al-Dolaymi, MD, FIBMS (ortho),
Pieter D'Hooghe, MD, PhD, MBA

KEYWORDS

- Ankle sprain • Ankle instability • Return to sports • Treatment • Rehabilitation
- Soccer • Football

KEY POINTS

- Ankle sprains show gender differences, with female competitors being 25% more likely to sustain such injuries compared with male competitors.
- Despite the high frequency of ankle sprains, the ideal management is controversial, and a significant percentage of patients sustaining an ankle sprain never fully recover.
- Studies show that around 70% of patients experiencing a first-time ankle sprain will recur in the future or may develop chronic ankle instability.
- The acronym POLICE (protection, rest, optimal loading, ice, compression, and elevation) can summarize the management of acute ankle sprains.
- A rehabilitation-based conservative program is the mainstream for lateral ankle sprain treatment but surgery can be considered in high-level athletes.

INTRODUCTION

The ankle joint is a synovial hinge joint with movements in the sagittal plane. The hinge is formed between the distal epiphyses of the tibia and fibula, interlocked like a mortise, and articulating with the talus in a highly congruent joint.[1]

Ankle and foot trauma is widespread, with ankle sprains in the leading. Most people have complete healing and recovery after them but some develop into chronic instability, causing impairments during physical activities.[2] The lateral collateral ankle complex is the most frequently affected. Approximately 85% of such injuries are due to

Funding: None.
No ethics approval was required for the presented study.
Aspetar Orthopaedic and Sports Medicine Hospital, Inside Aspire Zone, Sports City Street, Al Buwairda St, Doha 29222, Qatar
* Corresponding author.
E-mail address: theodorakysmarin@yahoo.com

inversion sprains of the lateral ligaments, 5% are eversion sprains of the medial collateral ligament, and 10% are inferior tibiofibular syndesmotic injuries. The anterior talofibular ligament (ATFL) is the most common component of the lateral collateral ankle complex to be injured in an ankle sprain.[3–5]

Epidemiology

Acute ankle sprains are underreported because they are usually self-treated, especially in nonathletic patients but can constitute up to 30% of injuries seen in sports medicine outpatient clinics.[6] Ankle sprains show gender differences, with female competitors being 25% more likely to sustain such injury than male competitors.[7–11] Female basketball players are more at risk of acute first-time inversion sprain than those participating in other sports (**Box 1**).[7]

Injury Biomechanics

The type of ankle injury depends on 2 factors: the foot's position at the time of impaction and the direction of the force. The typical mechanism of injury is an inversion of the plantarflexed foot (70%–91%).[17–19] Even more, in the presence of relative weakness of the lateral collateral ligament complex (90%–95%)[17,18] with a diminished ATFL load-to-failure (approximately 150 N).[20,21] Additionally, the calcaneofibular(CFL) ligament can be injured due to an adduction force when the foot is in dorsiflexion or neutral positions, as well as the posterior talofibular ligament, which can be torn due to forced dorsiflexion.

The injury mechanism can also guide the diagnosis of potentially associated lesions, including osteochondral injuries of the talar dome, fractures, and damage to the peroneus tendons or superficial nerve.

TREATING ANKLE SPRAINS

Despite the high frequency of ankle sprains, the ideal management is controversial, and a significant percentage of patients sustaining an ankle sprain never fully recover.[22–24] Studies show that around 70% of patients experiencing a first-time ankle sprain will recur in the future or may develop chronic ankle instability.[23,25–27]

A ligament tear remains the most crucial factor in determining the management and predicting the return to sport (RTS). The ankle sprain grading system is vital to

---

Box 1
Risk factors of ankle sprains

- Previous history of sprains or strains. Athletes who have had sprains in the past are at a higher risk of sustaining the same injury again than individuals who have never had it before.[12]

- Inappropriate footwear. Not wearing supportive footwear designed for a specific sport or surface increases the risk of ankle sprains. For example, wearing low-topped shoes instead of high-tops when playing basketball.[13,14]

- Poor athletic conditioning. Athletes attempting strenuous activities without prior conditioning, such as regular ankle and calf stretching and strengthening exercises, increase the risk of injury.[15,16]

- Fatigue. Fatigued athletes, at or near the end of vigorous activity, present a higher risk of injury, especially when they "push through" the fatigue in pursuit of performance instead of resting. For example, marathon runners are at a higher risk of ankle sprains during the last few miles of the race.

differentiate between grade I sprains, in which there is only stretching or microtears; from grade II and III sprains, in which there is a tear in addition to a varying degree of instability.[28] The treatment modalities for acute ankle sprain include the following.

Nonpharmacologic Treatment

The acronyms POLICE (protection, rest, optimal loading, ice, compression, and elevation) can summarize the management of acute ankle sprains.[29]

Protection and rest

A systematic review that studied the effectiveness of external ankle supports in preventing ankle sprains among athletes who had suffered a previous ankle injury showed that 70% had fewer ankle sprains with bracing or taping than those who did not wear prophylactic support.[30] Protective measures include cast splints, air or plastic splints, and Velcro or lace-up braces. Ankle taping can also increase ankle stability but taping is less effective than bracing in preventing ankle sprains because it is highly dependent on the expertise of the individual who performs the taping.[30–32]

Data about the ideal duration of protective measures are scarce. However, according to the biology of ligament healing, it is generally accepted that a minimum of 1 year of protective ankle bracing or taping during sports activities is needed for all athletes who have sustained partial or complete (grade II or III) ankle ligament tear.

Optimal loading

The preferred management of grade II and III lateral ankle sprains is immobilization with an external splint while allowing early weight-bearing. All studies recommend early weight-bearing in the treatment of acute ankle sprain. Even complete grade III ankle sprains show a better healing tendency with early weight-bearing.[33] Clinical researchers have shown that early weight-bearing optimizes the positioning of the torn collateral ligaments for healing while encouraging restoration of the "closed-pack" position of the ankle joint.[34]

Ice

The available literature has advocated cryotherapy in the form of ice cups, ice packs, chemical cold packs, and cooling unit devices. Ice decreases pain and presumably reduces swelling after an ankle sprain.[35] There is a controversy among researchers about the preferred cryotherapy protocol, with some recommending application for 20 to 30 minutes and others advising for 10 minutes and repeating the application at least 3 to 4 times per day during the first 5 days of treatment.[36]

Compression and elevation

It is used to control interstitial bleeding and swelling during the acute phases of the ankle sprain. This can be done by bandaging or using easy-to-apply compression sleeves that can be reused daily.[37]

Rehabilitation. The rehabilitation program is still mainstream in managing ankle injuries, and a good training program is essential. Functional rehabilitation comprises an organized and structured program for recovery of the physical and technical skills for optimal sports performance, focusing on pain relief and compensating functional impairment.[38] The rehabilitation program should include cryotherapy, edema relief, optimal weight-bearing management, range of motion exercises for ankle dorsiflexion improvement, triceps surae stretching, isometric exercises and peroneus muscles strengthening, balance and proprioception training, and bracing/taping. Despite the evidence showing no differences in outcomes comparing supervised and self-administered programs, the former may allow faster progression.[12,38] Following stricter protocols for treatment will hopefully reduce the high incidence of long-term disability that currently results from severe ankle sprains.

Pharmacologic treatment. Evidence supports using nonsteroidal anti-inflammatory drugs during the acute phase of ankle sprain.[39–41] The National Athletic Trainers' Association endorses using nonsteroidal anti-inflammatory drugs in managing ankle sprain as credible. These drugs reduce pain and swelling while improving short-term functional improvement.[42] However, some authors warn against using them, especially long-term use because it may lead to delayed ligament healing.[43]

Outcomes

Although ankle sprains are one of the most common injuries, especially in sport-related incidents, these patients' outcomes are often unclear. About 70% of patients report full recovery at 2 weeks to 36 months,[2] most occurring within the first 6 months.[44] However, 3% to 30% of patients who reported recurrent episodes at 2 weeks to 96 months after the initial sprain may develop longer-term residual pain and instability.[45–47] Moreover, participation in competitive sports has been correlated with residual ankle instability and dysfunction (**Table 1**).[44,48]

The management of ankle injuries varies and depends on the injury's severity and concomitant injuries.[49,50] Most cases are treated conservatively, mainly when there is no associated fracture. To date, no clinical indicator can be used to identify those who may develop recurrent instability or disability requiring a rehabilitation program

Table 1
Factors affecting the outcomes of ankle sprains

Factor	Description
Pathoanatomy of the injury	Single-ligament injuries have better outcomes than multiple and complex tears[51–54]
Imaging	Ottawa foot and ankle rules are valuable to determine the suitability of plain radiographs for investigating ankle sprains[55]
Participation in competitive sports	Sports activity at a high level (training >3 times a week) is a significant prognostic factor for residual symptoms
Swelling	Reflects the severity of the injury—persistent swelling (more than 3 mo) after the initial injury is associated with poorer outcomes Because ankle swelling is a primary contributing factor to a range of motion loss, patients are advised to use cryotherapy, compression, and elevation to decrease swelling and pain[56]
Range of motion	Restricted range of motion at the ankle can lead to functional dysfunction for patients with even daily physical activity. This is why gaining a full range of motion is considered by many authors as a sign of recovery[53,57,58]
Mechanical instability	Ligamentous laxity caused by tears[51,54]
Functional instability	This instability is due to neuromuscular dysfunction due to damage to the articular mechanoreceptors in the injured ligaments and deconditioning during the postinjury period[52]

or surgery. Furthermore, radiological findings do not necessarily reflect the severity of a patient's presentations and recovery time (**Box 2**).

HOW TO GET THE ATHLETE BACK TO THE GAME?

After an acute ankle sprain, it is hard to predict precisely when an athlete can RTS.[12] The current literature lacks formal criteria to assist in the decision to RTS of athletes with a ligamentous ankle injury.

There is strong evidence that residual disability of ankle joint injury is often caused by an inadequate rehabilitation and training program and early RTS.[59] Therefore, the athlete should start their criteria-based rehabilitation and gradually progress through the programmed activities. For example, the medical team focuses firstly on pain-free straightforward jogging or cycling before progressing to running with cutting or a change of direction (agility T-test or zigzag test).

Furthermore, medical teams must develop ankle-specific programs for athletes performing through pain. Skill-related activities such as pivoting and cutting must be added to the proposed training program when the athlete is pain-free or has mild symptoms with the previously programmed activities. It is helpful to evaluate the effectiveness of the rehabilitation protocol by using self-reported ankle scoring systems (e.g., Foot and Ankle Outcome Score [FAOS]).[60] However, functional performance tests are used to assess the athlete's ability to perform sport-specific skills and to prepare him for the next level of training.[42] Therefore, data from these outcomes must be evaluated during the rehabilitation protocol as a baseline to assess the progression contrasting with the contralateral normal side.[61–64] For an athlete to RTS, an ideal functional performance of a minimum of 90%, compared with the contralateral side, has been recommended.[65]

In general, athletes with ankle injuries may return to play depending on their signs and symptoms (**Box 3**).

The RTS in amateur and professional soccer players after an acute ankle sprain has been reported between 7 and 15 $\pm$ 19 days, respectively.[18,66] Nevertheless, the time required depends on several factors, including the following:

Box 2
Complications after an ankle sprain

- Chronic ankle instability: It is accompanied by a feeling of instability by the patient, swelling after activity, and prolonged recovery

- Impingement syndrome: Intra-articular localized fibrotic synovitis in the lateral gutter of the ankle following inversion injuries

- Fractures and osteochondral injuries include osteochondral injuries of the talar dome due to inversion and eversion mechanisms and fracture of the anterior calcaneal process due to inversion injuries. Patients with a fracture commonly complain of bony tenderness

- Recurrent peroneal tendon subluxation: It occurs due to injury and detachment of the peroneal retinaculum from the posterior aspect of the fibula

- Complex regional pain syndrome: It may develop after ankle injuries. The actual cause for this is unknown; however, it may develop from an unusual response of the ankle and foot to disuse and/or immobilization of the ankle and foot. Early, controlled weight-bearing and rehabilitation may prevent the development of complex regional pain syndrome

- Syndesmotic injury: This condition is diagnosed clinically by the presence of tenderness over the anterior aspect of the ankle and pain when squeezing the fibula against the tibia at the midshaft (squeeze test).

> **Box 3**
> **Return-to-play criteria after an ankle sprain**
>
> - No pain
> - Full active and passive range of motion
> - About 70%–90% of muscle strength compared with the uninjured ankle
> - Negative clinical examination
> - Balance on one leg for more than 30 s with eyes closed
> - Satisfactory functional examination ensuring that all dysfunctions resulting from the injury have been restored
> - Preinjury cardiorespiratory fitness status
> - No doubts about the athlete's health and safety

1. The severity of the injury and associated bony injuries
2. Athlete's compliance, cooperation, performance level, and baseline functional demands. Players with highly functional baseline demands may take longer to return to preinjury level if at all).[67] In fact, only 12% of competitive athletes returned to sport compared with 88% of recreational athletes
3. Rehabilitation program

WHAT IS THE ROLE OF SURGERY IN ACUTE ANKLE SPRAINS TREATMENT?

The surgical repair of acute ankle sprains is controversial. Most of the studies have methodological flaws and, thus, should be interpreted carefully.[68] Surgery can be done acutely or after failing conservative treatment because it does not seem to yield different outcomes.[69] Although conservative and surgical therapies produce satisfactory results, subtle differences favoring surgery on pain and recurrent instability have been reported.[70]

Surgical techniques can follow 2 principles.[71]

- Anatomic techniques: anatomical reinsertion of the ligament or reconstruction with a graft, for example, Bröstrom technique.
- Functional crutch techniques: improving the healing response of the native ligament to its normal length and tensile conditions by using a functional crutch, for example, InternalBrace technique.

The Bröstrom-Gould technique shares both principles and, similar to most techniques, can be performed in various approaches: open, percutaneous, and arthroscopically. At present, arthroscopic techniques are preferred because they allow for assessing and potentially addressing concomitant injuries, which can be present ranging from 42% to 93% of patients.[72–74]

RTS typically ranges between 12 weeks and 4 months following surgery.[75] In a case series including 42 professional athletes with an acute lateral ankle sprain, White and colleagues[76] reported a mean return to training time of 63 days (49–110) and an RTS of 77 days (56–127) with diagnostic ankle arthroscopy and open modified Bröstrom repair. Similarly, Sanchez and colleagues,[77] in their case series of 40 patients, reported more than 30 points of American Orthopaedic Foot & Ankle Society (AOFAS) improvement in function and pain control with an arthroscopy-assisted ATFL reconstruction. Although all patients had a preoperative diagnosis of chronic lateral ankle

---

Box 4
Criteria for surgical repair/reconstruction of acute lateral ankle sprain

- Failed conservative treatment[69,71]
- Athletes or high-demand patients[69]
- Grade III lateral ankle sprains[76]
- Combined ATFL and CFL ligament injury[76]
- Acute injuries with mechanical instability[71,76]
- Reconstruction with extensor retinaculum or tendon graft should be considered in the presence of an irreparable ATFL injury[77]

---

instability, 2 acute instability cases were of high-performance athletes who required an early RTS.

Finally, a recent systematic review by Goru and colleagues,[78] comprising 10 studies (343 athletes), showed that the modified Broström technique using an anchor provides satisfactory outcomes in athletes with lateral ankle instability. The technique is safe, and RTS can be expected at a mean of 16 weeks, with an 89% rate of return to pre-injury performance. However, associated injuries are correlated with delayed RTS (**Box 4**).[75,76,78]

SUMMARY

Ankle sprains treatment remains controversial. Although rehabilitation is mainstream in conservative treatment with a satisfactory RTS rate and time, many patients will still develop chronic ankle instability. Thus far, no clinical indicator can be used to identify those patients and when an athlete can RTS safely.

CLINICS CARE POINTS

- Early weight-bearing is recommended in the treatment of acute ankle sprain.
- The rehabilitation program should include cryotherapy, edema relief, optimal weight-bearing management, range of motion exercises for ankle dorsiflexion improvement, triceps surae stretching, isometric exercises and peroneus muscles strengthening, balance and proprioception training, and bracing/taping.
- To date, no clinical indicator can identify those who may develop recurrent instability or disability requiring a rehabilitation program or surgery.
- The current literature lacks formal criteria to assist in the decision to RTS of athletes with a ligamentous ankle injury.
- For an athlete to RTS, an ideal functional performance of a minimum of 90%, compared with the contralateral side, has been recommended.
- There is strong evidence that residual disability of ankle joint injury is often caused by an inadequate rehabilitation and training program and early return to sports.
- Surgical treatment is safe, and return to sports can be expected at a mean of 16 weeks with an 89% rate of return to preinjury performance.

DECLARATIONS OF INTEREST

None.

DATA AVAILABILITY STATEMENT

The data underlying this article are available in the article and its online supplementary material.

ACKNOWLEDGMENTS

None.

CONTRIBUTIONS

T. Marín Fermín: Conceptualization, Methodology, Validation, Investigation, Resources, Writing–Original Draft, Visualization, Project administration. A.A. Al-Dolaymi: Conceptualization, Validation, Writing–Review and Editing, Supervision. P, D'Hooghe: Conceptualization, Methodology, Validation, Investigation, Writing–Review and Editing, Supervision, Project administration.

All authors contributed to the conception and design of the study; acquisition, analysis, and interpretation of the data; drafting the work and revising it critically for important intellectual content; agreed to be accountable for all aspects of the study in ensuring that questions related to the accuracy or integrity of any part of the study were appropriately investigated and resolved. All authors read and approved the final article.

REFERENCES

1. Mohammed AA, Abbas KA, Mawlood AS. A comparative study in fixation methods of medial malleolus fractures between tension bands wiring and screw fixation. Springerplus 2016;5:530.
2. Hiller CE, Nightingale EJ, Raymond J, et al. Prevalence and impact of chronic musculoskeletal ankle disorders in the community. Arch Phys Med Rehabil 2012;93(10):1801–7.
3. Ivins D. Acute ankle sprain: an update. Am Fam Physician 2006;74(10):1714–20.
4. Gross MT, Liu HY. The role of ankle bracing for prevention of ankle sprain injuries. J Orthop Sports Phys Ther 2003;33(10):572–7.
5. LeBlanc KE. Ankle problems masquerading as sprains. Prim Care 2004;31(4): 1055–67.
6. Mahaffey D, Hilts M, Fields KB. Ankle and foot injuries in sports. Clin Fam Pract 1999;1(1):233–50.
7. Beynnon BD, Vacek PM, Murphy D, et al. First-time inversion ankle ligament trauma: the effects of sex, level of competition, and sport on the incidence of injury. Am J Sports Med 2005;33(10):1485–91.
8. Fernandez WG, Yard EE, Comstock RD. Epidemiology of lower extremity injuries among U.S. high school athletes. Acad Emerg Med 2007;14(7):641–5.
9. McKeon PO, Mattacola CG. Interventions for the prevention of first time and recurrent ankle sprains. Clin Sports Med 2008;27(3):371–viii.
10. Fong DT, Man CY, Yung PS, et al. Sport-related ankle injuries attending an accident and emergency department. Injury 2008;39(10):1222–7.
11. Nelson AJ, Collins CL, Yard EE, et al. Ankle injuries among United States high school sports athletes, 2005-2006. J Athl Train 2007;42(3):381–7.
12. D'Hooghe P, Cruz F, Alkhelaifi K. Return to play after a lateral ligament ankle sprain. Curr Rev Musculoskelet Med 2020;13(3):281–8.
13. Barrett J, Bilisko T. The role of shoes in the prevention of ankle sprains. Sports Med 1995 Oct;20(4):277–80.

14. Beynnon BD, Murphy DF, Alosa DM. Predictive factors for lateral ankle sprains: a literature review. J Athl Train 2002;37(4):376–80.
15. Flevas DA, Pappas E, Ristanis S, et al. Effect of laterality and fatigue in peroneal electromechanical delay. SICOT J 2022;8:22.
16. Grassi A, Alexiou K, Amendola A, et al. Postural stability deficit could predict ankle sprains: a systematic review. Knee Surg Sports Traumatol Arthrosc 2018; 26(10):3140–55.
17. Woods C, Hawkins R, Hulse M, et al. The Football Association Medical Research Programme: an audit of injuries in professional football-analysis of preseason injuries. Br J Sports Med 2002;36(6):436–41.
18. Kofotolis ND, Kellis E, Vlachopoulos SP. Ankle sprain injuries and risk factors in amateur soccer players during a 2-year period. Am J Sports Med 2007;35(3): 458–66.
19. Hawkins RD, Hulse MA, Wilkinson C, et al. The association football medical research programme: an audit of injuries in professional football. Br J Sports Med 2001;35(1):43–7.
20. Krips R, de Vries J, van Dijk CN. Ankle instability. Foot Ankle Clin 2006;11(2): 311, vi.
21. St Pierre RK, Rosen J, Whitesides TE, et al. The tensile strength of the anterior talofibular ligament. Foot Ankle 1983;4(2):83–5.
22. Brand RL, Black HM, Cox JS. The natural history of inadequately treated ankle sprain. Am J Sports Med 1977;5(6):248–9.
23. Verhagen RA, de Keizer G, van Dijk CN. Long-term follow-up of inversion trauma of the ankle. Arch Orthop Trauma Surg 1995;114(2):92–6.
24. Itay S, Ganel A. Clinical and functional status following lateral ankle sprains: follow-up of 90 young adults treated conservatively. Orthop Rev 1982;11:73–6.
25. Yeung MS, Chan KM, So CH, et al. An epidemiological survey on ankle sprain. Br J Sports Med 1994;28(2):112–6.
26. Gerber JP, Williams GN, Scoville CR, et al. Persistent disability associated with ankle sprains: a prospective examination of an athletic population. Foot Ankle Int 1998;19(10):653–60.
27. Braun BL. Effects of ankle sprain in a general clinic population 6 to 18 months after medical evaluation. Arch Fam Med 1999;8(2):143–8.
28. van den Bekerom MP, Kerkhoffs GM, McCollum GA, et al. Management of acute lateral ankle ligament injury in the athlete. Knee Surg Sports Traumatol Arthrosc 2013;21(6):1390–5.
29. Bleakley CM, Glasgow P, MacAuley DC. PRICE needs updating, should we call the POLICE? Br J Sports Med 2012;46(4):220–1.
30. Dizon JM, Reyes JJ. A systematic review on the effectiveness of external ankle supports in the prevention of inversion ankle sprains among elite and recreational players. J Sci Med Sport 2010;13(3):309–17.
31. Olmsted LC, Vela LI, Denegar CR, et al. Prophylactic ankle taping and bracing: a numbers-needed-to-treat and cost-benefit analysis. J Athl Train 2004;39(1): 95–100.
32. Rovere GD, Clarke TJ, Yates CS, et al. Retrospective comparison of taping and ankle stabilizers in preventing ankle injuries. Am J Sports Med 1988;16(3): 228–33.
33. Kerkhoffs GM, Rowe BH, Assendelft WJ, et al. Immobilisation for acute ankle sprain. A systematic review. Arch Orthop Trauma Surg 2001;121(8):462–71.
34. Smith RW, Reischl SF. Treatment of ankle sprains in young athletes. Am J Sports Med 1986;14(6):465–71.

35. Hubbard TJ, Aronson SL, Denegar CR. Does cryotherapy hasten return to participation? A systematic review. J Athl Train 2004;39(1):88–94.
36. Bleakley CM, McDonough SM, MacAuley DC, et al. Cryotherapy for acute ankle sprains: a randomised controlled study of two different icing protocols. Br J Sports Med 2006;40(8):700–5.
37. Wilkerson GB, Horn-Kingery HM. Treatment of the inversion ankle sprain: comparison of different modes of compression and cryotherapy. J Orthop Sports Phys Ther 1993;17(5):240–6.
38. Gaddi D, Mosca A, Piatti M, et al. Acute ankle sprain management: an umbrella review of systematic reviews. Front Med (Lausanne) 2022;9:868474.
39. Bleakley CM, McDonough SM, MacAuley DC. Some conservative strategies are effective when added to controlled mobilisation with external support after acute ankle sprain: a systematic review. Aust J Physiother 2008;54(1):7–20.
40. Slatyer MA, Hensley MJ, Lopert R. A randomized controlled trial of piroxicam in the management of acute ankle sprain in Australian Regular Army recruits: the Kapooka Ankle Sprain Study. Am J Sports Med 1997;25(4):544–53.
41. Mazières B, Rouanet S, Velicy J, et al. Topical ketoprofen patch (100 mg) for the treatment of ankle sprain: a randomized, double-blind, placebo-controlled study. Am J Sports Med 2005;33(4):515–23.
42. Kaminski TW, Hertel J, Amendola N, et al. National Athletic Trainers' Association position statement: conservative management and prevention of ankle sprains in athletes. J Athl Train 2013;48(4):528–45.
43. Mishra DK, Fridén J, Schmitz MC, et al. Anti-inflammatory medication after muscle injury. A treatment resulting in short-term improvement but subsequent loss of muscle function. J Bone Joint Surg Am 1995;77(10):1510–9.
44. van Rijn RM, van Os AG, Bernsen RM, et al. What is the clinical course of acute ankle sprains? A systematic literature review. Am J Med 2008;121(4):324–31.e6.
45. Kemler E, van de Port I, Backx F, et al. A systematic review on the treatment of acute ankle sprain: brace versus other functional treatment types. Sports Med 2011;41(3):185–97.
46. Hossain M, Thomas R. Ankle instability: presentation and management. Orthop Trauma 2015;29:145–51.
47. Houston MN, Hoch JM, Hoch MC. Patient-reported outcome measures in individuals with chronic ankle instability: a systematic review. J Athl Train 2015;50(10):1019–33.
48. Verhagen E, van der Beek A, Twisk J, et al. The effect of a proprioceptive balance board training program for the prevention of ankle sprains: a prospective controlled trial. Am J Sports Med 2004;32(6):1385–93.
49. Bridgman SA, Clement D, Downing A, et al. Population based epidemiology of ankle sprains attending accident and emergency units in the West Midlands of England, and a survey of UK practice for severe ankle sprains. Emerg Med J 2003;20(6):508–10.
50. Bleakley CM, O'Connor SR, Tully MA, et al. Effect of accelerated rehabilitation on function after ankle sprain: randomised controlled trial. BMJ 2010;340:c1964.
51. Hubbard TJ, Hicks-Little CA. Ankle ligament healing after an acute ankle sprain: an evidence-based approach. J Athl Train 2008;43(5):523–9.
52. Hertel J. Functional Anatomy, pathomechanics, and pathophysiology of lateral ankle instability. J Athl Train 2002;37(4):364–75.
53. Renström P, Lynch SA. Management of Acute Ankle Sprains. In: Nyska M, Mann G, editors. Human kinetics. Champaign, IL: The Unstable Ankle; 2002. p. 168–76.

54. Prado MP, Fernandes TD, Camanho GL, et al. Mechanical instability after acute ankle ligament injury: randomized prospective comparison of two forms of conservative treatment. Rev Bras Ortop 2013;48(4):307–16.
55. Stiell IG, Greenberg GH, McKnight RD, et al. A study to develop clinical decision rules for the use of radiography in acute ankle injuries. Ann Emerg Med 1992; 21(4):384–90.
56. Bleakley CM, Glasgow PD, Philips N, et al. Management of acute soft tissue injury using protection rest ice compression and elevation: recommendations from the association of chartered physiotherapists in sports an exercise medicine (ACPSM) executive summary. London, UK: Chartered Society of Physiotherapy; 2010.
57. Beynnon BD, Renström PA, Haugh L, et al. A prospective, randomized clinical investigation of the treatment of first-time ankle sprains. Am J Sports Med 2006;34(9):1401–12.
58. Kaikkonen A, Kannus P, Järvinen M. A performance test protocol and scoring scale for the evaluation of ankle injuries. Am J Sports Med 1994;22(4):462–9.
59. Renström PA, Konradsen L. Ankle ligament injuries. Br J Sports Med 1997;31(1): 11–20.
60. Roos EM, Brandsson S, Karlsson J. Validation of the foot and ankle outcome score for ankle ligament reconstruction. Foot Ankle Int 2001;22(10):788–94.
61. Pauole K, Madole K, Garhammer J, et al. Reliability and validity of the T-test as a measure of agility, leg power, and leg speed in college aged men and women. J Strength Cond Res 2000;14(4):443–50.
62. Gonell AC, Romero JA, Soler LM. Relationship between the y balance test scores and soft tissue injury incidence in a soccer team. Int J Sports Phys Ther 2015; 10(7):955–66.
63. McGuine TA, Greene JJ, Best T, et al. Balance as a predictor of ankle injuries in high school basketball players. Clin J Sport Med 2000;10(4):239–44.
64. Plisky PJ, Rauh MJ, Kaminski TW, et al. Star excursion balance test as a predictor of lower extremity injury in high school basketball players. J Orthop Sports Phys Ther 2006;36(12):911–9.
65. Hupperets MD, Verhagen EA, van Mechelen W. Effect of unsupervised home based proprioceptive training on recurrences of ankle sprain: randomised controlled trial. BMJ 2009;339:b2684.
66. Waldén M, Hägglund M, Ekstrand J. Time-trends and circumstances surrounding ankle injuries in men's professional football: an 11-year follow-up of the UEFA champions league injury study. Br J Sports Med 2013;47(12):748–53.
67. Colvin AC, Walsh M, Koval KJ, et al. Return to sports following operatively treated ankle fractures. Foot Ankle Int 2009;30(4):292–6.
68. Kerkhoffs GM, Handoll HH, de Bie R, et al. Surgical versus conservative treatment for acute injuries of the lateral ligament complex of the ankle in adults. Cochrane Database Syst Rev 2007;2:CD000380.
69. Hepple S, Guha A. The role of ankle arthroscopy in acute ankle injuries of the athlete. Foot Ankle Clin 2013;18(2):185–94.
70. Pijnenburg AC, Bogaard K, Krips R, et al. Operative and functional treatment of rupture of the lateral ligament of the ankle. A randomised, prospective trial. J Bone Joint Surg Br 2003;85(4):525–30.
71. Corte-Real N, Caetano J. Ankle and syndesmosis instability: consensus and controversies. EFORT Open Rev 2021;6(6):420–31.

72. Marín Fermín T, Macchiarola L, Zampeli F, et al. Osteochondral lesions of the talar dome in the athlete: what evidence leads to which treatment. J Cartilage Joint Preservation 2022;2(2):100065.
73. Joshy S, Abdulkadir U, Chaganti S, et al. Accuracy of MRI scan in the diagnosis of ligamentous and chondral pathology in the ankle. Foot Ankle Surg 2010;16(2):78–80.
74. O'Neill PJ, Van Aman SE, Guyton GP. Is MRI adequate to detect lesions in patients with ankle instability? Clin Orthop Relat Res 2010;468(4):1115–9.
75. Pearce CJ, Tourné Y, Zellers J, et al. Rehabilitation after anatomical ankle ligament repair or reconstruction. Knee Surg Sports Traumatol Arthrosc 2016;24(4):1130–9.
76. White WJ, McCollum GA, Calder JD. Return to sport following acute lateral ligament repair of the ankle in professional athletes. Knee Surg Sports Traumatol Arthrosc 2016;24(4):1124–9.
77. Sánchez CA, Briceño I, Robledo J. Outcomes of a modified arthroscopic-assisted reconstruction technique for lateral ankle instability. Rev Bras Ortop (Sao Paulo) 2022;57(4):577–83.
78. Goru P, Talha S, Majeed H. Outcomes and return to sports following the ankle lateral ligament reconstruction in professional athletes: a systematic review of the literature. Indian J Orthop 2021;56(2):208–15.

Chronic Lateral Ankle Instability

Can We Get Even Better with Surgical Treatment?

Jose Antonio Veiga Sanhudo, MD, PhD[a],*, Eric Ferkel, MD[b],
Kepler Alencar Mendes de Carvalho, MD[c]

KEYWORDS

- Ankle sprains • Ankle instability • Ankle reconstruction • Chronic instability
- Tendon augmentation

KEY POINTS

- Repetitive ankle sprains can lead to lateral ligament attenuation. "Laxity" and "giving way" are symptoms indicators of ankle instability.
- Lateral ankle ligament surgeries can be performed through an open approach, arthroscopically, arthroscopic-assisted, or percutaneously.
- The anatomic ankle reconstruction technique described by Broström is renowned for its excellent outcomes and high rate of return to sports.
- In skilled hands, arthroscopy-assisted or fully arthroscopic ligament reconstruction carries a high rate of good and excellent outcomes and returns to sports.

INTRODUCTION

Ankle sprains are the most common injuries in sports and are always a cause for concern because up to 74% of patients develop residual symptoms and many develop chronic ankle instability (CAI).[1] Despite the high prevalence of this injury, its treatment remains controversial, and many patients neglect its severity, returning to physical activity within a few days, increasing the chance of another sprain. Up to 34% of patients will have another sprain of the same ankle within 3 years.[2,3] Repetitive ankle sprains can lead to lateral ligament attenuation and an ever-increasing sensation of "giving way." "Laxity" is observed on physical examination, whereas "giving way" is

[a] Foot & Ankle Department, Hospital Moinhos de Vento, Avenida Juca Batista 8000, 18 Porto Alegre RS, Brazil CEP 91781-200; [b] Southern California Orthopedic Institute, 6815 Noble Avenue, Suite 200, Van Nuys, CA, USA; [c] Department of Orthopedics and Rehabilitation, University of Iowa, Carver College of Medicine, Iowa City, IA, USA
* Corresponding author.
E-mail address: sanhudotraumato@gmail.com

Foot Ankle Clin N Am 28 (2023) 321–332
https://doi.org/10.1016/j.fcl.2023.01.004
1083-7515/23/© 2023 Elsevier Inc. All rights reserved.

foot.theclinics.com

the symptom described by the patient. Both are indicators of ankle instability. These findings are associated with mechanical and functional instability, decreased performance in recreational and occupational activities, decreased global and regional functions, and impairment of quality of life.[1–5]

Although ankle instability is divided into mechanical and functional, both usually coexist. In classic functional instability, a patient with minimal laxity complains of the ankle giving way and reports a history of several previous sprains. The factors associated with functional instability include proprioceptive deficits, decreased neuromuscular control, loss of evertor strength, tight gastrocnemius–soleus complex, and decreased postural control. Hindfoot varus, midfoot cavus, and ligamentous laxity are predisposing factors for a lateral ankle sprain. Combining one or more of these factors with functional instability often results in an initial sprain followed by subsequent episodes of recurrence. Chronic lateral ankle instability is usually the result of an untreated or inadequately treated sprain. However, it is still possible that even after an appropriately treated sprain, the ankle cannot recover its preinjury function and will develop sequelae, including chronic instability. Once established, CAI leads to a feeling of giving way with decreased performance and long periods of inactivity after each injury. Additionally, chronic instability can lead to chondral damage intraarticularly, which can predispose a patient to tibio-talar joint arthritis.

Most experts agree that conservative treatment is the modality of choice initially after an acute ankle sprain, especially when it is the first such episode. However, the effect of nonsurgical treatment on already established chronic instability has yet to receive much research interest. However, there is a consensus that nonsurgical treatment is more effective for patients with significant functional instability. The cornerstone of ankle rehabilitation aimed at relieving symptoms and preventing future sprains is a combination of kinetic chain strengthening, evertor strength training, proprioceptive training, and lateral wedge insoles.[6–8] When conservative treatment is not effective, surgical treatment is indicated.

Surgical Treatment

The surgical techniques for treating chronic instability are divided into anatomic repair, anatomic reconstruction with a graft, and nonanatomic reconstruction. Anatomic repair is performed when the ligaments are in suitable condition to be restored without using other tissues to replace them. In this technique, the torn ligaments are tightened and repaired or reinserted into the fibula with anchors or tunnels to restore adequate tension and joint stability. Anatomic ligament reconstruction uses autogenous or allogenic graft due to the poor quality of the native ligaments that are injured beyond a point where primary repair is impossible. Nonanatomic reconstruction involves local tendon transfer to provide joint stabilization.

Anatomic ligament reconstruction with a graft and nonanatomic reconstruction is typically reserved for severe recalcitrant cases, patients with a significantly elevated Body Mass Index (BMI), hindfoot varus malalignment, and long-standing instability with comorbid ligament hyperlaxity.

Lateral ankle ligament surgeries can be performed through an open approach, arthroscopically, arthroscopic-assisted, or percutaneously. The traditional open approach for ankle ligament reconstruction involves larger or smaller incisions depending on the chosen technique. The Broström procedure and its numerous modifications are the most frequently performed. Many surgeons consider arthroscopy to be a helpful adjunct in identifying and treating intra-articular injuries but also the main procedure for fully arthroscopic reconstructions. However, it should be considered that fluid extravasation into the soft tissues may make it more challenging identifying the soft tissue planes in open procedures after ankle arthroscopy.[9] Although arthroscopy is justified by many surgeons as the initial approach to identify any comorbid lesions, it is essential to remember that every patient undergoing ligament reconstruction of the ankle must be initially investigated with plain radiography and MRI. MRI will detect most of these associated findings before surgery. In addition, it is estimated that iatrogenic injuries to the joint cartilage occur in 31% of procedures, with 6.7% of cases considered severe lesions.[10] A percutaneous approach to reconstruction of the lateral ligamentous complex aims to reduce the procedure's morbidity and is usually indicated in the absence of ankle deformity. The technique uses radiography instead of arthroscopy to find critical points for ligament stabilization. Arthroscopy has been used to assist the procedure in selected cases.[11–15]

Anatomic Repair

The anatomic ankle reconstruction technique described by Broström is renowned for its excellent outcomes and high rate of return to sports, even in the long term, with no difference in results between male and female patients. Technical details, such as imbrication and ligament fixation with or without anchors, vary among authors, and there is no established superiority of any one technique.[16–23] Bell and colleagues reported 91% of excellent functional results with the Broström-Gould technique after an average of 25 years of follow-up. Karlsson and colleagues achieved 87% good to excellent outcomes using a similar surgical technique.[16,17] Gould's modification of the original Broström technique with reinforcement of the extensor retinaculum, described in 1966, is performed by many authors whenever possible because it increases the strength of the repair by 60% and improves the contact area of the joint surface but good outcomes can be achieved even without this modification.[23,24]

Anatomic and Nonanatomic Reconstruction

Before surgery, it is sometimes difficult to estimate the quality of the ligaments accurately through physical examination and imaging, even with MRI. Stress radiography is helpful in demonstrating lateral ligament competence but it cannot demonstrate the quality of the tissue to be repaired. Therefore, the decision to migrate from an anatomic repair to a reconstruction is, and can occasionally be, made intraoperatively.

In cases of severe and long-standing instability, generalized ligament hyperlaxity, obesity, high-demand activity, hindfoot varus malalignment, revision of previous surgery, and poor quality of the lateral ligaments, anatomic repair may be impossible or insufficient. In these cases, reconstruction with tendon augmentation is the alternate choice (**Fig. 1**). However, this technique has the disadvantage of sacrificing a healthy tendon as a graft. When the peroneus brevis is used, it has been shown to lead to a loss in eversion strength, as well as prolonged operative times. Coupled with the need for bone tunnels and a donor site approach, this has been shown to increase the morbidity of the procedure and increase the chance of joint stiffness and degenerative joint changes.[25–27]

The Evans, Christmas-Snook, and Watson-Jones techniques are the most common approaches in this category.[25–27] The Watson-Jones procedure, in which the peroneus brevis tendon is passed through drill holes in the lateral malleolus and the neck of the talus, provides good long-term outcomes. Nevertheless, cutaneous nerve injury and recurrent instability are expected in 18% of cases.[27]

The procedure described by Evans is technically more straightforward than the traditional Watson-Jones ligament reconstruction because only part of the distally attached peroneus brevis graft is passed through a single oblique drill hole in the distal fibula. However, the site of fixation is not anatomic.[25] In this technique, the peroneal

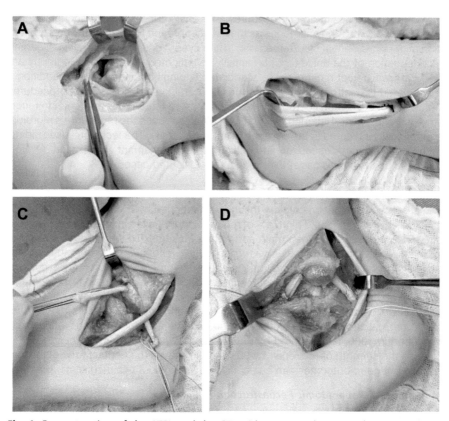

Fig. 1. Reconstruction of the ATFL and the CFL with peroneus brevis graft. Intraoperative images: (A) visualization of the injury degree level, (B) location and separation of the peroneus brevis and peroneus longus tendons, (C) passage of the peroneus brevis tendon through the peroneal tunnel, and (D) final reconstruction of the ATFL and CFL.

tendon graft is positioned between the attachments of the anterior talofibular ligament (ATFL) and the calcaneofibular ligament (CFL) and does not anatomically reconstitute the continuity of either.[28] The technique stabilizes the ankle and subtalar joint and restricts ankle inversion in the short term. However, studies show that there is a loss of efficiency in the long term, leading to inferior clinical outcomes compared with anatomic reconstruction.[25,28] Complications of the Evans technique are not uncommon. They include persistent swelling, decreased range of motion, persistent instability sensation, or a "too tight" repair feeling, leading 50% or more of patients to classify their outcome as unsatisfactory and report difficulty returning to their preinjury level of sports activity.[29,30] The Evans technique is also used as augmentation in combination with the Broström-Gould repair, with some studies describing good results and significant functional improvement.[31–36] Anatomic reconstruction using autologous free peroneus brevis or semitendinosus grafts aims to preserve the advantages of tendon reinforcement (greater strength) with a lower risk of decreased mobility.[37,38]

The Chrisman-Snook technique consists of using a split peroneus brevis graft, routed through bone tunnels in the fibula and calcaneus, to reconstruct the lateral ligaments. The procedure is not technically simple but it does provide good long-term outcomes and is an alternative for patients with low-quality connective tissue.

Nevertheless, one should be aware of the higher risk of incisional complications, sural nerve injury, a "too tight" repair feeling, and persistent instability with a "giving way" sensation.[26,39–41]

The use of an allograft is intended to reinforce the ligament reconstruction. The indications are the same as for an autograft but without the inconveniences of sacrificing a healthy structure and increasing operative time. This technique is advantageous in cases of previously failed reconstruction, mainly when an autologous graft was used. The use of nonautologous tissue, however, carries the disadvantages of a greater risk of local reaction and longer healing time.[42] Li and colleagues found in a systematic review and meta-analysis of outcomes after allograft reconstruction in patients with CLAI that there was an average American Orthopaedic Foot & Ankle Society (AOFAS) scores improved from 55.4 to 91.9, which was a 40% improvement. An 80% of the pooled proportion of patients returned to sports after surgery, and the total risk of recurrent instability after surgery was only 6%. Furthermore, no graft rejection was reported in any of the studies reviewed (Li H, Song Y, Li H, Hua Y. Outcomes After Anatomic Lateral Ankle Ligament Reconstruction Using Allograft Tendon for Chronic Ankle Instability: A Systematic Review and Meta-analysis. *J Foot Ankle Surg*. 2020;59(1):117 to 124. https://doi.org/10.1053/j.jfas.2019.07.008). Open or percutaneous anatomic reconstruction, using semitendinosus or posterior tibial allograft tendon, attached with bioabsorbable tenodesis screws, yields good functional outcomes.[43–45] Dierckman and Ferkel reported their results of this technique on 31 patients (Dierckman BD, Ferkel RD. Anatomic Reconstruction with a Semitendinosus Allograft for Chronic Lateral Ankle Instability. *Am J Sports Med*. 2015;43(8):1941-1950. https://doi.org/10.1177/0363546515593942). The authors found that 20% of patients with CLAI required allograft augmentation in addition to a direct primary repair. In their retrospective review, 100% of patients were completely satisfied at an average follow-up of 38 months. Results of Broström-Gould ligament repair versus anatomic reconstruction with a semitendinosus allograft demonstrated no difference in outcomes after a mean 2 years of follow-up.[46]

Suture Tape Augmentation

Immediately after lateral ligament reconstruction, the strength of the repaired ligaments is still limited, making cast or boot immobilization mandatory and preventing earlier rehabilitation. The use of tape augmentation in Broström-type ligament reconstruction aims to increase primary stability to the lateral ligaments, especially in patients with long-standing instability, obese patients, and high-performance athletes.

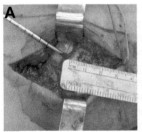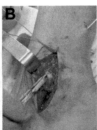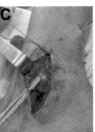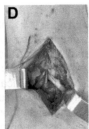

Fig. 2. Lateral ankle anatomic reconstruction using the autologous Gracilis tendon plus tape reinforcement. Intraoperative images: (*A*) location of the insertion point in the Fibula, (*B* and *C*) fibular stem tensioning thread, and (*D*) final reconstruction view (Gracilis tendon plus tape reinforcement).

Reinforcing the reconstruction with suture tape may allow for a shorter period of immobilization, permitting earlier, more intense functional rehabilitation and an earlier return to sports activities (**Fig 2**). However, the biomechanical consequences and the possibility of foreign body granulomatous reaction to placement of this inelastic device are still unknown.[47–53]

Case series have reported good outcomes with suture tape. Xu and colleagues recently compared modified Broström repairs with and without suture tape augmentation, with at least 2-year follow-up (Xu D-L, Gan K-F, Li H-J, et al. Modified Broström Repair With and Without Augmentation Using Suture Tape for Chronic Lateral Ankle Instability. *Orthop Surg*. 2019;11(4):671-678. https://doi.org/10.1111/os.12516). This study included 25 patients undergoing modified Broström repair with suture tape augmentation and 28 patients with isolated modified Broström repair. Both groups achieved satisfactory outcomes and significant improvements in terms of pain and functional outcome scores. There were no statistical differences between the 2 groups when comparing the range of motion, Visual Analog Scale (VAS), AOFAS scores, and radiologic outcomes. However, when comparing the Foot and Ankle Ability Measure surveys, the suture tape augmentation group had significantly better scores than the isolated Broström repair for the Sport (87.1 vs 78.2) and Total (93.1 vs 90.5) outcome surveys.

Nevertheless, other comparative studies have shown that superior results may be achieved only in the first weeks after surgery, with similar long-term outcomes. The possibility of more intense early rehabilitation is desirable for high-performance athletes but one must consider the approximately 30% increase in the cost of the procedure. There also is a greater risk of complications involving the peroneal nerve and tendons due to local tissue irritation.[51]

Arthroscopic and Arthroscopy-Assisted Reconstruction

CAI can be associated with many intra-articular conditions, including impingement, chondromalacia, osteochondral lesions of the talus, loose bodies, and osteophytes. These conditions can contribute to the clinical picture and surgical indication and, if not addressed, can be a cause of residual symptoms leading to less favorable outcomes after ligament stabilization.[1,2] Comorbid extra-articular lesions, such as peroneal tendinopathy, are not routinely treated arthroscopically, and surgeons should be aware of this limitation.[54,55] Arthroscopy can be helpful as a diagnostic and therapeutic tool for associated injuries alone but there are described techniques for fully arthroscopic ligament reconstruction (**Fig 3**). Interest in arthroscopic reconstruction stems from its minimally invasive nature and the possibility of reduced morbidity and faster recovery. In skilled hands, arthroscopy-assisted or fully arthroscopic ligament reconstruction carries a high rate of good and excellent outcomes and returns to sports, with no significant increase in complications, even in the presence of ligament hyperlaxity.[56] Arthroscopic techniques involve "Arthro-Broström" type anatomic repairs and autologous or allogeneic graft reconstructions.[47,57–66] These reconstructions require high arthroscopic skill to minimize the risk of iatrogenic injury to the cartilage. All carry a risk of complications, mainly neurovascular injury, due to the creation of portals and the passage of sutures, even under direct arthroscopic visualization. Incisional complications, tendon injuries, deep venous thrombosis, and recurrence of instability have also been described.[57–66] The higher cost of the procedure due to the use of more sophisticated instruments and materials must also be considered. Compared with the open technique, arthroscopic lateral ligament repair is technically more demanding. However, it leads to better AOFAS scores, less pain at 6 and 12 months, postoperatively, and earlier weight-bearing after surgery. Nonetheless, there does not

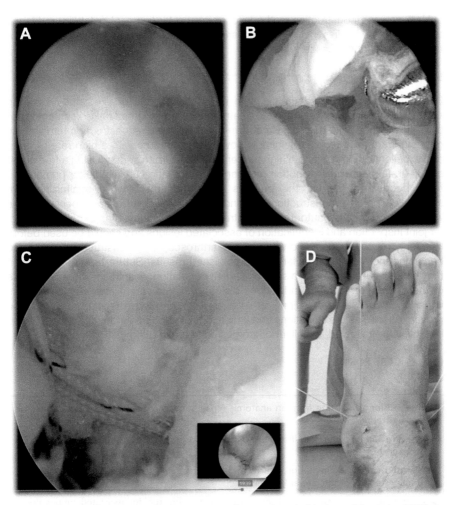

Fig. 3. Arthroscopic Bröstrom and treatment of osteochondral lesion of the talus (OLT). Intraoperative images: (*A*) Visualization of the injury degree level and arthroscopic loose body removal, (*B*) OLT treatment, (*C*) arthroscopic Bröstrom, and (*D*) external view.

seem to be any difference in long-term outcomes. Operative time and complication rate are statistically comparable.[67–71]

Comparative Studies Including All Techniques

Cao and colleagues performed a meta-analysis to compare the outcomes of different surgical techniques for treating CAI. Seven randomized clinical trials were included. The authors could not conclude the best surgical option for managing CAI due to a lack of statistical significance and low methodological quality. However, based on the existing evidence, Broström-type ligament reconstruction and its modifications lead to outstanding outcomes. Nonanatomic reconstructions should be used sparingly due to poor clinical outcomes and a high rate of sprain recurrence; nonanatomic reconstructions increase subtalar stiffness.[72] Lu and colleagues conducted a systematic review and meta-analysis to determine the overall effectiveness of various lateral ankle ligament reconstruction methods for chronic ankle ligament instability and found that, across 12 studies including 476 patients, good and excellent results were obtained in 85% of the cases.[73]

SUMMARY

During the past several decades there has been a great deal of study involving advanced techniques involved in the treatment of chronic lateral ankle ligament instability; however, open anatomic Broström-Gould ligament reconstruction remains the gold standard as a technically simple, low-cost procedure with a high rate of good and excellent outcomes and a high percentage of return to sports. Using a free autologous graft is an excellent option for ligament attenuation unsuitable for primary sutures because it carries the benefits of reinforcement while minimizing joint stiffness. Allograft reconstructions are indicated in revision cases, especially those with a history of failed autograft reconstruction. Arthroscopy is an excellent adjunct for joint inspection and identification of associated lesions and should be used before ligament reconstruction; however, fully arthroscopic reconstructions are also becoming increasingly popular due to published results. Suture-tape augmentation may be a useful adjuvant for a specific patient population, despite the increased costs of the procedure. Specific indications include patients where early rehabilitation is imperative, such as professional athletes, but its long-term benefits are yet to be proven. As long as the limitations and indications of each treatment option for chronic instability are followed, excellent outcomes can be expected in most cases.

CLINICS CARE POINTS

- The decision to migrate from an anatomic repair to a reconstruction can occasionally be made intraoperatively.
- In severe and long-standing instability, reconstruction with tendon augmentation could be necessary.
- The use of tape augmentation in Broström-type ligament reconstruction aims to increase primary stability of the lateral ligaments.
- Arthroscopy can be helpful as a diagnostic and therapeutic tool for associated injuries alone.
- Open anatomic Broström-Gould ligament reconstruction remains the gold standard as a technically simple with a high rate of good and excellent outcomes and a high percentage of return to sports.

DECLARATION OF INTERESTS

The authors have nothing to disclose.

REFERENCES

1. Krips R, de Vries J, van Dijk CN. Ankle instability. Foot Ankle Clin 2006;11(2): 311–29, vi.
2. Harrington KD. Degenerative arthritis of the ankle secondary to long-standing lateral ligament instability. J Bone Joint Surg Am. 1979;61(3):354–61.
3. Hedeboe J, Johannsen A. Recurrent instability of the ankle joint: Surgical repair by the Watson-Jones method. Acta Orthop Scand 1979;50:337–40.

4. Megan NH, Bonnie LV, Matthew C, et al. Health-related quality of life in individuals with chronic ankle instability. J Athl Train 2014;49(6):758–63.
5. Porter DA, Kamman KA. Chronic Lateral Ankle Instability: Open Surgical Management. Foot Ankle Clin 2018;23(4):539–54.
6. Drez D, Young JC, Waldman D, et al. Nonoperative treatment of double lateral ligament tears of the ankle. Am J Sports Med 1982;10(4):197–200.
7. Mann RA. In: Mann RA, Coughlin MJ, editors. Surgery of the foot and ankle, 2, 9th edition. St Louis (MO): Mosby; 1999. p. 1090–209.
8. Smith RW, Reischl SF. Treatment of ankle sprains in young athletes. Am J Sports Med 1986;14(6):465–71.
9. Aicale R, Maffulli N. Chronic Lateral Ankle Instability: Topical Review. Foot Ankle Int 2020;41(12):1571–81.
10. Vega J, Golanó P, Peña F. Iatrogenic articular cartilage injuries during ankle arthroscopy. Knee Surg Sports Traumatol Arthrosc 2016;24(4):1304–10.
11. Espinosa N, Smerek J, Kadakia AR, et al. Operative management of ankle instability: reconstruction with open and percutaneous methods. Foot Ankle Clin 2006; 11(3):547–65.
12. Youn H, Kim YS, Lee J, et al. Percutaneous Lateral Ligament Reconstruction with Allograft for Chronic Lateral Ankle Instability. Foot Ankle Int 2012;33(2):99–104.
13. Glazebrook M, Stone J, Matsui K, et al. ESSKA AFAS Ankle Instability Group. Percutaneous Ankle Reconstruction of Lateral Ligaments (Perc-Anti RoLL). Foot Ankle Int 2016;37(6):659–64.
14. Cao S, Wang C, Wang X, et al. Percutaneous Inferior Extensor Retinaculum Augmentation Technique for Chronic Ankle Instability. Orthop Surg 2022;14(5): 977–83.
15. Drakos M, Hansen O, Kukadia S. Ankle instability. Foot Ankle Clin N Am 2022; 27(2):371–84.
16. Bell SJ, Mologne TS, Sitler DF, et al. Twenty-six-year results after Brostrom procedure for chronic lateral ankle instability. Am J Sports Med 2006;34(6):975–8.
17. Karlsson J, Bergsten T, Lansinger O, et al. Reconstruction of the lateral ligaments of the ankle for chronic lateral instability. J Bone Joint Surg Am 1988;70(4):581–8.
18. Tourné Y, Mabit C, Moroney PJ, et al. Long-term follow-up of lateral reconstruction with extensor retinaculum flap for chronic ankle instability. Foot Ankle Int 2012; 33(12):1079–86.
19. Choi HJ, Kim DW, Park JS. Modified broström procedure using distal fibular periosteal flap augmentation vs anatomic reconstruction using a free tendon allograft in patients who are not candidates for standard repair. Foot Ankle Int 2017;38(11): 1207–14.
20. Xu HX, Choi MS, Kim MS, et al. Gender Differences in Outcome After Modified Broström Procedure for Chronic Lateral Ankle Instability. Foot Ankle Int 2016; 37(1):64–9.
21. Hu CY, Lee KB, Song EK, et al. Comparison of bone tunnel and suture anchor techniques in the modified Broström procedure for chronic lateral ankle instability. Am J Sports Med 2013;41(8):1877–84.
22. Cho BK, Kim YM, Park KJ, et al. A prospective outcome and cost-effectiveness comparison between two ligament reattachment techniques using suture anchors for chronic ankle instability. Foot Ankle Int 2015;36(2):172–9.
23. Aydogan U, Glisson RR, Nunley JA. Extensor retinaculum augmentation reinforces anterior talofibular ligament repair. Clin Orthop Relat Res 2006;442:210–5.

24. Jeong BO, Kim MS, Song WJ, et al. Feasibility and Outcome of Inferior Extensor Retinaculum Reinforcement in Modified Broström Procedures. Foot Ankle Int 2014;35(11):1137–42.

25. Evans DL. Recurrent instability of the ankle-a method of surgical treatment. Proc R Soc Med 1952;46(5):343–4.

26. Chrisman OD, Snook GA. Reconstruction of lateral ligament teras of the ankle. An experimental study and clinical evaluation of seven patients treated by a new modification of the Elmslie procedure. J Bone Joint Surg Am 1969;51(5):904–12.

27. Watson-Jones R. The classic: Fractures and joint injuries, by R Watson-Jones, Vol. II, 4th edition, Baltimore, Williams and Wilkins Company,1955. Clin Orthop 1974;(105):4–10.

28. Prisk VR, Imhauser CW, O'Loughlin PF, et al. Lateral ligament repair and reconstruction restore neither contact mechanics of the ankle joint nor motion patterns of the hindfoot. J Bone Joint Surg Am. 2010;92(14):2375–86.

29. Baumhauer JF, O'Brien T. Surgical Considerations in the Treatment of Ankle Instability. J Athl Train 2002;37(4):458–62.

30. Sammarco VJ. Complications of Lateral Ankle Ligament Reconstruction. Clin Orthop Relat Res 2001;391:123–32.

31. Bahr R, Pena F, Shine J, et al. Biomechanics of ankle ligament reconstruction. An in vitro comparison of the Brostrom repair, Watson-Jones reconstruction, and a new anatomic reconstruction technique. Am J Sports Med 1997;25(4):424–32.

32. Krips R, van Dijk CN, Halasi T, et al. Long-Term Outcome of Anatomical Reconstruction Versus Tenodesis for the Treatment of Chronic Anterolateral Instability of the Ankle Joint: A Multicenter Study. Foot Ankle Int 2001;22(5):415–21.

33. Krips R, Brandsson S, Swensson C, et al. Anatomical reconstruction and Evans tenodesis of the lateral ligaments of the ankle. Clinical and radiological findings after follow-up for 15 to 30 years. J Bone Joint Surg Br 2002;84(2):232–6.

34. Girard P, Anderson RB, Davis WH, et al. Clinical evaluation of the modified Brostrom-Evans procedure to restore ankle stability. Foot Ankle Int 1999;20(4):246–52.

35. Hsu AR, Ardoin GT, Davis WH, et al. Intermediate and long-term outcomes of the modified Brostrom-Evans procedure for lateral ankle ligament reconstruction. Foot Ankle Spec 2016;9(2):131–9.

36. Kaikkonen A, Lehtonen H, Kannus P. Jarvinen M. Long-term functional outcome after surgery of chronic ankle instability. A 5-year follow-up study of the modified Evans procedure. Scand J Med Sci Sports 1999;9(4):239–44.

37. Hashimoto T, Kokubo T. Anatomical Tenodesis Reconstruction Using Free Split Peroneal Brevis Tendon for Severe Chronic Lateral Ankle Instability. Keio J Med 2022;71(2):44–9.

38. Wang B, Xu XY. Minimally invasive reconstruction of lateral ligaments of the ankle using semitendinosus autograft. Foot Ankle Int 2013;34(5):711–5.

39. Allen T and Kelly M. Modern Open and Minimally Invasive Stabilization of Chronic Lateral Ankle Instability. Foot Ankle Clin, Volume 26(1): 87–101.

40. Snook GA, Chrisman OD, Wilson TC. Long-term results of the Chrisman-Snook operation for reconstruction of the lateral ligaments of the ankle. J Bone Joint Surg 1985;67-A:1–7.

41. Hennrikus WL, Mapes RC, Lyons PM, et al. Outcomes of the Chrisman-Snook and modified-Brostrom procedures for chronic lateral ankle instability. A prospective, randomized comparison. Am J Sports Med 1996;24(4):400–4.

42. Xu X, Hu M, Liu J, et al. Minimally invasive reconstruction of the lateral ankle ligaments using semitendinosus autograft or tendon allograft. Foot Ankle Int 2014; 35(10):1015–21.
43. Miller AG, Raikin SM, Ahmad J. Near-anatomic allograft tenodesis of chronic lateral ankle instability. Foot Ankle Int 2013 Nov;34(11):1501–7.
44. Jung HG, Shin MH, Park JT, et al. Anatomical Reconstruction of Lateral Ankle Ligaments Using Free Tendon Allografts and Biotenodesis Screws. Foot Ankle Int 2015;36(9):1064–71.
45. Ferkel E, Nguyen S, Kwong C. Chronic Lateral Ankle Instability: Surgical Management. Clin Sports Med 2020;39(4):829–43.
46. Matheny LM, Johnson NS, Liechti DJ, et al. Lateral Ankle Ligament Repair Versus Reconstruction. Am J Sports Med 2016;44(5):1301–8.
47. Yoo JS, Yang EA. Clinical results of an arthroscopic modified Brostrom operation with and without an internal brace. J Orthop Traumatol 2016;17(4):353–60.
48. Cho B-K, Park K-J, Kim S-W, et al. Minimal Invasive Suture-Tape Augmentation for Chronic Ankle Instability. Foot Ankle Int 2017;38(4):405–11.
49. Cho BK, Park JK, Choi SM, et al. A randomized comparison between lateral ligaments augmentation using suture-tape and modified Broström repair in young female patients with chronic ankle instability. Foot Ankle Surg 2019;25(2):137–42.
50. Ollivere BJ, Bosman HA, Bearcroft PW, et al. Foreign body granulomatous reaction associated with polyethelene 'Fiberwire(®)' suture material used in Achilles tendon repair. Foot Ankle Surg 2014;20(2):e27–9.
51. Martin KD, Andres NN, Robinson WH, et al. Suture Tape Augmented Broström Procedure. Foot Ankle Int 2021;42(2):145–50.
52. Ulrike W, Gloria H, Martin O, et al. Improved Outcome and Earlier Return to Activity After Suture Tape Augmentation Versus Brostrom Repair for Chronic Lateral Ankle Instability? A Systematic Review. Arthrosc J Arthrosc Relat Surg 2022; 38(2):597–608.
53. Cho Byung-Ki. MD1, Kyoung-Jin Park, MD1, Ji-Kang Park, MD1, and Nelson F. SooHoo, MD2 Procedure Augmented With Suture-Tape for Ankle Instability in Patients With Generalized Ligamentous Laxity. J Orthop Traumatol 2016;17(4): 353–60.
54. Sandlin MI, Taghavi CE, Charlton TP, et al. Lateral Ankle Instability and Peroneal Tendon Pathology. Instr Course Lect 2017;66:301–12.
55. Komenda GA, Ferkel RD. Arthroscopic Findings Associated with the Unstable Ankle. Foot Ankle Int 1999;20(11):708–13.
56. Yeo ED, Park JY, Kim JH, et al. Comparison of Outcomes in Patients With Generalized Ligamentous Laxity and Without Generalized Laxity in the Arthroscopic Modified Broström Operation for Chronic Lateral Ankle Instability. Foot Ankle Int 2017;38(12):1318–23.
57. Vega J, Golanó P, Pellegrino A, et al. All-inside arthroscopic lateral collateral ligament repair for ankle instability with a knotless suture anchor technique. Foot Ankle Int 2013;34(12):1701–9.
58. Feng SM, Sun QQ, Wang AG, et al. Arthroscopic Anatomical Repair of Anterior Talofibular Ligament for Chronic Lateral Instability of the Ankle: Medium and Long-Term Functional Follow-Up. Orthop Surg 2020;12(2):505–14.
59. Yang Y, Han J, Wu H, et al. Arthro-Broström with endoscopic retinaculum augmentation using all-inside lasso-loop stitch techniques. BMC Musculoskelet Disord 2022;23(1):795.
60. Acevedo JI, Mangone P. Arthroscopic Brostrom technique. Foot Ankle Int 2015; 36(4):465–73.

61. Guillo S, Archbold P, Perera A, et al. Arthroscopic anatomic reconstruction of the lateral ligaments of the ankle with gracilis autograft. Arthrosc Tech 2014;3(5): e593–8.

62. Vilá-Rico J, Cabestany-Castellà JM, Cabestany-Perich B, et al. All-inside arthroscopic allograft reconstruction of the anterior talo-fibular ligament using an accesory transfibular portal. Foot Ankle Surg 2019;25(1):24–30.

63. Maffulli N, Del Buono A, Maffulli GD, et al. Isolated anterior talofibular ligament Broström repair for chronic lateral ankle instability: 9-year follow-up. Am J Sports Med 2013;41(4):858–64.

64. Allegra F, Boustany SE, Cerza F, et al. Arthroscopic anterior talofibular ligament reconstruction in chronic ankle instability. Two years results. Injury 2020; 51(suppl 3):S56–62.

65. Corte-Real NM, Moreira RM. Arthroscopic repair of chronic lateral ankle instability. Foot Ankle Int. 2009;30(3):213–217.

66. Cordier G, Ovigue J, Dalmau-Pastor M, et al. Endoscopic anatomic ligament reconstruction is a reliable option to treat chronic lateral ankle instability. Knee Surg Sports Traumatol Arthrosc 2020;28(1):86–92.

67. Attia AK, Taha T, Mahmoud K, et al. d'Hooghe P. Outcomes of Open Versus Arthroscopic Broström Surgery for Chronic Lateral Ankle Instability: A Systematic Review and Meta-analysis of Comparative Studies. Orthop J Sports Med 2021; 9(7). 23259671211015207.

68. Woo BJ, Lai MC, Koo K. Arthroscopic Versus Open Broström-Gould Repair for Chronic Ankle Instability. Foot Ankle Int 2020;41(6):647–53.

69. Guelfi M, Zamperetti M, Pantalone A, et al. Open and arthroscopic lateral ligament repair for treatment of chronic ankle instability: A systematic review. Foot Ankle Surg 2018;24(1):11–8.

70. Brown AJ, Shimozono Y, Hurley ET, et al. Arthroscopic versus open repair of lateral ankle ligament for chronic lateral ankle instability: a meta-analysis. Knee Surg Sports Traumatol Arthrosc 2020;28(5):1611–8.

71. Yeo ED, Lee KT, Sung IH, et al. Comparison of All-Inside Arthroscopic and Open Techniques for the Modified Broström Procedure for Ankle Instability. Foot Ankle Int 2016;37(10):1037–45.

72. Cao Y, Hong Y, Xu Y, et al. Surgical management of chronic lateral ankle instability: a meta-analysis. J Orthop Surg Res 2018 Jun 25;13(1):159.

73. Lu A, Wang X, Huang D, et al. The effectiveness of lateral ankle ligament reconstruction when treating chronic ankle instability: A systematic review and meta-analysis. Injury 2020;51(8):1726–32.

Ankle Joint Microinstability
You Might Have Never Seen It but It Has Definitely Seen You

Jordi Vega, MD[a,b,c,d,*], Miki Dalmau-Pastor, PhD[a,c]

KEYWORDS

- Ankle sprain • Ankle microinstability • Ankle pain • Ligament fascicles
- Anterior talofibular ligament

KEY POINTS

- Ankle microinstability results from the superior fascicle injury of an anterior talofibular ligament (ATFL) and is a potential cause of chronic pain and disability after an ankle sprain.
- In contrast to the inferior fascicle of ATFL, the superior fascicle of ATFL is an intra-articular but extrasynovial structure, and it is relaxed in dorsiflexion and tightened in plantarflexion.
- The superior fascicle of ATFL is observed on the lateral gutter floor during an ankle dorsiflexion and nondistraction arthroscopic technique.
- Ankle microinstability is usually asymptomatic. When symptoms appear, patients describe a subjective ankle instability feeling, recurrent symptomatic ankle sprains, anterolateral pain, or a combination of them.
- The diagnosis of ankle microinstability is based primarily on the patient's medical history and physical examination. A subtle anterior drawer test can usually be observed, with no talar tilt.
- Ankle microinstability should be initially treated conservatively. If this fails, and because the superior fascicle of ATFL is an intra-articular ligament, an arthroscopic procedure is recommended in order to address the superior fascicle injury of ATFL.

INTRODUCTION

Ankle microinstability is a potential cause of chronic pain and disability that occurs after an ankle sprain. Although a young concept in the ankle,[1–3] microinstability of the hip and shoulder are recognized clinical entities.[4,5]

[a] Laboratory of Arthroscopic and Surgical Anatomy, Department of Pathology and Experimental Therapeutics (Human Anatomy Unit), University of Barcelona, Feixa Llarga s/n. 08907 Hospitalet del Llobregat, Spain; [b] Foot and Ankle Unit, iMove Traumatology-Clinica Tres Torres, Barcelona, Spain; [c] MIFAS by GRECMIP, Merignac, France; [d] Foot and Ankle Consultant, Clinique Montchoisi, Lausanne, Switzerland
* Corresponding author. iMove Traumatology, Via Augusta 281, 1st-3rd floor, 08017 Barcelona, Spain.
E-mail address: jordivega@hotmail.com

Foot Ankle Clin N Am 28 (2023) 333–344
https://doi.org/10.1016/j.fcl.2023.01.008
1083-7515/23/© 2023 Elsevier Inc. All rights reserved.

foot.theclinics.com

Although it has been popularized with the name of *ankle microinstability*, other names such as "occult ankle instability," "minor ankle instability," "initial ankle instability," or "functional ankle instability with morphological ligament changes" have been used to define it. A consensus will be required in the future to clarify the best way to name this pathologic condition but for the purpose of this article, ankle microinstability will be used.

The main pathomechanism of ankle microinstability is an isolated injury to the superior fascicle of ATFL after an inversion ankle sprain.[1] Until the emergence of the ankle microinstability concept, the superior fascicle of ATFL was a neglected structure because ATFL was not commonly separated in 2 fascicles, superior and inferior, and therefore no specific anatomical or functional characteristics were attributed to it. However, now it is recognized as a key structure in the development of ankle pathologic condition.

Therefore, a thorough knowledge of the anatomy and function of the superior fascicle of ATFL is mandatory to understand the ankle microinstability concept. It can clinically run asymptomatic or with a subjective instability feeling, cause repetitive ankle sprains, anterolateral ankle pain or complaints, or a combination of any of them. In addition, as a mechanical instability, secondary tibiotalar injuries can be observed in chronic presentations. These secondary lesions can be the origin of symptoms in many patients, therefore covering or occulting ankle microinstability as the origin of the problem.

For these reasons, underdiagnosing the superior fascicle injury of ATFL is easy.

Finally, imaging diagnosis have traditionally not been focused in the superior fascicle of ATFL as a different structure, and therefore, its normal and pathological characteristics have not been defined; for those reasons, ATFL injuries are diagnosed as whole, without differentiating between its superior and inferior fascicles.

The aim of this article is to provide insights on the superior fascicle of ATFL and its injury and to point the clinical, diagnostic, and treatment aspects of ankle microinstability.

ANATOMY OF THE SUPERIOR FASCICLE OF ANTERIOR TALOFIBULAR LIGAMENT

The lateral collateral ligament complex of the ankle has been described as being formed by the anterior talofibular ligament (ATFL), the calcaneofibular ligament (CFL), and the posterior talofibular ligament (PTFL).

The ATFL runs from the anterolateral aspect of the fibular malleolus to the anterolateral part of the talus, immediately anterior to its triangular lateral articular surface. The ATFL was classically described as a ligament formed by 1, 2, or 3 fascicles[6]; however, recent studies have determined that the ATFL has 2 fascicles, one superior and one inferior.[7,8] More importantly, the superior fascicle was found to be an intra-articular but extrasynovial structure, whereas the inferior fascicle was found to be connected to the CFL, forming the lateral fibulotalocalcaneal ligament (LFTCL) complex, an extra-articular structure[7] (**Fig. 1**). The superior fascicle of ATFL was also shown to relax in dorsiflexion and to tighten in plantarflexion and inversion, whereas the LFTCL was shown as an isometric structure (**Fig. 2**). In a separate study, the connecting fibers between the inferior fascicle of ATFL and the CFL were shown to be robust enough to transmit tension between both structures.[9] Additionally, a study looking at the medial aspect of the lateral ligaments was able to find constant connections between ATFL, CFL, and PTFL: the inferior fascicle of ATFL and CFL were found to be connected in all cases, as were CFL and PTFL; the inferior fascicle of ATFL and PTFL were also connected in all cases, whereas the superior fascicle of ATFL and

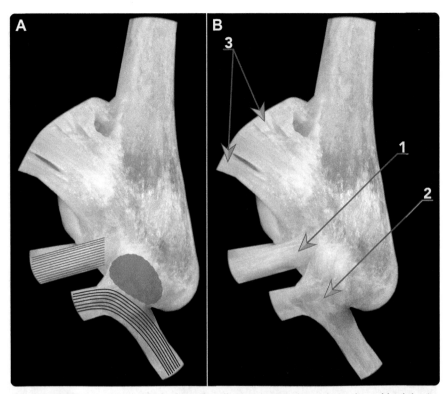

Fig. 1. The LFTCL complex with the lateral malleolus disarticulated from the ankle. (*A*). View with the lateral ankle ligaments highlighted: ATFL superior fascicle (*blue lines*), LFTCL complex (*black lines*) and area showing the common origin of the LFTCL complex (*red area*). (*B*). Classic view of the LFTCL complex. 1. ATFL superior fascicle. 2. LFTCL complex. 3. ATiFL and distal fascicle. (Figure reproduced with permission from Vega J, Malagelada F, Manzanares Céspedes MC, Dalmau-Pastor M. The lateral fibulotalocalcaneal ligament complex: an ankle stabilizing isometric structure. Knee Surg Sports Traumatol Arthrosc. 2020 Jan;28(1):8-17. https://doi.org/10.1007/s00167-018-5188-8.)

PTFL were connected in 42.5% of cases[8] (**Fig. 3**). Normally, a perforating artery is present between superior and inferior fascicles of ATFL, accounting for the postsprain hematoma that is observed in patients.

These new findings on the ankle ligaments have major implications for ankle instability. Probably, the most important finding is the superior fascicle of ATFL being an intra-articular structure, and how this can affect its healing capability (**Fig. 4**). It was proved that the anterior cruciate ligament (ACL) of the knee is not able to heal after injury because it is an intra-articular but extrasynovial structure. After an ACL rupture, the synovial membrane that covers it ruptures as well, the ligament becoming intrasynovial. It is known that synovial fluid prevents collagen synthesis, thus explaining why intra-articular ligaments do not heal.[10] When this is translated to the ankle joint, and with the evidence available today, it is fair to hypothetize that the superior fascicle of ATFL will remain ruptured unless it is surgically repaired, which is consistent with arthroscopic observations. However, partial or even complete ruptures of the superior fascicle of ATFL will not translate clinically into a major instability but rather into ankle microinstability.

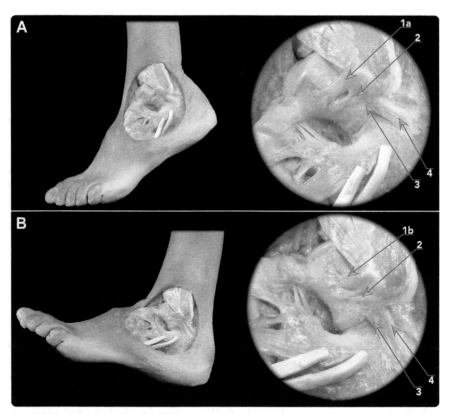

Fig. 2. Comparison of the morphology of the lateral ankle ligaments in plantarflexion (*A*) and dorsal flexion (*B*). Note how the structures forming the LFTCL complex maintain tension throughout the range of motion while the ATFL superior fascicle does not. 1a. Taut ATFL superior fascicle. 1b. Lax ATFL superior fascicle. 2. ATFL inferior fascicle. 3. Arciform fibers of the LFTCL complex. 4. CFL. (Figure reproduced with permission from Vega J, Malagelada F, Manzanares Céspedes MC, Dalmau-Pastor M. The lateral fibulotalocalcaneal ligament complex: an ankle stabilizing isometric structure. Knee Surg Sports Traumatol Arthrosc. 2020 Jan;28(1):8-17. https://doi.org/10.1007/s00167-018-5188-8.)

ARTHROSCOPIC ANATOMY OF THE SUPERIOR FASCICLE OF ANTERIOR TALOFIBULAR LIGAMENT

As an intra-articular structure, the superior fascicle of ATFL can be observed forming the floor of the lateral gutter during an ankle dorsiflexion and nondistraction arthroscopic technique (**Fig. 5**). It cannot be observed using distraction arthroscopy, as the lateral gutter collapses and prevents its visualization[11] (**Fig. 6**).

The superior fascicle of ATFL is observed as a horizontal hammock covered by a thin layer of synovial tissue. This fascicle can be followed from its fibular origin to its talar insertion. The distal portion of the fibula is observed occupying the lateral gutter, and the superior fascicle of ATFL origin can be recognized in continuity with the fibular insertion of the anterior tibiofibular ligament (ATiFL) distal fascicle. Lateral to the ligament, the joint capsule is observed. The sinovial layer that covers the joint capsule is in continuity with the one covering the superior fascicle of ATFL. When the ankle is plantarflexed, the superior fascicle of ATFL becomes vertical. However, if plantarflexion

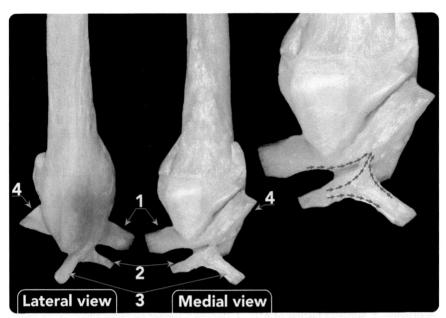

Fig. 3. Lateral and medial views of the fibular malleolus in a specimen with superior fascicle of ATFL (ATFLsf), inferior fascicle of ATFL (ATFLif), CFL, and PTFL connections. 1. ATFLsf. 2. AT-FLif. 3. CFL. 4. PTFL. (Figure reproduced with permission from Dalmau-Pastor M, Malagelada F, Calder J, Manzanares MC, Vega J. The lateral ankle ligaments are interconnected: the medial connecting fibres between the anterior talofibular, calcaneofibular and posterior talofibular ligaments. Knee Surg Sports Traumatol Arthrosc. 2020 Jan;28(1):34-39. https://doi.org/10.1007/s00167-019-05794-8.)

continues, or when distraction is applied, the joint capsule becomes taut. As a result, the lateral gutter becomes tightly closed and the ligament is not visible.[11]

Recognition of lateral gutter normality is mandatory to arthroscopically diagnose the superior fascicle injury of ATFL.[12]

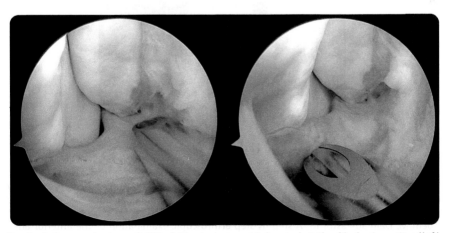

Fig. 4. Arthroscopic view of ATFLsf. The instrument is located at the fibular insertion (*left*), and then at the talar insertion (*right*).

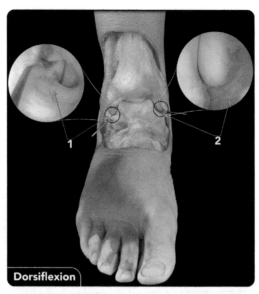

Fig. 5. Anterior ankle view of a dissection. Correlation of both gutters observed in ankle dorsiflexion. 1. Superior fascicle of ATFL. 2. Deltoid ligament (anterior tibiotalar ligament). (Figure reproduced with permission from Vega J, Malagelada F, Karlsson J, Kerkhoffs GM, Guelfi M, Dalmau-Pastor M. A step-by-step arthroscopic examination of the anterior ankle compartment. Knee Surg Sports Traumatol Arthrosc. 2020 Jan;28(1):24-33. https://doi.org/10.1007/s00167-019-05756-0.)

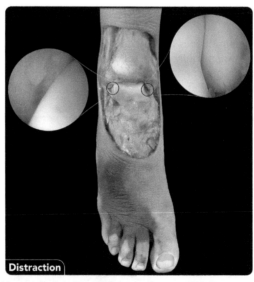

Fig. 6. Anterior ankle view of a dissection. Correlation of both gutters observed in ankle distraction. The superior fascicle of ATFL and deltoid ligament are not visible. (Figure reproduced with permission from Vega J, Malagelada F, Karlsson J, Kerkhoffs GM, Guelfi M, Dalmau-Pastor M. A step-by-step arthroscopic examination of the anterior ankle compartment. Knee Surg Sports Traumatol Arthrosc. 2020 Jan;28(1):24-33. https://doi.org/10.1007/s00167-019-05756-0.)

PATHOMECHANISM OF ANKLE MICROINSTABILITY

The pathomechanism of ankle microinstability is an isolated injury to the superior fascicle of ATFL.[1] The origin of any superior fascicle injury of ATFL is an ankle sprain or traumatism provoking an ankle inversion.

Ankle sprains are one of the most common injuries in both sports and daily activities. Probably due to its high incidence and apparently minor immediate clinical consequences, ankle sprains were considered to be a minor problem with little impact.[13] However, a major or minor ligament injury usually occurs after any ankle sprain. Because of its anatomical location, the superior fascicle of ATFL is the first ligament injured after an ankle sprain, and in a light-to-moderate sprain, the superior fascicle of ATFL is commonly the only ligament injured.

Because of anatomical characteristics, an ATFL injury is normally found at its fibular attachment, as a ligament disinsertion.[14] The superior fascicle injury of ATFL can be partial or complete; the injury starts at the medial side of the fascicle as just an attenuation of its structure; it then progresses to a medial or proximal partial disinsertion, to a complete disinsertion, and finally a complete resorption in very chronic cases[12] (**Fig. 7**). Because its intra-articular location, the superior fascicle of ATFL has an impaired capacity to heal; therefore, once the injury process has started, only prevention of new ankle sprains can avoid progression to more severe injury types because the ligament will remain deficient after the first moderate–severe ankle sprain.

A recent ankle biomechanical study has observed that the superior fascicle of ATFL mainly controls not only talar internal rotation but also a minimal anterior talar translation.[15] As a result, the superior fascicle of ATFL deficit will mainly increase the internal talar rotation and, secondarily, anterior talar translation.

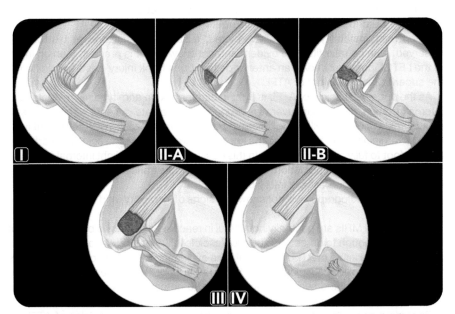

Fig. 7. Superior fascicle injury types of ATFL. (Figure reproduced with permission from Vega J, Malagelada F, Dalmau-Pastor M. Ankle microinstability: arthroscopic findings reveal four types of lesion to the anterior talofibular ligament's superior fascicle. Knee Surg Sports Traumatol Arthrosc. 2021 Apr;29(4):1294-1303. https://doi.org/10.1007/s00167-020-06089-z.)

The abnormal increased talar motion can also cause impingement syndromes due to pathological soft-tissue or osteophyte creation, or a combination of both.[12] The internal rotation of the talus poses stress on the medial side of the ankle,[16] which could cause damage to the articular cartilage at the medial talar aspect, and/or to the anterior part of the deltoid ligament.[17] When the anterior part of the deltoid is injured, it is observed separated from the medial malleolus as an open book injury, and a lack of external talar rotation and anterior translation exist as the consequence.

CLINICAL SYMPTOMS OF ANKLE MICROINSTABILITY

Although the superior fascicle injury of ATFL can be observed in most patients after an ankle sprain, ankle microinstability is usually asymptomatic. When patients become symptomatic, they describe a subjective feeling of ankle instability, or recurrent symptomatic ankle sprains, or anterolateral pain, or a combination of these symptoms.[1,3] Probably, many patients with a diagnosis of anterolateral soft tissue impingement syndrome present an ankle microinstability, this is, the superior fascicle injury of ATFL as the source of their pain. Similarly, patients with symptomatic osteochondral talar defects, deltoid ligament injury, or anterior tibia osteophyte can also present an asymptomatic ankle microinstability. If we assume that a partial or total superior fascicle injury of ATFL is present since the first episode of ankle inversion sprain, the resulting undiagnosed microinstability can cause medial and lateral articular pathologic condition, which in turn explains the association between chronic ankle instability and intra-articular pathologic condition.[18,19]

DIAGNOSIS OF ANKLE MICROINSTABILITY

The diagnosis of ankle microinstability is based primarily on the patient's medical history and physical examination to rule out the presence of chronic ankle instability as classically described, or other ankle disorders.[2,3,12]

When microinstability is clinically explored, a subtle anterior drawer test can be observed, with no talar tilt. If an evident anterior drawer test is present, then an injury of the LFTCL complex and/or an anterior deltoid open book injury exists in addition to the superior fascicle injury of ATFL.

As the superior fascicle of ATFL is tight in plantar flexion and it mainly restricts talar internal rotation, a new maneuver was proposed to evaluate patients with high suspicion of ankle microinstability: the tibiotalar posterior drawer test. With the patient lying on the examining table, the hip and the knee are flexed allowing the ankle plantarflexed and the foot to fully rest on the table. In this position, and with a slight internal foot rotation, the tibia is pushed posteriorly. If the tibia and fibula translate to posterior, the test indicates the superior fascicle injury of ATFL.[20]

Stress ankle radiographs will not show any signs of instability, and we do not recommend its use.

Conventional MRIs are generally not useful in reaching a diagnosis because they are not sensitive enough to detect the superior fascicle injury of ATFL, especially if a minor superior fascicle injury of ATFL is present. The evaluating radiologist or surgeon needs to have a high level of suspicion to detect the superior fascicle lesion of ATFL. The presence of augmented synovial fluid can help to detect the lesion as the liquid can be placed in the area of the injury.

Regarding separate identification of the superior and inferior fascicles of ATFL on MRI, a study performed using isotropic 3D volume acquisition demonstrated that it is possible to observe both ATFL fascicles, as well as the intra-articular and extra-articular connections among ATFL, CFL, and PTFL[21] (**Fig. 8**).

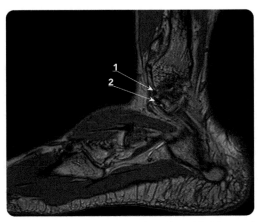

Fig. 8. Sagittal MRI images showing the 2 ATFL fascicles with (1) superior ATFL fascicle and (2) inferior ATFL fascicle. (Figure reproduced with permission from Hong CC, Lee JC, Tsuchida A, Katakura M, Jones M, Mitchell AW, Dalmau-Pastor M, Calder J. Individual fascicles of the ankle lateral ligaments and the lateral fibulotalocalcaneal ligament complex can be identified on 3D volumetric MRI. Knee Surg Sports Traumatol Arthrosc. 2022 Dec 20. https://doi.org/10.1007/s00167-022-07275-x.)

The use of other imaging techniques can be helpful in reaching a diagnosis of ankle microinstability, especially ultrasound or MRI with intra-articular contrast but more studies are required to evaluate the value of these imaging studies.

In consequence, as current imaging studies are not yet capable of accurately detecting the superior fascicle injury of ATFL, arthroscopy is currently the gold standard to identify the ligament injury when the diagnosis of microinstability is suspected.[12] Through a dorsiflexion and nondistraction ankle arthroscopy technique, the superior fascicle injury of ATFL can be diagnosed in the lateral gutter. The presence of pathological soft tissue in the area is a common finding and when removed, the ligament injury can be observed, and classified according to the 4 types of injuries described.[12]

TREATMENT OF ANKLE MICROINSTABILITY

As with other joints, ankle microinstability should be initially treated through a conservative therapy.

Although symptoms can be successfully relieved, and the ankle instability feeling disappear after a program of muscle strengthening and neuromuscular training, symptoms can recidivate in the short term and treatment effects disappear over time.[22–24] In addition, ankle instability has been shown to be a predisposing factor in the generation of arthrosis and other intra-articular disorders, and restoration of tibio-talar joint stability is critical to avoid such joint alterations. Although conservative treatment can reduce the symptomatology, it usually does not fix the mechanical instability, and in many cases, a surgical treatment to obtain a correct articular stabilization will be needed (**Box 1**).

When indicated, surgical treatment should focus on addressing the ligamentous injury and associated intra-articular pathologic condition if any. The superior fascicle injury of ATFL can be repaired through an open procedure; however, as an intra-articular ligament, an arthroscopic procedure is recommended, and the all-inside arthroscopic ligament repair is the technique of choice by the authors[25] (**Fig. 9**).

Box 1
Indications of surgical superior fascicle repair of ATFL

Indications of surgical superior fascicle repair of ATFL:
- Failed conservative treatment or recidivation of symptoms after a successful conservative treatment period
- Presence of concomitant chondral or osteochondral lesion that needs to be addressed
- Presence of concomitant and symptomatic soft-tissue and/or bony impingement
- Presence of concomitant intra-articular loose body that needs to be removed
- Symptomatic microinstability in young and/or active patients
- Symptomatic rotational ankle instability
- Asymptomatic ankle, but more than one ankle sprain a year in a young and/or active patient
- Asymptomatic ankle, but presence of initial articular degenerative changes in imaging studies, in a young patient

---

According to the different types of the superior fascicle injury of ATFL, types I, II, and III can be treated through an all-inside arthroscopic ligament repair procedure.[12]

When there is no ligament remnant to repair, type IV, then a ligament reconstruction with a plastia is required. The arthroscopic all inside ATiFL transfer is a viable technique to substitute the superior fascicle of ATFL.[26] A recent biomechanical study shows no differences between the transferred ATiFL and the noninjured superior fascicle of ATFL.[27]

On the other side, depending of the quality ligament remnant, and regardless of the type of injury, the superior fascicle of ATFL can be difficult to repair when its quality is poor.[28] Some authors recommend a ligamentplasty with autograft in these cases,[28] whereas others recommend to augment the ligament repair.[29,30]

SUMMARY

Ankle microinstability is a potential cause of chronic ankle pain and instability feeling after an ankle sprain. An injury of the superior fascicle of ATFL, an intra-articular ligament, is the cause. A high index of suspicion is required in order to diagnose ankle microinstability, as normally only a subtle anterior talar translation can be observed during clinical exploration. Current imaging studies are not sensitive enough to detect the ligament injury causing ankle microinstability. Although conservative treatment is usually performed as the first line of treatment, arthroscopic all-inside ligament repair is the most common surgical treatment to address the superior fascicle injury of ATFL.

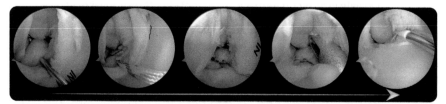

Fig. 9. Steps of the arthroscopic all inside the superior fascicle repair of ATFL with a knotless anchor. After fibular footprint debridement, the ligament is penetrated with a suture-passer. The nitinol of the suture-passer is changed by a suture that will grasp the ligament. Next, the tunnel for the anchor is performed, and the ligament is reattached after introduction of the anchor charged with the sutures.

CLINICS CARE POINTS

- After a moderated ankle sprain, the superior fascicle of ATFL is injured, and a lack of stability could be observed as the consequence.
- Anterolateral ankle pain, instability feeling, repetitive ankle sprain, or a combination of them is usually observed in patients with ankle microinstability.
- Current standard imaging studies are not sensitive enough to detect the superior fascicle injury of ATFL.
- After a failed conservative therapy, arthroscopic all-inside ligament repair is recommended.

DECLARATION OF INTERESTS

The authors have nothing to disclose.

REFERENCES

1. Vega J, Peña F, Golanó P. Minor or occult ankle instability as a cause of antero-lateral pain after ankle sprain. Knee Surg Sports Traumatol Arthrosc 2016;24(4): 1116–23.
2. Vega J, Dalmau M, Malagelada F, et al. Ankle arthroscopy: an update. J Bone Joint Surg Am 2017;99:1395–407.
3. Vega J, Guelfi M, Heyrani N, et al. Ankle microinstability. Tech Foot Ankle Surg 2019;18:73–9.
4. Reinold MM, Curtis AS. Microinstability of the shoulder in the overhead athlete. Int J Sports Phys Ther 2013;8(5):601–16.
5. Safran MR. Microinstability of the Hip-Gaining Acceptance. J Am Acad Orthop Surg 2019;27(1):12–22.
6. Milner CE, Soames RW. Anatomy of the collateral ligaments of the human ankle joint. Foot Ankle Int 1998;19:757–60.
7. Vega J, Malagelada F, Manzanares MC, et al. The lateral fibulotalocalcaneal ligament complex: An ankle stabilizing isometric structure. Knee Surg Sports Traumatol Arthrosc 2020;28(1):8–17.
8. Dalmau-Pastor M, Malagelada F, Calder J, et al. The lateral ankle ligaments are interconnected: The medial connecting fibres between the anterior talofibular, calcaneofibular and posterior talofibular ligaments. Knee Surg Sports Traumatol Arthrosc 2020;28(1):34–9.
9. Cordier G, Nunes GA, Vega J, et al. Connecting fibers between ATFL's inferior fascicle and CFL transmit tension between both ligaments. Knee Surg Sports Traumatol Arthrosc 2021;29(8):2511–6.
10. Murray MM. Current status and potential for primary ACL repair. Clin Sports Med 2009;28(1):51–61.
11. Vega J, Malagelada F, Karlsson J, et al. A step-by-step arthroscopic examination of the anterior ankle compartment. Knee Surg Sports Traumatol Arthrosc 2020; 28(1):24–33.
12. Vega J, Malagelada F, Dalmau M. Ankle microinstability: Arthroscopic findings reveal four types of anterior talofibular ligament's superior fascicle lesion. Knee Surg Sports Traumatol Arthrosc 2021;29(4):1294–303.
13. Kerkhoffs GM, Kennedy JG, Calder JD, et al. There is no simple lateral ankle sprain. Knee Surg Sports Traumatol Arthrosc 2016;24(4):941–3.

14. Kumai T, Takakura Y, Rufai A, et al. The functional anatomy of the human anterior talofibular ligament in relation to ankle sprains. J Anat 2002;200(5):457–65.
15. Dalmau-Pastor M, El-Daou H, Stephen J, et al. Clinical relevance and function of different fascicles of the anterior talofibular ligament: a robotic study. Am J Sports Med: In review process.
16. Van den Bogert AJ, Smith GD, Nigg BM. In vivo determination of the anatomical axes of the ankle joint complex: an optimization approach. J Biomech 1994; 27(12):1477–88.
17. Vega J, Allmendinger J, Malagelada F, et al. Combined arthroscopic all-inside repair of lateral and medial ankle ligaments is an effective treatment for rotational ankle instability. Knee Surg Sports Traumatol Arthrosc 2020;28(1):132–40.
18. Hintermann B, Boss A, Schäfer D. Arthroscopic findings in patients with chronic ankle instability. Am J Sports Med 2002;30(3):402–9.
19. Choi WJ, Lee JW, Han SH, et al. Chronic lateral ankle instability: The effect of intra-articular lesions on clinical outcome. Am J Sports Med 2008;36(11): 2167–72.
20. Vega J, Montesinos E, Malagelada F, et al. Microinstability of the ankle. Lateral ankle instability: an international approach by Ankle Instability Group. Berlin, Germany: Springer, ESSKA-AFAS; 2021. p. 55–62.
21. Hong CC, Lee JC, Tsuchida A, et al. Individual fascicles of the ankle lateral ligaments and the lateral fibulotalocalcaneal ligament complex can be identified on 3D volumetric MRI. Knee Surg Sports Traumatol Arthrosc 2022. https://doi.org/10.1007/s00167-022-07275-x. On line ahead of print.
22. Lentell G, Baas B, Lopez D, et al. The contributions of proprioceptive deficits, muscle function, and anatomic laxity to functional instability of the ankle. J Orthop Sports Phys Ther 1995;21:206–15.
23. Gerber JP, Williams GN, Scoville CR, et al. Persistent disability associated with ankle sprains: a prospective examination of an athletic population. Foot Ankle Int 1998;19:653–60.
24. De Vries JS, Krips R, Sierevelt IN, et al. Interventions for treating chronic ankle instability. Cochrane Database Syst Rev 2011;10(8):CD004124.
25. Vega J, Golanó P, Pellegrino A, et al. All-inside arthroscopic lateral collateral ligament repair for ankle instability with a knotless suture anchor technique. Foot Ankle Int 2013;34(12):1701–9.
26. Vega J, Poggio D, Heyrani N, et al. Arthroscopic all-inside ATiFL's distal fascicle transfer for ATFL's superior fascicle reconstruction or biological augmentation of lateral ligament repair. Knee Surg Sports Traumatol Arthrosc 2020;28(1):70–8.
27. Xiao L, Zheng B, Zhou Y, et al. Biomechanical study of arthroscopic all-inside anterior talofibular ligament suture augmentation repair, plus suture augmentation repair and anterior tibiofibular ligament's distal fascicle transfer augmentation repair. J Clin Med 2022;11:5235.
28. Thès A, Odagiri H, Elkaïm M, et al. Arthroscopic classification of chronic anterior talo-fibular ligament lesions in chronic ankle instability. Orthop Traumatol Surg Res 2018;104(8):S207–11.
29. Vega J, Montesinos E, Malagelada F, et al. Arthroscopic all-inside anterior talo-fibular ligament repair with suture augmentation gives excellent results in case of poor ligament-tissue remnant quality. Knee Surg Sports Traumatol Arthrosc 2020;28(1):100–7.
30. Cordier G, Lebecque J, Vega J, et al. Arthroscopic ankle lateral ligament repair with biological augmentation gives excellent results in case of chronic ankle instability. Knee Surg Sports Traumatol Arthrosc 2020;28(1):108–15.

The Role of Needle Arthroscopy in the Assessment and Treatment of Ankle Sprains

James J. Butler, MB, BCh, Andrew I. Brash, MD,
Mohammad T. Azam, BS, Brittany DeClouette, MD,
John G. Kennedy, MD, MCh, FFSEM, FRCS (Orth)*

KEYWORDS

- Lateral ankle ligament complex • ATFL • In-office needle arthroscopy

KEY POINTS

- Nonoperative management is the mainstay treatment option for acute lateral ligament sprains.
- Following failure of conservative modalities, surgical intervention is warranted.
- Concerns have been raised regarding complication rates and prolonged return to play rates following both open repair and arthroscopic repair.
- In-office needle arthroscopic (IONA) ATFL repair augmented with suture tape facilitates repair of the lateral ligament complex under local anaesthesia with minimal soft tissue disruption providing accelerated return to daily and sporting activities.
- In addition, IONA facilitates diagnosis and treatment of any concomitant intra-articular pathologic condition.

INTRODUCTION

Lateral ankle ligament sprains following an acute ankle inversion injury are a commonly encountered pathologic condition, sustained by 27,000 Americans on a daily basis.[1] Patients often present with acute lateral ankle pain, swelling, and instability.[2] Diagnosis can be made solely based on the findings from the patient's clinical history and physical examination. Plain film radiographs are typically obtained to rule out a fracture at the malleoli, navicular bone, or base of the fifth metatarsal, provided the patient satisfies the criteria of the Ottawa ankle rules.[2] MRI can be a useful diagnostic tool in the subacute setting to identify osteochondral lesions of the ankle joint,

Foot and Ankle Division, Department of Orthopedic Surgery, NYU Langone Health, 1/1 Delancey Street, 2nd Floor, New York, NY 10002, USA
* Corresponding author.
E-mail address: john.kennedy@nyulangone.org

Foot Ankle Clin N Am 28 (2023) 345–354
https://doi.org/10.1016/j.fcl.2023.01.005
1083-7515/23/© 2023 Elsevier Inc. All rights reserved.
foot.theclinics.com

syndesmotic injuries, and injuries to the surrounding tendinous structures.[3] Between 50% and 80% of patients are treated successfully with conservative management, which entails rest, icing, compression, and elevation in the initial days following the index injury, followed by early weight-bearing and referral to physical therapy for ankle strengthening, range of motion, and proprioceptive exercises.[4]

When conservative measures have failed, surgical intervention is warranted. In patients with adequate remnants of the anterior talo-fibular ligament (ATFL), surgical repair of the lateral ligament complex is indicated.[5] For patients with poor-quality ATFL remnants, patients with an elevated body mass index and patients with generalized ligamentous laxity, reconstruction of the lateral ligament complex is required.[5] The mainstay reparative technique for chronic lateral ankle instability (CLAI) has historically been the open modified Broström repair.[6] However, high complication rates with prolonged return to sporting activities have been reported. To address these deficiencies, minimally invasive arthroscopic techniques have been developed. Although there has been promising data from various case series suggesting improved outcomes with standard arthroscopic intervention,[7] multiple systematic reviews and meta-analyses have found comparable complication and revision rates between open and arthroscopic repair cohorts.[8]

The reemergence of in-office needle arthroscopy (IONA) under local anaesthesia in recent years provides the opportunity to repair the disrupted lateral ligament complex with minimal soft tissue trauma facilitating earlier weight-bearing and rapid return to daily and sporting activities.[9] In addition, IONA avoids the risks associated with sedation and has reduced costs compared with traditional arthroscopic treatment in a full operating suite.[9]

The purpose of this review is to discuss the role of IONA in the assessment and repair of the lateral ligament complex in the context of the surgical procedures currently available for lateral ankle ligament repair.

CURRENT MANAGEMENT STRATEGIES

Nonoperative management is the mainstay treatment option for patients with lateral ligament complex tears.[10] Treatment modalities include a short period of rest, icing, compression, and elevation of the joint supplemented with oral nonsteroidal anti-inflammatories as required.[11] The degree of immobilization is dependent on the severity of the injury and physician preference. Grade 1 tears require no immobilization. Grade 2 tears require support provided by a flexible wrap with immobilization for 3 to 5 days. Grade 3 tears require the use of rigid ankle support for approximately 1 week. After the initial few days from the index injury, patients are be referred for formal physical therapy with an emphasis on ankle strength, range of motion, proprioception, and balance exercises.[12-14] Formal physical therapy is recommended for 4 to 8 weeks, before consideration of more invasive surgical intervention.

Following failure of conservative management, surgical intervention is often warranted to address the CLAI. Numerous surgical techniques have been described and can be broadly classified as anatomical repair and nonanatomical repair, which can be approached in an open or arthroscopic fashion.[6,15-17]

Nonanatomical repair through the Evans procedure in 1953 was the first surgical technique proposed to address CLAI.[15] Other nonanatomical procedures include the Chrisman-Snook,[18] Castaing,[16] and Watson-Jones procedures,[19] all of which involve sacrificing a portion of the peroneal tendon to enhance the stability at the lateral aspect of the ankle. These procedures have fallen out of favor in recent years due to loss of eversion strength and development of degenerative, deforming forces across the ankle joint following sacrifice of the peroneal tendons.[20] In addition, the extensive operative exposure together with the requirement for prolonged postoperative immobilization makes this an unattractive surgical treatment option.

To address the deficiencies associated with nonanatomical repair, Broström developed the first anatomical repair in 1966, which involves shortening of the Anterior talofibular ligament (ATFL) and CFL followed by placement of a pants-over-vest suture.[21] Baraza and colleagues[22] reported no cases of instability in 20 patients who underwent Broström repair at 30.3 months follow-up. However, a moderate secondary surgical procedure rate (15%) was reported. Furthermore, a long-term follow-up study by Bell and colleagues[23] reported excellent foot and ankle outcome score (FAOS) scores at 26.3 years after Broström repair in a young military cohort. However, this data must be interpreted with caution due to a 29.1% loss to follow-up rate in addition to the authors not reporting the number of complications observed.

The Broström procedure was modified by Gould in 1980 whereby the repair construct is augmented by attaching the inferior edge of the extensor retinaculum to the fibula.[6] Multiple retrospective case series have demonstrated excellent outcomes at short-to-mid term follow-up. Rigby and colleagues[24] demonstrated substantial improvement in FAOS scores and visual analog scale (VAS) scores along with a 97% return to sport rate following open Broström-Gould procedure at 44.4 months follow-up.

Further alterations to the original Broström repair include the Karlsson procedure. This was first proposed in 1989 and described sectioning the ATFL 3 to 5 mm from its insertion onto the fibula, excision of the surrounding scar tissue, and reattaching the ATFL to the fibula through drill holes or, more recently, suture anchors.[17] Concerns have been raised regarding postoperative lengthening of the ATFL and CFL following Broström and Broström-Gould procedures, predisposing patients to ligamentous laxity and, ultimately, recurrence of ankle instability.[25] Reattaching the ATFL to the fibula with drill holes or suture anchors via the Karlsson technique effectively eliminates the risk of developing postoperative laxity. A systematic review and meta-analysis by Deng and colleagues[26] found superior American orthopedic foot and ankle society (AOFAS) scores, Tegner scores, and lower operation times in the Karlsson cohort compared with the modified Broström cohort.

Although improvements in subjective clinical scoring tools and low revision rates have been reported at midterm follow-up following open anatomical repair for CLAI, concerns have been raised regarding postoperative wound complications and the risk of recurrent ankle instability.

To reduce the risk of wound complications and prolonged immobilization following open repair for CLAI, arthroscopic techniques have been developed.[27] Arthroscopic anatomical repair for CLAI was first introduced in the 1990s but significant difficulties were initially encountered including high complication rates, surgical complexity, poorly defined indications, and longer operative times. However, with the emergence of improved arthroscopic technology, arthroscopic intervention has become a more popular technique. Arthroscopic repair preserves the soft tissue envelope and provides more adequate visualization of the ankle joint to identify and treat any concomitant intra-articular pathologic condition.[27] Patients with an acute ankle inversion injury often develop ankle osteochondral lesions, peroneal tendon dysfunction, bony anteromedial impingement, or soft tissue-related anterolateral ankle impingement.[28] The presence of these concomitant pathologic conditions is a harbinger for poor postoperative outcomes, thus, must be addressed before repair of the injured lateral ligament complex. Batista and colleagues[29] reported outcomes following a 2 portal arthroscopic lateral ligament repair in 22 patients at a mean follow-up of 25 months. The mean AOFAS improved from a preoperative score of 63.0 to a postoperative score of 90.0. In addition, neither complications nor recurrences were noted. Furthermore, a meta-analysis by Attia and colleagues[27] compared outcomes between open and arthroscopic Broström repair in patients with CLAI. Following pooling of the data, the authors found statistically significant superior AOFAS and VAS scores, lower wound complication rates, and quicker return to full weight-bearing in the arthroscopic cohort.

Although good results have been reported following both arthroscopic and open lateral ankle ligament repair, a consensus has not been reached regarding the optimal surgical technique for CLAI. Furthermore, despite improvements in subjective clinical outcomes and low revision rates following arthroscopic repair, a concerning complication rate has been reported throughout multiple systematic reviews.[27] As a result, new technological advances have been developed.

In-office Needle Arthroscopy

There has been a growing trend during the last number of years in orthopedic surgery to promote further minimally invasive surgical techniques to reduce complication rates and operative costs. In-office needle arthroscopy (IONA) is a minimally invasive surgical technique that facilitates arthroscopic inspection and treatment with the patient wide-awake under local anaesthetic that has gained prominence during the last number of years.[30] IONA was first introduced in the 1990s but was never widely adopted due to the poor resolution of the arthroscopic camera, lack of precise indications for the procedure, and inability to treat any pathologic conditions that were identified during arthroscopic examination. However, recent advancements in IONA technology have led to its resurgence in use during the last number of years.[31] A new disposable chip-on-tip camera system provides 400 × 400 pixel resolution together with a 120° field of view using a 1.9-mm cannula sheath, which can be viewed on a 1300 high-definition monitor (Arthrex, Inc., Naples, Florida, United States of America). A major benefit provided by IONA is the identification of pathologic conditions that may not have been captured on MRI, such as osteochondral lesions of the ankle joint and degeneration of the peroneal and posterior tibialis tendons. IONA technology provides not only arthroscopic examination but also simultaneous treatment of any identified pathologic condition via a litany of surgical instruments that are available including shavers, burrs, graspers, scissors, probes, resectors, thermal ablators, and punches.[32] IONA can be performed in the office setting, which mitigates against the significant costs associated with arthroscopic examination under sedation in the operating room setting.

IONA has been used to identify and treat various pathologies across multiple joints, including the ankle, foot, first metatarsophalangeal joint, knee, and shoulder.[30,33–35] Numerous case series have been published in the literature assessing outcomes following IONA including anterior ankle impingement, posterior ankle impingement, meniscal tears, and anterior cruciate ligament repair.[30,33,36,37] A retrospective review by Colasanti and colleagues[30] examined outcomes at 15.5-month follow-up for 31 patients who underwent IONA for anterior ankle impingement. There was a statistically significant improvement in FAOS and Patient-Reported Outcomes Measurement Information System (PROMIS) scores at final follow-up. In addition, 100% of patients returned to work at a mean time of 1.98 days and 96% of patients return to sporting activities at a mean time of 3.9 weeks. Furthermore, in 45.2% of patients, IONA was able to identify some aspect of ankle pathologic condition that was missed on MRI.

In patients with lateral ligament complex injuries that have failed conservative management, IONA offers the ability to repair the torn ligament and identify and treat any other concomitant pathologic condition that has been found or potentially missed on MRI.

IN-OFFICE NEEDLE ARTHROSCOPIC ANTERIOR TALO-FIBULAR LIGAMENT REPAIR TECHNIQUE

Below, we describe our technique for ATFL repair with augmentation with suture tape via IONA[31] (**Boxes 1** and **2**). We use suture tape for augmentation for numerous reasons. High stresses placed on the ATFL during the early, aggressive rehabilitation phase may elongate the repaired ligament increasing the risk for subsequent instability at the joint. Furthermore, patients with underlying conditions that overload the lateral ligament complex such as joint hyperlaxity, cavovarus hindfoot deformity, and obesity require significant stability of the repaired construct in order to counteract the additional forces acting on the lateral ankle.[38] Thus, we think it is critical to provide as much additional stability to the lateral aspect of the ankle as possible, without compromising normal, anatomical motion at the ankle.

In the office setting, the patient is positioned supine on the examination table, and the ankle is prepped with a solution of chlorhexidine gluconate mixed with isopropyl alcohol. The ankle is draped so as to provide a sterile operative field. The locations for the standard anteromedial, anterolateral, and accessory portals are identified and marked with a surgical marking pen. The accessory portal is located 1 cm anterior to the tip of the fibula and is made adjacent to the footprint of the ATFL on the talus, which is identified intraoperatively. The skin and subcutaneous tissues at the site of the portals are anesthetized using a solution of 1% lidocaine with 1 in 100,000 epinephrine. The course of the superficial peroneal nerve and sural nerve are also identified and marked. A resting period of 5 to 10 minutes is observed, following which 5 mL of 0.5% bupivacaine with epinephrine mixed with 1% lidocaine with 1 in 100,000 epinephrine in a 1:1 ratio is injected into the ankle. Epinephrine is used to promote local hemostasis. A number 11 blade is used to make a small, 2-mm stab incision followed by spreading of the subcutaneous tissues and then insertion of a blunt trocar. The 1.9-mm needle arthroscope is exchanged over the trocar while connected to the system provided by the manufacturer (Dual Wave, Arthrex Inc, Naples, Florida) with integrated inflow and outflow fluid management system at a modifiable pressure of 35 mm Hg. Inflow consists of a solution of 1 liter of 0.9% normal saline and 5 mL of epinephrine.

Box 1
Pearls and pitfalls

Pearls
    Add epinephrine to lidocaine and bupivacaine to promote hemostasis
    To confirm physiological laxity, insert an instrument under the suture tape construct
    Position the ankle in 30° of plantarflexion to prevent overtightening
    Ensure that the patient is given adequate head and leg support to mitigate against lower extremity movement during the procedure

Pitfalls
    Inadvertent overtightening of the suture tape construct may restrict motion at both the ankle and subtalar joints
    Injury to the sural nerve may occur following incorrect placement of the superior and inferior portals
    Debridement before a comprehensive diagnostic evaluation may lead to iatrogenic injury

---

Box 2
Step-by-step approach to the technique

Step 1: The patient is positioned supine on the examination table

Step 2: The ankle is prepped with chlorhexidine gluconate/isopropyl alcohol and subsequently draped to create a sterile field

Step 3: The portals are injected with a solution of lidocaine, bupivacaine, and epinephrine

Step 4: Establish the standard anteromedial and anterolateral portals followed by insertion of the arthroscope into the anteromedial portal and the shaver into the anterolateral portal

Step 5: Resect the AITFL to expose the anatomic footprint of the ATFL on the fibula

Step 6: Lift the attachment of the ATFL off of the distal fibula

Step 7: Mark the anatomic footprint of the talar attachment of the ATFL

Step 8: Establish the accessory portal 1 cm anterior to the distal tip of the fibula

Step 9: Insert a guide pin through the accessory portal at the talar footprint and overdrill with a cannulated 3.5-mm drill to the laser line

Step 10: Introduce the suture anchor and overdrill to seat it into the talus. Tap the suture anchor until the treads engage the underlying subchondral bone

Step 11: Shave the fibular periosteum down to the subchondral bone

Step 12: Place a guidewire and overdrill with a 3.5-mm cannulated drill to the laser line

Step 13: Insert a knotless suture anchor and suture tape with appropriate tension into the prepped fibular site

Step 14: Assess the tension of the construct with a probe and cut any excess suture tape

Step 15: Instruct the patient to range the ankle to assess for potential overtightening of the repaired construct

Step 16: Use the arthroscope to identify and treat any concomitant intra-articular pathologic condition

---

Initially, a portion of the anterior inferior tibiofibular ligament (AITFL) is resected to identify the anatomical footprint of the ATFL on the fibula. Further debridement of the surrounding region is required to improve visualization of the area. The attachment of the ATFL is lifted off of the distal fibula. The anatomic footprint of the talar attachment of the ATFL is marked, which serves as the accessory portal site. A guide pin is placed through the accessory portal at the talar footprint, which is subsequently overdrilled with a cannulated 3.5-mm drill to the laser line. Next, FiberTape suture anchor (Arthrex Inc, Naples, Florida, USA) is introduced and seated into the talus. The suture anchor is then tapped until the threads engage the underlying subchondral bone. A shaver is introduced through the anteromedial portal to shave the fibular periosteum down to the subchondral bone. Following placement of a guide wire in the prepped fibular site, a 3.5-mm cannulated drill is overdrilled to the laser line. Next, a knotless suture anchor and suture tape is placed with appropriate tension. A probe is used to assess for overtightening of the repair construct. Concomitant treatment of any intra-articular pathologic condition identified on preoperative imaging can be managed during the procedure, if indicated. Inspection of the ankle joint is performed intraoperatively to identify any pathology that may not have been captured on preoperative imaging.

When the procedure is completed, the patient actively ranges the ankle to ensure adequate motion, tendon gliding, and stability. The portal sites are closed with wound closure strips and a soft, sterile dressing is applied. Patients are instructed to commence ankle range of motion exercises and to weight bear as tolerated immediately after procedure. Patients are prescribed prophylactic oral cephalexin 250 mg 4 times daily for 1 day. For analgesia, oral nonsteroidal anti-inflammatory medications can be taken as required for up to 4 days postoperatively and are encouraged to ice and elevate the leg when not ambulating. Patients are instructed to keep the dressings dry for the first 3 days postoperatively and are then encouraged to use an Ace compression bandage for an additional week. Patients are referred for formal physical therapy for strengthening, proprioceptive, balance, and range of motion exercises.

Early Clinical Data

IONA ATFL repair with augmentation with suture tape is an attractive alternative to traditional open and/or arthroscopic repair under sedation in light of the rapid return to daily activities, minimal soft tissue trauma, and significantly reduced operative fees. Improvements in patient-reported outcome measurements and subjective ankle stability have been recorded, although more detailed statistical analysis is required to determine significance. In addition, no complications have been observed to date, which is a major issue encountered by traditional arthroscopic repair techniques.

The first IONA ATFL repair with augmentation with suture tape that we performed was in a 17-year-old male who presented with a 1-year history of left lateral ankle pain and subjective instability following recurrent ankle sprains during his martial arts training. His examination revealed tenderness to palpation along the left lateral ankle gutter together with a soft endpoint on passive inversion of the left ankle and a positive anterior drawer test. His MRI demonstrated tearing of the ATFL and a mild sprain of the CFL. He subsequently underwent left IONA ATFL repair with augmentation with suture tape. He began weight-bearing as tolerated immediately following the procedure and commenced physical therapy 2 days postoperatively. He reported subjective ankle stability at 4 weeks postoperatively and could unilaterally heel raise at 6 weeks postoperatively, and subsequently returned to martial arts training. All 5 domains of his PROMIS scores improved from postoperatively and no complications were observed.

The second case is of a 22-year-old woman who presented with a 2-week history of left lateral ankle pain and subjective instability following an acute inversion injury during lacrosse practice. She initially managed this conservatively with rest, icing, compression, and elevation but her pain did not subside. Her physical examination demonstrated tenderness at the left ATFL and along the distribution of the left peroneal tendons. In addition, there was a soft endpoint on left ankle inversion with a positive anterior drawer test. Her MRI demonstrated a grade 2 ATFL tear with mild peroneus longus tenosynovitis with anterolateral subcutaneous edema. She subsequently underwent IONA ATFL repair with augmentation with suture tape and peroneal tendoscopy and debridement of the degenerated tendon. Her FAOS improved from a preoperative score of 52.6 to a postoperative score of 91.0 and returned to lacrosse at 6 weeks postoperatively. No complications were reported.

SUMMARY

ATFL repair with augmentation with suture tape in the office setting facilitates rapid recovery and return to daily activities at a reduced operative cost compared with open and traditional arthroscopic repair. In addition, the minimal soft tissue trauma by the IONA instrumentation significantly reduces the extensive complication rate associated with traditional arthroscopic and open techniques. Further research is warranted to identify the precise role of IONA in the management of lateral ankle ligament complex injuries.

CLINICS CARE POINTS

- Acute injury to the lateral ankle ligament complex is most frequently managed conservatively.
- Surgical intervention is warranted following failure of nonoperative treatment modalities.
- Although good outcomes have been reported following both open and arthroscopic anatomical lateral ligament repair, a concerning complication rate has been noted.
- IONA ATFL repair augmented with suture tape facilitates repair of the lateral ligament complex under local anaesthesia providing rapid return to daily and sporting activities,
- In addition, IONA facilitates diagnosis and treatment of any concomitant intra-articular pathologic condition.

DECLARATION OF INTERESTS

The authors report the following potential conflicts of interest or sources of funding: J.G. Kennedy is a consultant to Arteriocyte Industries (Isto Biologics) and Arthrex Inc, and receives support from Ohnell Family Foundation, United States and Mr and Mrs Michael J. Levitt. J.G. Kennedy reports as a board or committee member for the American Orthopaedic Foot and Ankle Society, European Society of Sports Traumatology, Knee Surgery and Arthroscopy, Ankle and Foot Associates, and International Society for Cartilage Repair of the Ankle.

REFERENCES

1. Renstrom PA. Persistently Painful Sprained Ankle. J Am Acad Orthop Surg 1994; 2(5):270–80.
2. D'Hooghe P, Cruz F, Alkhelaifi K. Return to Play After a Lateral Ligament Ankle Sprain. Curr Rev Musculoskelet Med 2020;13(3):281–8.
3. Martin B. Ankle sprain complications: MRI evaluation. Clin Podiatr Med Surg 2008;25(2):203–47, vi.
4. Delahunt E, Coughlan GF, Caulfield B, et al. Inclusion criteria when investigating insufficiencies in chronic ankle instability. Med Sci Sports Exerc 2010;42(11): 2106–21.
5. Feng SM, Maffulli N, Ma C, et al. All-inside arthroscopic modified Broström-Gould procedure for chronic lateral ankle instability with and without anterior talofibular ligament remnant repair produced similar functional results. Knee Surg Sports Traumatol Arthrosc 2021;29(8):2453–61.
6. Gould N, Seligson D, Gassman J. Early and late repair of lateral ligament of the ankle. Foot Ankle 1980;1(2):84–9.
7. Hou ZC, Su T, Ao YF, et al. Arthroscopic modified Broström procedure achieves faster return to sports than open procedure for chronic ankle instability. Knee Surg Sports Traumatol Arthrosc 2022. https://doi.org/10.1007/s00167-022-06961-0.
8. Song YJ, Hua YH. Similar Outcomes At Early Term After Arthroscopic Or Open Repair Of Chronic Ankle Instability: A Systematic Review And Meta-Analysis. J Foot Ankle Surg 2019;58(2):312–9.

9. Shimozono Y, Hoberman A, Kennedy JG, et al. Arthroscopic anterior talofibular ligament repair with use of a 2-portal technique. JBJS Essent Surg Tech 2019; 9(4). https://doi.org/10.2106/JBJS.ST.18.00104.

10. Physical therapy after an ankle sprain: using the evidence to guide physical therapist practice. J Orthop Sports Phys Ther 2021;51(4):159-60.

11. Halabchi F, Hassabi M. Acute ankle sprain in athletes: CLINICAL aspects and algorithmic approach. World J Orthop 2020;11(12):534-58.

12. JU Wester, Jespersen SM, Nielsen KD, et al. Wobble board training after partial sprains of the lateral ligaments of the ankle: a prospective randomized study. J Orthop Sports Phys Ther 1996;23(5):332-6.

13. Kerkhoffs GMMJ, Struijs PAA, Marti RK, et al. Functional treatments for acute ruptures of the lateral ankle ligament: a systematic review. Acta Orthop Scand 2003; 74(1):69-77.

14. Smith BI, Docherty CL, Simon J, et al. Ankle strength and force sense after a progressive, 6-week strength-training program in people with functional ankle instability. J Athl Train 2012;47(3):282-8.

15. Evans DL. Recurrent instability of the ankle; a method of surgical treatment. Proc R Soc Med 1953;46(5):343-4.

16. Castaing J, Falaise B, Burdin P. [Ligamentoplasty using the peroneus brevis in the treatment of chronic instabilities of the ankle. Long-term review]. Rev Chir Orthop Reparatrice Appar Mot 1984;70(8):653-6.

17. Karlsson J, Bergsten T, Lansinger O, et al. Surgical treatment of chronic lateral instability of the ankle joint. A new procedure. Am J Sports Med 1989;17(2): 268-73 [discussion: 273-274].

18. Chrisman OD, Snook GA. Reconstruction of lateral ligament tears of the ankle. An experimental study and clinical evaluation of seven patients treated by a new modification of the Elmslie procedure. J Bone Joint Surg Am 1969;51(5):904-12.

19. Watson-Jones R. The classic: "Fractures and Joint Injuries" by Sir Reginald Watson-Jones, taken from "Fractures and Joint Injuries," by R. Watson-Jones, Vol. II, 4th ed., Baltimore, Williams and Wilkins Company, 1955. Clin Orthop Relat Res 1974;(105):4-10.

20. Baumhauer JF, O'Brien T. Surgical considerations in the treatment of ankle instability. J Athl Train 2002;37(4):458-62.

21. Broström L. Sprained ankles. VI. Surgical treatment of "chronic" ligament ruptures. Acta Chir Scand 1966;132(5):551-65.

22. Baraza N., Re-operation rates following Brostrom repair, JSM Foot and Ankle, 2 (1), 2017, 1019.

23. Bell SJ, Mologne TS, Sitler DF, et al. Twenty-six-year results after broström procedure for chronic lateral ankle instability. Am J Sports Med 2006;34(6):975-8.

24. Rigby RB, Cottom JM. A comparison of the "All-Inside" arthroscopic Broström procedure with the traditional open modified Broström-Gould technique: a review of 62 patients. Foot Ankle Surg 2019;25(1):31-6.

25. Kirk KL, Campbell JT, Guyton GP, et al. ATFL elongation after brostrom procedure: a biomechanical investigation. Foot Ankle Int 2008;29(11):1126-30.

26. Deng X, Zou M, Zhu H, et al. A comparison of the modified Broström procedure and modified Karlsson procedure in treating chronic lateral ankle instability: a systematic review and meta-analysis. Ann Palliat Med 2021;10(7):7534-42.

27. Attia AK, Taha T, Mahmoud K, et al. Outcomes of open versus arthroscopic broström surgery for chronic lateral ankle instability: a systematic review and meta-analysis of comparative studies. Orthop J Sports Med 2021;9(7). https://doi.org/10.1177/23259671211015207.

28. Odak S, Ahluwalia R, Shivarathre DG, et al. Arthroscopic evaluation of impingement and osteochondral lesions in chronic lateral ankle instability. Foot Ankle Int 2015;36(9):1045–9.
29. Batista JP, Del Vecchio JJ, Patthauer L, et al. Arthroscopic lateral ligament repair through two portals in chronic ankle instability. Open Orthop J 2017;11:617–32.
30. Colasanti CA, Mercer NP, Garcia JV, et al. In-office needle arthroscopy for the treatment of anterior ankle impingement yields high patient satisfaction with high rates of return to work and sport. Arthroscopy 2022;38(4):1302–11.
31. Mercer NP, Azam MT, Davalos N, et al. Anterior talofibular ligament augmentation with internal brace in the office setting. Arthrosc Tech 2022;11(4):e545–50.
32. Np M, Al G, Dj K, et al. Achilles Paratenon Needle Tendoscopy in the Office Setting. Arthroscopy techniques 2022;11(3). https://doi.org/10.1016/j.eats.2021.10.024.
33. Annibaldi A, Monaco E, Daggett M, et al. In-office needle arthroscopic assessment after primary ACL repair: short-term results in 15 patients. J Exp Orthop 2022;9(1):89.
34. Daggett MC, Stepanovich B, Geraghty B, et al. Office-based needle arthroscopy: a standardized diagnostic approach to the shoulder. Arthrosc Tech 2020;9(4):e521–5.
35. Kaplan DJ, Chen JS, Colasanti CA, et al. Needle arthroscopy cheilectomy for hallux rigidus in the office setting. Arthrosc Tech 2022;11(3):e385–90.
36. DiBartola AC, Rogers A, Kurzweil P, et al. In-office needle arthroscopy can evaluate meniscus tear repair healing as an alternative to magnetic resonance imaging. Arthrosc Sports Med Rehabil 2021;3(6):e1755–60.
37. Mercer NP, Samsonov AP, Dankert JF, et al. Improved clinical outcomes and patient satisfaction of in-office needle arthroscopy for the treatment of posterior ankle impingement. Arthrosc Sports Med Rehabil 2022;4(2):e629–38.
38. Choi SM, Cho BK, Kim SH. The influence of suture-tape augmentation on biological healing of the anterior talofibular ligament in chronic ankle instability: a quantitative analysis using MRI. J Foot Ankle Surg 2022;61(5):957–63.

Sprain of the Medial Ankle Ligament Complex

Patrick Pflüger, MD[a], Victor Valderrabano, MD, PhD[b],*

KEYWORDS

- Foot • Ankle • Ankle sprain • Deltoid ligament • Medial ankle instability
- Spring ligament

KEY POINTS

- The medial ligament complex of the ankle is essential for ankle joint stability.
- Injuries to the medial ankle ligaments can result in significant changes of biomechanics of the ankle and may result in ligamentous ankle osteoarthritis, mainly lateral valgus ankle osteoarthritis.
- Prevalence of sprain of the medial ligament ankle complex might be significantly higher, occurring in up to half of all ankle sprains.
- Isolated partial ligament injuries with physiologic or varus hindfoot can be managed conservatively, but patients with higher-grade lesions, or in the presence of concomitant lesions, or with hindfoot valgus, may benefit from surgical reconstruction.

INTRODUCTION

The medial ankle ligament complex (MALC) is the functional unit of the deltoid and spring ligament, connected by the tibiospring ligament and acting together biomechanically.[1] Sprains of the MALC are reported to occur far less frequently than lateral ankle ligamentous injuries.[2–4] This might be attributed to the bony anatomy of the talus with a larger radius lateral and smaller radius medial and the biomechanical strength of the deltoid ligament complex, and difficulties with diagnosis.[5] Because of a growing understanding of the important role of the MALC for ankle stability, advanced imaging technologies, as MRI and ankle arthroscopy, there is a greater awareness of MALC lesions. In a prospective study, arthroscopy revealed a deltoid ligament lesion in 40% of patients undergoing surgery for lateral chronic ankle instability (LCAI).[6] Another study of patients with LCAI even reported a prevalence of deltoid ligament injuries of 72%.[7] In acute ankle sprains, MRI revealed a deltoid ligament lesion in almost half of the cases, and the risk of MALC lesions increased significantly with complete

[a] Department of Orthopedics, Balgrist University Hospital, University of Zurich, Zurich, Switzerland; [b] SWISS ORTHO CENTER, Swiss Medical Network, Schmerzklinik Basel, University of Basel, Hirschgässlein 15, Basel 4010, Switzerland
* Corresponding author.
E-mail address: vvalderrabano@swissmedical.net

Foot Ankle Clin N Am 28 (2023) 355–367
https://doi.org/10.1016/j.fcl.2023.01.009
1083-7515/23/© 2023 Elsevier Inc. All rights reserved.

anterior talofibular ligament (ATFL) ruptures.[8] Considering these findings and the high prevalence of acute lateral ankle sprains, the incidence of MALC injuries is probably underreported.

The deltoid ligament maintains the medial ankle stability and also contributes significantly to the rotational stability of the ankle joint.[9,10] One severe ankle sprain or the development of a chronic ankle instability can lead to a ligamentous posttraumatic ankle osteoarthritis (OA),[11] representing the second most common cause for ankle OA.[12] The goal is therefore to correctly diagnose the injury and prevent persistent chronic ankle instability. In literature, there is still controversy about the optimal therapy.[13] This article serves to increase awareness for the prevalence of acute medial ankle sprains and how to successfully address it.

ANATOMY AND BIOMECHANICS

The most accepted description of the anatomy agrees on 6 fascicles contributing to a superficial and deep layer of the deltoid ligament (**Fig. 1**). Because of the close structural and functional connection, the spring (calcaneonavicular) ligament is often included with the deltoid ligament complex, therefore the term medial ankle ligament complex (MALC).[10,14]

The MALC contributes significantly to the medial and rotational ankle joint stability: rotational meaning lateral and medial combined. Depending on the position of the foot, different parts of the deltoid ligament can stabilize against varying movements.[15] The deltoid ligament significantly restrains anterior and posterior translation of the

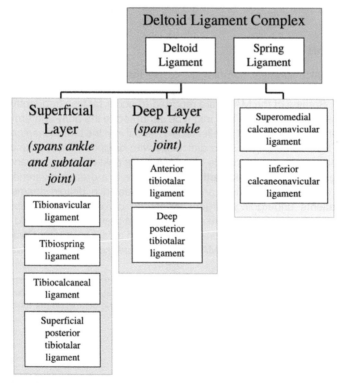

Fig. 1. The MALC.

unloaded ankle.[15,16] In the neutral and dorsiflexed position, the deltoid ligament is the primary restraint for internal rotation. The superficial layers contribute to both external and, together with the ATFL, internal rotation of the talus.[15,17,18] In conclusion, for rotational ankle stability, the cooperative function of both the lateral ankle ligaments and the MALC is essential.

In the coronal plane, the deltoid ligament resists valgus stress of the ankle as well as ankle eversion and anterolateral migration of the talus.[19,20] Considering the coupling mechanism between the foot and the leg, the resection of the deltoid ligament highly changes the movement transfer, especially during dorsiflexion/plantarflexion.[21,22] Therefore, insufficiency of the MALC can significantly change the physiologic gait pattern. A cadaver study found that sectioning of the superficial deltoid ligament will reduce the contact area up to 43%, and peak pressure will increase up to 30%.[23]

The spring ligament in conjunction with the superficial deltoid ligament supports the talar head and thereby stabilizes the medial ankle and the peritalar joints. Besides the posterior tibial tendon as dynamic support, the MALC is crucial for the maintenance of the plantar arch.[10,24]

MECHANISMS OF INJURY

Considering the biomechanical properties of the deltoid ligament complex, eversion/pronation, external rotation, and abduction may lead to MALC lesions.[25] Isolated simple deltoid injuries usually involve the superficial part. Complete disruptions of both layers, superficial and deep, are almost always associated with concomitant lesions.[8,13] Besides injuries to the lateral ankle ligament complex, osteochondral lesions of the talus, injuries to the syndesmotic complex, ankle fractures, or even posterior tibial tendon lesions are commonly seen with MALC lesions. [8,26–29]

DIAGNOSTICS
Clinical Examination

Depending on the position of the foot during injury and the deforming force, an injury to the MALC is more or less likely. Because of the high probability of concomitant lesions, a detailed clinical examination is essential to distinguish between the different injuries and to delineate further diagnostic steps. Accordingly, on the lateral/anterolateral ankle, examination should be performed to exclude injuries to the syndesmotic complex, lateral ankle ligaments and fibula (ligamentous/tendons injuries, fractures). Special attention needs to be taken, keeping in mind that a lateral injury of the ankle can contribute to overlook associated medial ligamentous injuries.[30,31]

Following an acute ankle sprain, patients typically present with a painful and swollen ankle sometimes leading to the inability to bear weight. A differentiated clinical assessment is necessary to detect pathologic conditions that are predictive for an MALC lesion, as, for example, medial hematoma and medial tenderness (**Fig. 2**). Valderrabano and Hintermann[32] also proposed a clinical classification system to further specify the medial chronic ankle instability (MCAI) (**Table 1**).

Imaging

Radiographs
Conventional radiographs should include anterior-posterior (AP), mortise, and lateral views to visualize bony avulsion of the deltoid ligament and exclude ankle fractures. If possible, weight-bearing radiographs can help to further distinguish between stable and unstable injuries, but the reliability to detect ligamentous ankle injuries is low.[13,33] In addition, one needs to keep in mind that in a 2-dimensional investigation it is nearly

Clinical examination of medial ankle instability

1. (Bilateral) Inspection	2. Palpation	3. Clinical Tests
• Swelling/hematoma on the medial side	• Medial pain	• Positive external rotation test (superificial layer)
• Malalignment	• Tenderness (medial gutter/deltoid ligament/spring ligament)	• Positive eversion stress test (deep layer)
• Deformity	• Pain/tenderness along the posterior tibial tendon	• Positive anteromedial drawer test
If able to bear weight:		• Negative single heel rise test (hindfoot valgus on tiptoe)
• asymmetrical planovalgus and abductus of the affected ankle/foot		

Fig. 2. Clinical symptoms and signs for medial ankle instability. (*Adapted from* Ref.[1])

impossible to detect a 3-dimensional (rotational-coronal-sagittal) instability. Radiographic cutoff values are also dependent on the quality of the radiographs (mortise, AP view) and prone to bias.[33,34]

Magnetic Resonance Imaging (MRI)

MRI is the most sensitive noninvasive diagnostic tool to diagnose an MALC lesion and its additional injuries as well as is usually recommended if clinical tests are positive for a medial ankle sprain.[13,31,35,36] However, reported sensitivity of MRI to detect any injury to MALC is about 84%.[37] Tears of the superficial deltoid can be detected with a sensitivity of 83%, and tears of the deep deltoid can be detected with a sensitivity of 96%.[38] Considering concomitant lesions such as osteochondral lesions, MRI findings can match only in two-thirds of the cases with arthroscopic findings.[39] Furthermore, MRI is a static examination and thus does not allow a direct conclusion regarding the ankle stability.

Sonography

Ultrasonography (US) is a helpful tool to assess acute ankle injuries and can be used also to dynamically assess ankle function.[40,41] A study reported a sensitivity of 87% of

Table 1
Clinical classification for medial chronic ankle instability according to Valderrabano and Hintermann[32]

			Clinical Classification			
			Medial Chronic Ankle Instability (MCAI)			
	Giving Way	Hindfoot Valgus/ Pronation	Medical Ankle Pain	Anterolateral Ankle Pain	Posterior Tibial Dysfunction	Flexibility of Deformity
Grade I	+	+	+	(+)	-	Yes
Grade II	++	+	+++	(+)	-	Yes
Grade III	+++	++	+++	+	+	Yes
Grade IV	++++	+++	++++	++	++	No

US for detecting an anterior talofibular lesions, but did not evaluate the accuracy for deltoid lesions.[41] In a study of 12 patients with supination external rotation fractures, sensitivity of US for deltoid rupture was 100%.[42] US is useful for detecting any lesion to the deltoid ligament, but inferior to MRI in terms of classification of the type of injury.[43] Furthermore, US is investigator dependent and a requires a trained examiner.[44]

Computed tomography

Computed tomography (CT) can help to further visualize the bony geometry of the ankle and foot. Despite the feasibility of assessing ankle ligaments via standard CT, there are some restrictions concerning the medial collateral ligaments, especially in acute injuries.[45] With the increasing use of weight-bearing cone-beam CT (CBCT), research defined reference values for normal ankles and evaluated especially the reliability to predict syndesmotic instability.[46,47] A meta-analysis showed excellent interobserver agreement and significant difference between uninjured and injured ankles regarding the mean area of the tibiofibular syndesmosis. The authors concluded that the accuracy of CBCT is not yet validated and serves more as an adjunct tool.[46] No reliable data are available regarding the significance of the CBCT for acute medial ankle injuries.

Diagnostic ankle arthroscopy

Ankle arthroscopy allows the verification of the MALC and assesses possible lateral and syndesmotic ligamentous injuries, cartilage status, and the presence of osteochondral lesions.[1,27,48] MCAI can be classified according to the arthroscopic findings (**Table 2**).[32]

THERAPEUTIC OPTIONS OF MEDIAL ANKLE LIGAMENT COMPLEX INJURIES

High-quality evidence regarding the optimal therapy for medial injuries is sparse. Therapeutic recommendations are based on the consensus for the treatment of lateral ligamentous injuries.[13]

Decisive for the treatment of medial ankle sprains is the type of injury (partial/complete) and the presence of concomitant lesions.[1]

Nonoperative

Isolated deltoid injuries with no instability can be treated nonoperatively with a short period (1–2 weeks) of immobilization following the PRICE (protection, rest, ice, compression, and elevation) scheme with nonsteroidal anti-inflammatory drug patches/cremes/medication to reduce pain and swelling. For simple sprains (grade I), soft ankle orthosis is indicated for 4 to 6 weeks. More severe sprains (grades II–III) may require a stronger ankle brace, walker, or stabilizing shoe. Rehabilitation should be initiated as soon as possible, and physical therapy aims at improving proprioception, range of motion, and muscle force (posterior tibial muscle). In cases of a preinjury concomitant pes planovalgus, an insole with medial arch support deloads the injured MALC. The goal is to prevent medial or rotational ankle instability with recurrent ankle sprains that can lead to ligamentous ankle OA.[1,49,50]

Operative

Indication for operative treatment is highly dependent on the stability of the ankle joint, the presence of concomitant lesions, and functional demand of the patient. In cases of medial and lateral ligamentous injuries, usually the first-line treatment is conservative as outlined before, but selected cases with relevant instability and grade II to III lesions

Table 2
Arthroscopic classification for medial chronic ankle instability according to Valderrabano and Hintermann[32]

		Arthroscopic Classification				
		Medial Chronic Ankle Instability (MCAI)				
	Superficial/Ventral Deltoid	Deep/Posterior Deltoid	Medial Malleolar Periosteal Scar	Medial Malleolar Osteophytes	Tibiotalar Distance (mm)	Lateral Ligament Lesion
Grade I	Elongated/partial ruptured/avulsion	Normal	+	+	2–5	No
Grade II	Ruptured	Elongated/partial ruptured	++	+	2–5	No
Grade III	Ruptured	Elongated/partial ruptured	+++	+	>5	Yes
Grade IV	Ruptured	Elongated/partial ruptured	++++	++	>5	Yes

may profit from early operative intervention.[13] The spring ligament and the quality of posterior tibial tendon should be inspected and evaluated. Operative strategy is also dependent on the hindfoot alignment. In patients with a severe MALC injury and chronic (flexible) flatfoot, beside the MALC reconstruction, the posterior tibial tendon may need to be augmented/reconstructed and the medial soft tissues supported by calcaneal osteotomy (lateral lengthening calcaneal osteotomy if additional abductus deformity, medial sliding calcaneal osteotomy in isolated valgus deformity) in a primary setting.[1]

If the syndesmotic complex is injured as well, the presence of an ATFL and deltoid injury is predictive for a dynamically unstable ankle (West Point IIb), and athletes may benefit from surgery: syndesmotic stabilization. A pathologic clinical examination (squeeze test, external rotation) in conclusion with verified ligamentous lesions in the MRI correlates significantly with an instability of the ankle and then forms the basis for an operative intervention.

In the presence of preoperatively verified osteochondral lesion (OCL), the type and location of the OCL and patient factors (age, body mass index, preoperative level of activity) as well as ankle pathologic conditions (alignment, OA) define the type of OCL reconstructive surgery: shaving, microfracturing, Autologous Matrix-Induced Chondrogenesis (AMIC), Autologous Chondrocyte Implantation (ACI), and others. Depending on the type of location of the OCL lesion (medial vs lateral, anterior vs posterior), different surgical approaches (eg, medial malleolar osteotomy) with additional surgeries are necessary for a successful treatment.[51,52]

The indication for deltoid ligament repair in ankle fractures remains controversial. A current meta-analysis of comparative studies of deltoid ligament repair and nonrepair in acute ankle fractures reported a superiority regarding the medial clear space, rate of complications, and American Orthopaedic Foot & Ankle Society (AOFAS) score for the deltoid repair group.[53] Taking especially into consideration the relative short follow-up time of the included studies and cause of ankle OA, the repair of the medial ankle stabilizer may prevent rapid deterioration of the ankle function and avoid sequelae. Therefore, the authors of this article advocate a deltoid ligament repair in unstable Weber type B/C fractures.

Probably the most challenging task is to differentiate between stable and unstable injuries. Static diagnostics, that is, MRI or weight-bearing radiographs/CT scans, can help to raise the positive predictive value for a dynamically unstable ankle, but a thorough clinical examination is indispensable. In acute injuries, it is therefore recommended to initially immobilize the ankle and reassess the patient. This is also important after conservative treatment to detect persistent instability and select patients who will profit from surgical therapy (**Fig. 3**).

Surgical Technique

The authors strongly recommend starting with a diagnostic ankle arthroscopy to detect concomitant injuries and verify the MALC injury and the type of ankle instability. Arthroscopy is performed with the patient supine and the knee flexed 90°, putting the foot in a hanging position. A detailed description of the authors' preferred technique was outlined before.[1] Here, the authors want to emphasize the importance of a systematic arthroscopic examination and evaluation of the deltoid ligament complex. The rupture of the deltoid ligament and the significant medial gapping during eversion/pronation and/or external rotation are proving a deltoid ligament insufficiency.[4,54]

After diagnostic arthroscopy, open surgery starts with a slightly curved 8- to 10-cm incision, starting 2 to 4 cm proximal to the tip of the medial malleolus and aiming toward the tuberosity of the navicular bone. The deltoid ligament is exposed and more

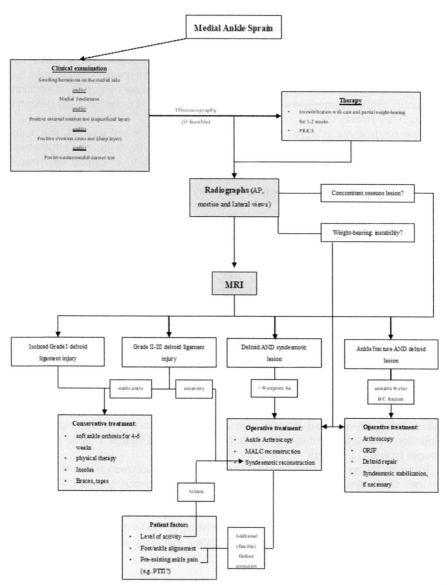

Fig. 3. The treatment of medial ankle sprains. ORIF, open reduction and internal fixation; PRICE, protection, rest, ice, compression, and elevation; PTTI, posterior tibial tendon insufficiency.

plantar the PTT as well as the spring ligament visualized. The type of injury of the MACL is evaluated. There is an anatomic classification according to the injury location: proximal, intermediate, and distal MACL tear (**Box 1**).[32,55]

In the case of concomitant lateral instability and detected ATFL lesion, an additional lateral approach can be performed for a lateral ligament repair.

Depending on the level of deltoid lesion and local soft tissue status, the deltoid ligament is reconstructed. If feasible, the deltoid can be tensioned from distal to proximal

> **Box 1**
> **Surgical locoanatomic classification of medial ankle ligament complex[32,55]**
>
> Surgical locoanatomic classification
>   Type I lesion: Proximal tear/avulsion of the deltoid ligament; most common
>   Type II lesion: Intermediate tear of the deltoid ligament
>   Type III lesion: Distal tear/avulsion of the deltoid and spring ligament

and attached to the medial malleolus by transosseous sutures or anchors. Alternatively, and more probable in subacute/chronic injuries, augmented reconstructions with periosteal flaps and free autograft reconstruction with plantaris longus, hamstring tendon, or the flexor digitorum longus (FDL) are possible surgical options.[10,54,56–58]

If in the standing clinical examination there was an asymmetric pes valgus/planovalgus/planovalgus et abductus deformity, a calcaneal osteotomy is needed: lateral lengthening calcaneal osteotomy for pes planovalgus and pes planovalgus et abductus deformity, medial sliding calcaneal osteotomy for isolated valgus deformity.[59] The calcaneal osteotomy reduces the strain in the reconstructed MALC.[60,61]

The postoperative treatment protocol comprises 15 kg partial weight-bearing for 6 weeks in a walker with limited range of motion (free dorsiflexion, plantarflexion of maximum 10°, no inversion) and physiotherapy.

Pitfalls in the Treatment of Medial Ankle Ligament Complex Injuries

Because of the importance of the MALC for 3-dimensional ankle stability, MALC injuries may cause consequential damages for the patient. If overlooked or inadequately treated, acute MALC injuries can lead to MCAI with rotational chronic ankle instability and ultimately in valgus ankle OA.[9,62] In progressive collapsing foot deformity (PCFD), the spring and deltoid ligaments are almost always compromised. An acute MACL lesion can therefore be the cause of the development of PCFD or significantly contribute to a progression of a subtle or nonsymptomatic PCFD.[63] In addition, lesions to the deltoid ligament can destabilize the syndesmosis and result in chronic syndesmotic insufficiency.[64,65]

DISCUSSION

Medial ankle sprains are more commonly reported in current literature owing to a rising awareness. In acute ankle sprains, an MALC lesion can be present in almost half of the cases, and the risk of MALC lesions increases significantly with complete ATFL ruptures.[8] The deltoid-spring ligament complex is the main static restraint of the tibiotalar, talocalcaneal, and talonavicular joint. Biomechanical investigations stressed the importance of the deltoid ligament complex for 3-dimensional ankle stability, and medial ankle insufficiency can lead to ligamentous ankle OA.[9–11,15] Despite the growing understanding of the physiologic function of the deltoid ligament complex, there is still controversy regarding the optimal therapy. This can be attributed to 2 main problems associated with these kinds of injuries. First, following a (medial) ankle sprain, the lesion needs to be diagnosed correctly and ankle stability thoroughly evaluated. There is no noninvasive imaging that is highly sensitive detecting the lesion as well as for the evaluation of ankle stability. Clinical examination is essential but requires experience. The correct diagnosis can therefore only be the sum of different noninvasive imaging modalities and clinical experience. Second, medial ankle injuries are commonly associated with concomitant lesions. Studies investigating the outcome following conservative and operative treatment need to take these factors into consideration for correctly interpreting the results. High-quality evidence regarding the optimal therapy for MALC injuries is sparse. Therapeutic recommendations are mainly delineated from studies in athletes and based on the consensus of experts.[13] Only in ankle fractures with associated deltoid ligament lesion is there rising evidence for a superiority of an operative treatment of deltoid injuries.[53]

CLINICS CARE POINTS

- Deltoid/medial ankle ligament complex injuries are more common and present in up to half of the cases following an ankle sprain.
- Concomitant lesions (lateral ankle ligament, osteochondral lesion, syndesmotic injury, posterior tibial tendon lesion, fractures) are common and decisive for the correct management.
- Assessment of medial ankle stability is essential for an adequate and successful treatment.
- Unstable and multiple injuries (concomitant lesion) benefit from surgical medial ankle ligament complex reconstruction with repair of the additional lesions.

DISCLOSURE

The authors have nothing to disclose.

REFERENCES

1. Alshalawi S, Galhoum AE, Alrashidi Y, et al. Medial Ankle Instability: The Deltoid Dilemma. Foot Ankle Clin 2018;23(4):639–57.
2. Waterman BR, Owens BD, Davey S, et al. The epidemiology of ankle sprains in the United States. JBJS 2010;92(13):2279–84.
3. Doherty C, Delahunt E, Caulfield B, et al. The incidence and prevalence of ankle sprain injury: a systematic review and meta-analysis of prospective epidemiological studies. Sports Med 2014;44(1):123–40.
4. Czajka CM, Tran E, Cai AN, et al. Ankle sprains and instability. Med Clin North Am 2014;98(2):313–29.
5. Savage-Elliott I, Murawski CD, Smyth NA, et al. The deltoid ligament: an in-depth review of anatomy, function, and treatment strategies. Knee Surg Sports Traumatol Arthrosc 2013;21(6):1316–27.
6. Hintermann B, Boss A, Schäfer D. Arthroscopic findings in patients with chronic ankle instability. Am J Sports Med 2002;30(3):402–9.
7. Crim JR, Beals TC, Nickisch F, et al. Deltoid ligament abnormalities in chronic lateral ankle instability. Foot Ankle Int 2011;32(9):873–8.
8. Roemer FW, Jomaah N, Niu J, et al. Ligamentous Injuries and the Risk of Associated Tissue Damage in Acute Ankle Sprains in Athletes: A Cross-sectional MRI Study. Am J Sports Med 2014;42(7):1549–57.
9. Longo UG, Loppini M, Fumo C, et al. Deep deltoid ligament injury is related to rotational instability of the ankle joint: a biomechanical study. Knee Surg Sports Traumatol Arthrosc 2021;29(5):1577–83.
10. Hintermann B, Ruiz R. Biomechanics of Medial Ankle and Peritalar Instability. Foot Ankle Clin 2021;26(2):249–67.
11. Valderrabano V, Hintermann B, Horisberger M, et al. Ligamentous posttraumatic ankle osteoarthritis. Am J Sports Med 2006;34(4):612–20.
12. Valderrabano V, Horisberger M, Russell I, et al. Etiology of ankle osteoarthritis. Clin Orthopaedics Relat Research®. 2009;467(7):1800–6.

13. McCollum GA, van den Bekerom MP, Kerkhoffs GM, et al. Syndesmosis and deltoid ligament injuries in the athlete. Knee Surg Sports Traumatol Arthrosc 2013; 21(6):1328–37.
14. Golanó P, Vega J, De Leeuw PA, et al. Anatomy of the ankle ligaments: a pictorial essay. Knee Surg Sports Traumatol Arthrosc 2010;18(5):557–69.
15. Takao M, Ozeki S, Oliva XM, et al. Strain pattern of each ligamentous band of the superficial deltoid ligament: a cadaver study. BMC Musculoskelet Disord 2020; 21(1):289.
16. Harper MC. Deltoid ligament: an anatomical evaluation of function. Foot Ankle 1987;8(1):19–22.
17. Stormont DM, Morrey BF, An KN, et al. Stability of the loaded ankle. Relation between articular restraint and primary and secondary static restraints. Am J Sports Med 1985;13(5):295–300.
18. Rasmussen O, Kromann-Andersen C, Boe S. Deltoid ligament. Functional analysis of the medial collateral ligamentous apparatus of the ankle joint. Acta Orthop Scand 1983;54(1):36–44.
19. Milner CE, Soames RW. The medial collateral ligaments of the human ankle joint: anatomical variations. Foot Ankle Int 1998;19(5):289–92.
20. Close JR. Some applications of the functional anatomy of the ankle joint. JBJS 1956;38(4):761–81.
21. Hintermann B, Sommer C, Nigg BM. Influence of ligament transection on tibial and calcaneal rotation with loading and dorsi-plantarflexion. Foot Ankle Int 1995;16(9):567–71.
22. Sommer C, Hintermann B, Nigg BM, et al. Influence of ankle ligaments on tibial rotation: an in vitro study. Foot Ankle Int 1996;17(2):79–84.
23. Earll M, Wayne J, Brodrick C, et al. Contribution of the deltoid ligament to ankle joint contact characteristics: a cadaver study. Foot Ankle Int 1996;17(6):317–24.
24. Cifuentes-De la Portilla C, Larrainzar-Garijo R, Bayod J. Biomechanical stress analysis of the main soft tissues associated with the development of adult acquired flatfoot deformity. Clin Biomech (Bristol, Avon) 2019;61:163–71.
25. Lauge-Hansen N. Fractures of the ankle: II. Combined experimental-surgical and experimental-roentgenologic investigations. Arch Surg 1950;60(5):957–85.
26. Yu GR, Zhang MZ, Aiyer A, et al. Repair of the acute deltoid ligament complex rupture associated with ankle fractures: a multicenter clinical study. J Foot Ankle Surg 2015;54(2):198–202.
27. Calder JD, Bamford R, Petrie A, et al. Stable versus unstable grade II high ankle sprains: a prospective study predicting the need for surgical stabilization and time to return to sports. Arthrosc The J Arthroscopic Relat Surg 2016;32(4): 634–42.
28. Gerber JP, Williams GN, Scoville CR, et al. Persistent disability associated with ankle sprains: a prospective examination of an athletic population. Foot Ankle Int 1998;19(10):653–60.
29. Çabuk H, Çelebi F, İmren Y, et al. Compatibility of Lauge-Hansen Classification Between Plain Radiographs and Magnetic Resonance Imaging in Ankle Fractures. J Foot Ankle Surg 2018;57(4):712–5.
30. van den Bekerom MP, Mutsaerts EL, van Dijk CN. Evaluation of the integrity of the deltoid ligament in supination external rotation ankle fractures: a systematic review of the literature. Arch Orthop Trauma Surg 2009;129(2):227–35.
31. Crim J. Medial-sided Ankle Pain: Deltoid Ligament and Beyond. Magn Reson Imaging Clin N Am 2017;25(1):63–77.

32. Valderrabano V, Hintermann B. Diagnostik und Therapie der medialen Sprungge-lenkinstabilität. Arthroskopie 2005;18(2):112–8.
33. Krähenbühl N, Weinberg MW, Davidson NP, et al. Imaging in syndesmotic injury: a systematic literature review. Skeletal Radiol 2018;47(5):631–48.
34. van Leeuwen CAT, Sala M, Schipper IB, et al. The additional value of weight-bearing and gravity stress ankle radiographs in determining stability of isolated type B ankle fractures. Eur J Trauma Emerg Surg 2022;48(3):2287–96.
35. Joshy S, Abdulkadir U, Chaganti S, et al. Accuracy of MRI scan in the diagnosis of ligamentous and chondral pathology in the ankle. Foot Ankle Surg 2010;16(2):78–80.
36. Staats K, Sabeti-Aschraf M, Apprich S, et al. Preoperative MRI is helpful but not sufficient to detect associated lesions in patients with chronic ankle instability. Knee Surg Sports Traumatol Arthrosc 2018;26(7):2103–9.
37. Chun KY, Choi YS, Lee SH, et al. Deltoid Ligament and Tibiofibular Syndesmosis Injury in Chronic Lateral Ankle Instability: Magnetic Resonance Imaging Evalua-tion at 3T and Comparison with Arthroscopy. Korean J Radiol 2015;16(5):1096–103.
38. Crim J, Longenecker LG. MRI and surgical findings in deltoid ligament tears. AJR Am J Roentgenol 2015;204(1):W63–9.
39. Bae S, Lee HK, Lee K, et al. Comparison of arthroscopic and magnetic reso-nance imaging findings in osteochondral lesions of the talus. Foot Ankle Int 2012;33(12):1058–62.
40. Ergün T, Peker A, Aybay MN, et al. Ultrasonography view for acute ankle injury: comparison of ultrasonography and magnetic resonance imaging. Arch Orthop Trauma Surg 2022. https://doi.org/10.1007/s00402-022-04553-8.
41. Baltes TPA, Arnáiz J, Geertsema L, et al. Diagnostic value of ultrasonography in acute lateral and syndesmotic ligamentous ankle injuries. Eur Radiol 2021;31(4):2610–20.
42. Henari S, Banks LN, Radovanovic I, et al. Ultrasonography as a diagnostic tool in assessing deltoid ligament injury in supination external rotation fractures of the ankle. Orthopedics 2011;34(10):e639–43.
43. Margetic P, Salaj M, Lubina IZ. The Value of Ultrasound in Acute Ankle Injury: Comparison With MR. Eur J Trauma Emerg Surg 2009;35(2):141–6.
44. Peetrons PA, Silvestre A, Cohen M, et al. Ultrasonography of ankle ligaments. Can Assoc Radiol J 2002;53(1):6–13.
45. Sterzik A, Mueck F, Wirth S, et al. Evaluation of ankle ligaments with CT: A feasi-bility study. Eur J Radiol 2021;134:109446.
46. Raheman FJ, Rojoa DM, Hallet C, et al. Can Weightbearing Cone-beam CT Reli-ably Differentiate Between Stable and Unstable Syndesmotic Ankle Injuries? A Systematic Review and Meta-analysis. Clin Orthop Relat Res 2022;480(8):1547–62.
47. Patel S, Malhotra K, Cullen NP, et al. Defining reference values for the normal ti-biofibular syndesmosis in adults using weight-bearing CT. Bone Joint J 2019;101-b(3):348–52.
48. Vega J, Guelfi M. Arthroscopic Assessment and Treatment of Medial Collateral Ligament Complex. Foot Ankle Clin 2021;26(2):305–13.
49. Høiness P, Glott T, Ingjer F. High-intensity training with a bi-directional bicycle pedal improves performance in mechanically unstable ankles–a prospective ran-domized study of 19 subjects. Scand J Med Sci Sports 2003;13(4):266–71.
50. Eils E, Rosenbaum D. A multi-station proprioceptive exercise program in patients with ankle instability. Med Sci Sports Exerc 2001;33(12):1991–8.

51. Rikken QGH, Kerkhoffs G. Osteochondral Lesions of the Talus: An Individualized Treatment Paradigm from the Amsterdam Perspective. Foot Ankle Clin 2021; 26(1):121–36.
52. Bruns J, Habermann C, Werner M. Osteochondral Lesions of the Talus: A Review on Talus Osteochondral Injuries, Including Osteochondritis Dissecans. Cartilage 2021;13(1_suppl):1380s–401s.
53. Guo W, Lin W, Chen W, et al. Comparison of deltoid ligament repair and non-repair in acute ankle fracture: A meta-analysis of comparative studies. PLoS One 2021;16(11):e0258785.
54. Hintermann B, Valderrabano V, Boss A, et al. Medial ankle instability: an exploratory, prospective study of fifty-two cases. Am J Sports Med 2004;32(1):183–90.
55. Hintermann B, Knupp M, Pagenstert GI. Deltoid ligament injuries: diagnosis and management. Foot Ankle Clin 2006;11(3):625–37.
56. Boyer MI, Bowen V, Weiler P. Reconstruction of a severe grinding injury to the medial malleolus and the deltoid ligament of the ankle using a free plantaris tendon graft and vascularized gracilis free muscle transfer: case report. J Trauma 1994;36(3):454–7.
57. Ellis SJ, Williams BR, Wagshul AD, et al. Deltoid ligament reconstruction with peroneus longus autograft in flatfoot deformity. Foot Ankle Int 2010;31(9):781–9.
58. Deland JT, de Asla RJ, Segal A. Reconstruction of the chronically failed deltoid ligament: a new technique. Foot Ankle Int 2004;25(11):795–9.
59. CS L, de Cesar Netto C, Day J, et al. Consensus for the Indication of a Medializing Displacement Calcaneal Osteotomy in the Treatment of Progressive Collapsing Foot Deformity. Foot Ankle Int 2020;41(10):1282–5.
60. Otis JC, Deland JT, Kenneally S, et al. Medial arch strain after medial displacement calcaneal osteotomy: an in vitro study. Foot Ankle Int 1999;20(4):222–6.
61. Arangio GA, Salathé EP. Medial displacement calcaneal osteotomy reduces the excess forces in the medial longitudinal arch of the flat foot. Clin Biomech 2001;16(6):535–9.
62. Barg A, Pagenstert GI, Hügle T, et al. Ankle Osteoarthritis: Etiology, Diagnostics, and Classification. Foot Ankle Clin 2013;18(3):411–26.
63. Krautmann K, Kadakia AR. Spring and Deltoid Ligament Insufficiency in the Setting of Progressive Collapsing Foot Deformity. An Update on Diagnosis and Management. Foot Ankle Clin 2021;26(3):577–90.
64. Massri-Pugin J, Lubberts B, Vopat BG, et al. Role of the Deltoid Ligament in Syndesmotic Instability. Foot Ankle Int 2018;39(5):598–603.
65. Corte-Real N, Caetano J. Ankle and syndesmosis instability: consensus and controversies. EFORT Open Rev 2021;6(6):420–31.

High-Ankle Sprain and Syndesmotic Instability

How Far Have We Come with Diagnosis and Treatment?

Nacime Salomao Barbachan Mansur, MD, PhD[a,b,*],
Alexandre Leme Godoy-Santos, MD, PhD[c], Tim Schepers, MD, PhD[d]

KEYWORDS

- Syndesmosis • Tibiofibular • Instability • Lesion • High-ankle sprain • Diagnose
- Diagnostic • Treatment

KEY POINTS

- Syndesmotic instability is one of the most challenging diagnoses in orthopedics, particularly in the chronic and subtle scenarios.
- A full clinical and imaging evaluation can place assessors closer to the most appropriate conclusions while providing solid information for proper treatment.
- Several instability patterns might occur at the syndesmosis, what should be considered when diagnosing and treating patients.
- Implant choice depends on the injury configuration and syndesmotic behavior.
- Surgical stabilization in different planes sets tibiofibular interactions to conditions that approach native states.

BACKGROUND

Although lesions to the distal tibiofibular (TF) ligaments can be noted in approximately 25% of the sprains occurring at the ankle, the real incidence of the ones provoking syndesmosis instability is still uncertain, ranging from 1% to 16%.[1,2] This can be attributed to the fact that not all mechanical failures can be translated into an unstable joint, which is influenced by many anatomic aspects.[3] Several authors dedicated substantial research to the theme in the last three decades, contributing to the broader

[a] Escola Paulista de Medicina – Universidade Federal de São Paulo, Brazil; [b] University of Iowa, Carver College of Medicine, USA; [c] Universidade de Sao Paulo, R. Dr. Ovídio Pires de Campos, 333, 3rd floor, 05403-010, Sao Paulo, Brazil; [d] Trauma Unit, Department of Surgery, Amsterdam UMC Location J1A-214 Meibergdreef 9, 1105 AZ, Amsterdam, The Netherlands
* Corresponding author. University of Iowa, Carver College of Medicine, 200 Hawkins Drive, John PappaJohn Pavillion (JPP), Room 01066, Lower Level, Iowa City, IA 52242.
E-mail address: nacime@uol.com.br

Foot Ankle Clin N Am 28 (2023) 369–403
https://doi.org/10.1016/j.fcl.2023.01.006
1083-7515/23/© 2023 Elsevier Inc. All rights reserved.

foot.theclinics.com

knowledge we have today.[4] The fact that instability can present in different patterns and planes, gathering rotational, coronal, and sagittal abnormal motions was a landmark for this condition.[5] Tenths of millimeters might be responsible for an unstable and symptomatic joint, whereas "normality" population values for reference might not be feasible due to the high anatomic variance between individuals.[6] Moreover, the occurrence of the disease seems to be increasing, mostly due to the fact physicians are now more able to reach this challenging diagnose using good clinical judgment and new technology.[7] Treatment is also evolving rapidly, supported by good data demonstrating the advantages of early surgical intervention as well as the use of flexible and anatomic reconstructions.[8,9]

DIAGNOSING SYNDESMOSIS INSTABILITY

The literature on the diagnostic instruments for syndesmosis instability focused on the ligamentar (nonfractured) scenario can be found in **Table 1**.

History

Although syndesmotic injuries have always been highly associated with a history of ankle sprain with an ankle dorsiflexion, external rotation or eversion moment, data provided by previous studies showed it can occur with different mechanisms.[2,10–12] Sman and colleagues[10] prospectively evaluated 87 patients with an ankle sprain and found moderate accuracy values for pain out of proportion (72.6%), pain at the shank (61.4%), dorsiflexion with external rotation trauma (48.8%) and inability to hop (55.2%). Tenderness over the TF anterior topography extending proximally was observed in all 60 patients evaluated by Nussbaum and colleagues[12] and the length of tenderness (mean 8.5 cm) was correlated with the days lost in competition (13.4 days).

Physical Examination

Pain when palpating the anterior inferior TF ligament and the proximal syndesmosis topography is common, with reports from occurring in 83% to 100%, having a 56% accuracy (Acc), 83% to 92% sensitivity (Sn), and 29% to 63%% specificity (Sp).[10,12–15] The squeeze test has been described as happening in 33% to 100%, with Sn values from 26% to 36% and Sp values from 88% to 93.5%.[10,12,13,16,17] Calder and colleagues[18] found a 9.47 odds ratio (OR) for instability when athletes presented a positive squeeze test. Previous descriptions of the external rotational (ER) test portrayed a 75% to 100% occurrence, whereas more recent studies showed a 20% to 71% Sn and a 63% to 84% Sp.[10,12–14,17,19] Kiter and colleagues[20] described the crossed-leg test a being positive in 9 of 9 their patients. Fibular translation, also described as fibular drawer test, was only verified by Wagener and colleagues[13] as being existent in 100% of his cohort.

The different diagnostic accuracies from clinical presentations and physical examinations might not be able to unambiguously define instability, but they can grant a good background when the diagnose is suspected. The use of different tests in combination and in different timeframes might give the provider good confidence to warrant further investigation.[2,21]

Conventional Radiographs and Fluoroscopy

Syndesmotic investigation through weight-bearing (WB) conventional radiographs (CRs) is a historical landmark and continues to be the only available imaging option in many services and countries.[22] Yet still an essential part in the evaluation of an ankle

Table 1
Literature review of diagnostic tests for syndesmosis lesions and instabilities

Study	Sample	Tests	Results	Gold Standard
Hopkinson et al,[16] 1990	8 patients	Squeeze test Stress CR	8/8 positive 1/7 positive	None
Harper & Keller,[22] 1989	12 cadavers	CR	Normal AP TFCS<6 mm Normal AP TFO>6 mm Normal Mortise TFO>1 mm	Direct measurements
Ogilvie-Harris & Reed,[19] 1994	13 patients	ER test	13/13 positive	Arthroscopy
Xenos et al,[30] 1995	25 cadavers	CR	Posterior dislocation (lateral view) had a higher correlation (r = 0.81)	Direct measurements
Ebraheim et al,[24] 1997	12 cadavers	CR vs CT	CT superior in detecting 1 mm to 3 mm diastasis	Direct visualization
Teitz & Harrington,[78] 1998	7 cadavers	Squeeze test	No significant opening	Displacement transducer
Nussbaum et al,[12] 2001	60 patients	ER test Squeeze test Medial tenderness	55/60 positive 20/60 positive 24/60 positive	Not described
Beumer et al,[79] 2003	10 cadavers	ER test (7.5 Nm)	Lateral CR were not able to identify	Radiostereometric analysis
Takao et al,[26] 2003	23 patients	CR MRI	AP: 43.5% Sn, 100% Sp, and 75.0% Acc. Mortise: 65.2% Sn, 100% Sp, and 84.6% Acc. MRI: 100% Sn, 93.1% Sp, and 96.2% Acc.	Arthroscopy for ligament injury
Oae et al,[46] 2003	28 patients	MRI	AITFL discontinuity: 100% Sn, 70% Sp, 84% Acc PITFL Discontinuity: 100% Sn, 94% Sp, 95% Acc AITFL Lesion: 100% Sn, 93% Sp, 97% Acc PITFL Lesion: 100% Sn, 100% Sp, 100% Acc	Arthroscopy for ligament injury

(continued on next page)

Table 1
(continued)

Study	Sample	Tests	Results	Gold Standard
Candal-Couto et al,[29] 2004	7 cadavers	Hook test	Sagittal CR translation is higher than coronal	Ruler
Kiter & Bozkurt,[20] 2005	9 patients	Crossed-leg test	9/9 positive	Not described
Taser et al,[56] 2006	6 cadavers	Volume in CT	1mm increased volume in 43% and 20% for every additional 1 mm	Direct visualization
Han et al,[49] 2007	20 patients	MRI	90.0% Sn, 94.8% Sp, and 93.4% Acc	Arthroscopy
Kim et al,[80] 2007	45 patients	MRI	Higher overall Acc with contrast. Recess height: 16.2 mm injured vs 12.6 mm noninjured	Arthroscopy
Mei-Dan et al,[38] 2009	9 patients	US with stress	100% Sn and Sp for 0.9 mm difference between sides. 89% Sn and Sp for 0.4 mm difference between ER and N on the same side.	MRI for ligament injury (AITFL)
Wagener et al,[13] 2011	12 patients	CR, AITFL pain, FT, ER test, Squeeze test, Impaired DF	TFCS 4/12 positive, MCS 1/12 positive, AITFL: 10/12 positive, FT: 12/12 positive, ER: 9/12 positive, Squeeze: 6/12 positive, DF: 6/12 positive	Arthroscopy
de César et al,[17] 2011	56 patients	Squeeze test, ER test	30% Sn, 93.5% Sp, 20% Sn, 84.8% Sp	MRI for ligament injury
Dikos et al,[55] 2012	60 ankles	CT	Normality: TF intervals<2.3 mm and fibular rotation<6.5° when compared with CL	None

Study	Population	Test	Results	Reference standard
Femino et al,[81] 2013	6 cadavers	Varus ER test Valgus ER test	10.7 mm MG widening 5.4 mm MG widening Not significant for syndesmosis	Direct visualization
Sman et al,[10] 2015	87 patients	ER test DF Lunge Squeeze Squeeze test Palpation	71% Sn, 63% Sp 69% Sn, 41% Sp 26% Sn, 88% Sp 92% Sn, 29% Sp	MRI for ligament injury
Malhotra et al,[57] 2014	14 patients	CT	TF angle: 63.4° injured vs 68.4° CL 11/14 smaller angles Area: 1.71 cm² vs 1.21 cm² 14/14 higher area	Intraoperative Cotton and ER test
Ryan et al,[14] 2014	23 injured 40 controls	Syndesmosis pain Squeeze test ER test CR MRI	83% Sn, 63% Sp 36% Sn, 89% Sp 68% Sn, 83% Sp Mortise MCS > 6 mm: 27% Sn, 90% Sp AP MCS > 6 mm: 27% Sn, 69% Sp AP TFO < 6 mm: 50% Sn, 68% Sp AITFL injury: 50% Sn, 72% Sp PITFL injury: 13% Sn, 100% Sp Lambda: 75% Sn, 63% Sp	Arthroscopy
Schoennagel et al,[27] 2014	84 patients	CR	TFCS: 5.3 mm, 82% Sn, 75% Sp TFO: 2.8 m, 36% Sn, 78% Sp MCS: 2.8 m, 73% Sn, 59% Sp	MRI for ligament injury
Clanton et al,[47] 2016	21 patients 10 controls	MRI	AITFL: 87.5% Sn, 100% Sp PITFL: 95.2% Sp ITFL: 66.7% Sn, 86.7% Sp Recess: 82.4% Sn, 0.0% Sp	Arthroscopy for ligament injury
Chun et al,[48] 2015	50 patients	MRI	91% Sn, 100% Sp	Arthroscopy for ligament injury
Calder et al,[18] 2016	36 patients	Squeeze test MRI	9.47 OR for surgery Deltoid 11.04 OR for surgery	Arthroscopy

(continued on next page)

Table 1
(continued)

Study	Sample	Tests	Results	Gold Standard
Lepojärvi et al,[59] 2016	32 controls	WBCT	Normality: anteriorly located in 88% ER: 1.5 mm AP motion and 3° of fibula rotation	None
Feller et al,[32] 2017	10 cadavers	Stress Fluoro	Unable to detect progressive injuries	Arthroscopy
Guyton et al,[45] 2017	10 cadavers	Arthroscopy	ER and a 3 mm sphere: high likelihood	Direct visualization
Massri-Pugin et al,[76] 2017	14 cadavers	Arthroscopy	Coronal diastasis only noted when all ligaments were transected	Direct visualization
Lubberts et al,[82] 2017	14 cadavers	Arthroscopy	Distraction decreased TF diastasis	Direct visualization
Ahn et al,[58] 2017	78 patients	CT	Narrowest TF > 2 mm: AUC 0.86, 76% Sn, 81% Sp	Arthroscopy
LaMothe et al,[31] 2018	9 cadavers	Fluoroscopy	AP Incisura: 63% Sn, 100% Sp in lateral stress AP Incisura: 23% Sn, 100% Sp in ER Lateral: 63% Sn, 95% Sp in sagittal stress Lateral: 67% Sn, 89% Sp in ER stress	Motion capture
Osgood et al,[60] 2019	14 controls	WBCT CT	Difference in traditional CT measurements	None
Gosselin-Papadopoulos et al,[83] 2019	10 cadavers	Torque test ER test LT test	Torque test >3.5 mm: 90% Sn, 100% Sp Torque test superior	Direct visualization
Mousavian et al,[84] 2019	10 controls	4DCT	Syndesmotic translation changed during ankle motion (−0.70 mm)	None
Gosselin-Papadopoulos et al,[28] 2019	10 cadavers	CR	Syndesmotic view 66% and 61% Sn vs 27% and 33% in mortise	Direct visualization
Randell et al,[50] 2019	164 patients	MRI	PITFL lesion or PM edema: 93.5% until week 6; 54.2% after week 12	Arthroscopy

Study	Sample	Imaging	Findings	Reference standard
Hagemeijer et al,[85] 2019	12 patients, 24 controls	WBCT	Area: 118 mm² stable vs 164.8 mm² unstable; Anterior diff: 6.0 vs 8.4 mm; Middle: 4.6 vs 6.0 mm; Posterior: 9.14 vs 11.6 mm	Arthroscopy
Lubberts et al,[73] 2020	22 cadavers	Arthroscopy	Arthroscopy syndesmotic assessment tool >3.11 mm	Direct visualization
Hamard et al,[62] 2020	19 patients	CT, WBCT	Anterior TF: AUC 0.869 CT vs 0.555 WBCT; Minimal TF: 0.883 CT vs 0.608 WBCT; AP translation: 0.894 CT vs 0.467 WBCT	Arthroscopy
Del Rio et al,[65] 2020	39 patients	WBCT	Area 22.9 mm² higher in the injured side; From NWB to WB: 13.7% increase in the injured area vs 3.1% in noninjured	Arthroscopy
Hagemeijer et al,[39] 2020	28 controls	US with stress	AP translation: 0.89 mm; PA translation: 0.49 mm	None
Bhimani et al,[66] 2020	12 patients, 24 controls	WBCT	Volume from plafond to 5 cm proximal: higher ratio; 7.99 mm³ noninjured to 14.1 mm³ injured; 3D more sensitive than 2D	Arthroscopy
Burssens et al,[63] 2020	14 cadavers	WBCT	ER with load was superior to isolated load; PT: −3.1 mm; ER: −4.7°	Direct visualization
Hagemeijer et al,[75] 2021	8 studies	Arthroscopy	Coronal: 2.9 mm anterior, 3.4 mm posterior; Sagittal: 2.2 mm AP, 2.6 mm PA	Direct visualization
Ashkani Esfahani et al,[67] 2022	24 patients, 24 controls	WBCT	At 1 cm > 1.4 cm² area: 70% Sn, 81% Sp, 75% Acc; At 3 cm > 2.5 cm² area: 62% Sn, 80% Sp, 72% Acc; At 5 cm > 3.2 cm² area: 60% Sn, 79% Sp, 70% Acc; At 10 cm > 4.6 cm² area: 50% Sn, 71% Sp, 60% Acc	Arthroscopy

(continued on next page)

Table 1
(continued)

Study	Sample	Tests	Results	Gold Standard
			At 1 cm > 1.5 cm³: 62% Sn, 80% Sp, 70% Acc	
			At 3 cm > 5.3 cm³: 76% Sn, 81% Sp, 82% Acc	
			At 5 cm > 11.6 cm³: 95% Sn, 83% Sp, 90% Acc	
			At 10 cm > 29.2 cm³: 83% Sn, 79% Sp, 81% Acc	
Bhimani et al,[74] 2021	21 cadavers	Arthroscopy	PA and AP combined: 0.91 AUC Coronal combined: 0.73 AUC	Direct visualization
Shoji et al,[40] 2022	5 cadavers	US	Detectable TF distance increase even with no stress	Direct visualization
Hagemeijer et al,[41] 2022	10 cadavers	US Fluoroscopy	US: TFCS increases (2.6 mm) with ER, not detected by fluoroscopy	Direct visualization

Abbreviations: 4DCT, four-dimensional computed tomography; Acc, accuracy; AITFL, anterior inferior tibiofibular ligament; AP, anteroposterior; AUC, area under the curve; CL, contralateral; CR, conventional radiographs; CT, computed tomography; DF, dorsiflexion; ER, external rotation; FT, fibula translation; ITFL, interosseous tibiofibular ligament; MCS, medial clear space; MG, medial gutter; MRI, magnetic resonance imaging; N, neutral; NWB, non-weight-bearing; OR, odds ratio; PA, posteroanterior; PITFL, posterior inferior tibiofibular ligament; PM, posterior malleolus; Sn, sensitivity; Sp, specificity; TCO, tibiofibular overlap; TF, tibiofibular; TFCS, tibiofibular clear space; US, ultrasound; WB, weight-bearing; WBCT, weight-bearing computed tomography.

trauma, its capability in detecting subtle or chronic injuries is very limited (**Fig. 1**).[23–25] The anteroposterior (AP) and Mortise views, when using different thresholds for tibiofibular clear space (TFCS) or tibiofibular overlap (TFO), was able to have a 27% to 82% Sn and a 68% to 100% Sp.[14,26–28] The lateral view has been described as good tool to identify instability, especially when considering different planes.[29,30] Its accuracy was only depicted by LaMothe and colleagues[31] as having 63% and 67% Sn as well as 95% and 87% Sp when sagittal and ER stress were applied, respectively. The use of stress radiographs or fluoroscopy did not improve diagnostic capacity according to previous studies.[16,32,33]

Even when considering "nonfractured" syndesmotic injuries, a leg radiographical evaluation must not be forgotten.[34] The Maisonneuve fracture is prone to be missed at the first visit, with a neglected diagnosis rate of 14.28% to 44.4%.[34,35]

Ultrasound

Technological improvement, training, and feasibility are changing the perspective of ultrasound (US) in the musculoskeletal practice.[36] This includes the assessment of syndesmotic injuries and instabilities by the use of this dynamic instrument.[37] Mei-Dan and colleagues[38] found 100% Sn and 100% Sp when the TFCS was greater than 0.9 mm from the noninjured side or 0.4 mm from a neutral to external rotation stress state. When applying manual stress to control subjects, Hagemeijer and colleagues[39] found physiologic 0.89 mm mean AP translation and 0.49 mm mean PA translation. Shoji and colleagues[40] used five cadaveric models and were able to demonstrate increasing TF distances even when no stress was applied (4.9 to 8.4 mm with no stress; 6.7 to 9.9 mm with ER). Hagemeijer and colleagues[41] later compared US with fluoroscopy. The authors were able to detect TFCS increases

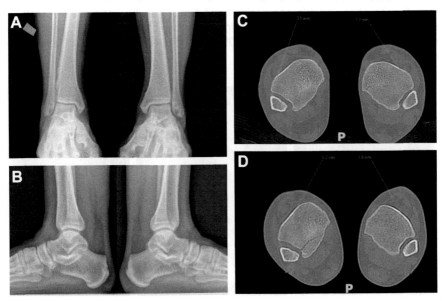

Fig. 1. Example of a patient that sustained a right ankle sprain and a clinical suspicion of syndesmosis instability was established. Conventional weight-bearing radiographs in the AP (*A*) and lateral views (*B*) do not display any significant changes. In this case, a non-WBCT (*C*) with an added ER protocol (*D*) was performed, not only demonstrating the tibiofibular instability but also an occult posterior malleolar fracture.

under ER stress through US (eg, 2.6 mm with 4.5 Nm) that were not captured by fluoroscopic images.[41] The use of US is progressively growing in clinical practice and in the body of literature, and can be safely used in a sideline evaluation or during an ankle sprain evaluation.[36,42,43] Its mobility, ease of use, dynamic capability, and potentially lower cost can make US a generalized technology.[43] However, assessor dependency and low interobserver reliabilities hinder its diffusiveness.[43] Science still needs to better support US's proper use in syndesmotic injuries, but the possibilities are open.

Magnetic Resonance

MRI provides structural soft tissue assessment (**Fig. 2**) like no other.[43,44] Nevertheless, anatomic injuries cannot be directly correlated to the instability of the syndesmosis.[23,45] Takao and colleagues[26] observed that MRI had a 96.2% Acc (100% Sn; 93.1% Sp) when ligament lesions were assessed by arthroscopy. The same arthroscopic evaluation was used by Oae and colleagues[46] that found 97% and 100% Acc for any sign of AITFL and posterior inferior tibiofibular ligament (PITFL) lesions. Clanton and colleagues (66.7% to 87.5% Sn; 0% to 100% Sp) and Chun and colleagues (91% Sn; 100% Sp) also employed arthroscopic ligament assessment as the reference to MRI findings.[47,48]

When arthroscopic instability was compared with MRI, different values were presented in the literature. Han and colleagues reported 93.4% Acc (90% Sn; 94.8% Sp), whereas Ryan and colleagues found Sn values from 13% (PITFL) to 75% (Lambda sign) and Sp values from 63% (Lambda) to 100% (PITFL).[14,49] Calder and colleagues depict an 11.04 OR for surgery in athletes with a high ankle sprain when the deltoid was found ruptured in the MRI.[18] Imaging acquisition timing was argued important according to Randell and colleagues who noticed an instability rate of 93.5% in PITFL injuries at 6 weeks, but only 54.2% at 12 weeks.[50] Even though presenting variable accuracies, useful data can be interpreted from these studies. Positive predictive values for instability near 100% for PITFL lesions and negative predictive values more than 70% for AITFL lesions in MRI can be valuable in decision-making.[14,47]

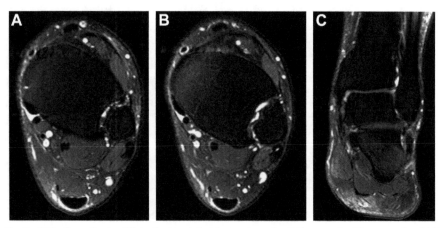

Fig. 2. MRI of a college athlete that sustained an external rotation sprain. More proximal (*A*) and distal (*B*) axial T2 views depicts a complete rupture of the anterior inferior tibiofibular ligament and injuries to the interosseous and PITFL. The coronal view (*C*) also demonstrates liquid at the most proximal aspect of the tibiofibular joint. This patient had an intraoperative arthroscopic confirmation of the syndesmosis instability and was treated accordingly.

Computed Tomography

A substantial scientific background was able to place computed tomography (CT) as the gold-standard when evaluating an unstable and malreduced syndesmosis in the ankle fracture setting.[23] Conversely, this is not the case when considering nonfractured syndesmotic instabilities.[7] That could be explained by the fact that subtle conditions or chronic states might need some degree of stress to produce bone motion in a static environment.[51] Much of the parameters studied today were defined by CT studies as well as what would be the normal (populational) values.[52] Normality might not apply to the syndesmotic evaluation once anatomic variability is vast and prone to changes according to foot positioning and image acquisition.[53,54]

Assessment through CT is superior to CR when identifying diastasis from 1 to 3 mm according to Ebraheim and colleagues[24] Dikos and colleagues investigated normal relations using CT and found TF intervals under 2.3 mm and fibular rotations below 6.5° in noninjured ankles.[55] A 43% increase in volume for 1 mm of TF opening followed by 20% for every additional millimeter was observed by Taser and colleagues in unstable cadavers.[56] Malhotra and colleagues compared injured and noninjured syndesmosis, finding smaller TF angles (63.4 vs 68.4) and higher areas (1.71 cm^2 vs 1.21 cm^2).[57] Interestingly, syndesmotic area and volume would become important parameters when evaluating the TF relation several years later. Ahn and colleagues showed that the narrowest TF above 2 mm had 76% of Sn and 81% of Sp for instability perceived by arthroscopy.[58]

Weight-Bearing Computed Tomography

As an emerging technique, capable of yielding physiologic load to the foot and ankle, weight-bearing computed tomography (WBCT) was quickly introduced in the syndesmosis instability environment with expectations that it could bring responses to the challenging instability question.[4] In the last few years, several studies tested the different characteristics and aspects of WBCT.[6] Lepojärvi and colleagues described that fibulas were found anteriorly located in 88% of control subjects and ER stress produced 1.5 mm in AP motion and 3° of rotation.[59] Changes on traditional CT parameters for syndesmosis when using WBCT were reported by Osgood and colleagues in terms of distance, diastasis, and angular values.[60] Shakoor and colleagues showed no changes in CT parameters when WB was applied.[61] That idea was sustained by Hamard and colleagues who compared accuracies between CT and WBCT, finding higher areas under the curve (AUC) for the non-WB status (0.869 to 0.894 vs 0.467 to 0.608).[62] The authors argued that a physiologic contralateral (CL) widening when standing could explain lower differences.[62] Burssens and colleagues tested cadavers with a syndesmotic injury model and found that external torque combined with load was superior to load in isolation to detect instability, particularly sagittal translation (−3.1 mm) and rotation (−4.7°).[63] Single load was capable of identifying coronal translation (−0.9 mm), which was noted in the submillimeter scale.[63]

The use of the CL noninjured segment as control and reference for pathologic findings is now the pattern due to the already commented population anatomic variability Using more specific and detailed metrics, allowed due to the development of bone segmentation, area (**Fig. 3**), and volume acquisitions, following studies challenged previous reported data.[64] Del Rio and colleagues used area (22.9 mm^2 higher in the injured side) to demonstrate unstable joints had a 13.7% increase (vs 3.1%) when WB was applied.[65] Using volume, Bhimani and colleagues, found that measurements taken from the plafond to 5 cm proximal had a higher change ratio from noninjured

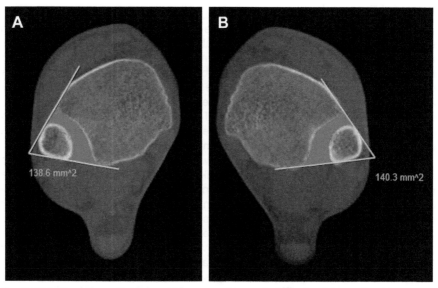

Fig. 3. WBCT syndesmotic area assessment using a dedicated software. Semi-automatic demarcation of the most proximal aspect of the tibial plafond joint takes the area measurement 1 cm proximal to the ankle (*A*) right ankle; (*B*) left ankle. In this case, the patient had an left ankle (*B*) sprain (140.3 mm^2) with a clinical syndesmotic instability suspicion that subsequently was confirmed by arthroscopy. The right normal side (*A*: 148.6mm) is compared to the injured side (*B*: 140.3mm^2) that displays an increase in area.

(7.99 mm^3) to injured (14.1 mm^3).[66] They also found three-dimensional (3D) measures to be more sensitive than two-dimensional (2D).[66] Ashkani Esfahani and colleagues tested the diagnostic capabilities of volume and area to diagnose syndesmotic instability in WBCT.[67] The authors found a higher accuracy for volumes taken up to 5 cm proximal (>11.6 cm^3: 95% Sn, 83% Sp, 90% Acc) in comparison to other levels or area measurements (eg, at 1 cm: >1.4cm2 area had 70% Sn, 81% Sp, 75% Acc).[67]

An exciting new horizon to the study of this complex condition was also possible secondary to the development of semi-automatic and automatic bone segmentation from WBCT.[68] Distance and coverage mapping technology were developed in an attempt to provide more objective and measurable data, potentially capable of recognizing minimal changes in the interactions between two bones (**Fig. 4**).[63,69,70] Future is still uncertain, but these innovations might help even more in finding the missing links among clinical presentation, subsidiary imaging, and proper diagnosis.[71]

Gold Standard

The assessment of any diagnostic capability is based on a reference standard test.[72] Many cadaveric studies used direct visualization to determine instability.[30,73] Clinically, arthroscopy is the gold-standard for most of the studied tests, although it is an invasive procedure.[5,10] In parallel, its ability to identify an unstable joint in all directions and patterns is still a matter of debate.[54] Further, the traditional arthroscopic syndesmotic assessment has been challenged and a more complete and detailed evaluation was developed (and supported by good literature) in the last years.[74]

Hagemeijer and colleagues, in a systematic review (SR) of cadaveric studies, found that the 2 mm established threshold in arthroscopy assessment was not supported by

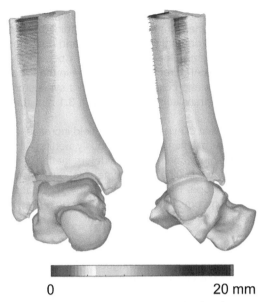

0   20 mm

Fig. 4. Bone segmentation from WBCT images allows the development of distances maps and coverage maps between two structures of interest. In this case, the syndesmosis is represented by the distance three-dimensional interaction amid tibia and fibula. The color pattern translates smaller distances as being red and higher distances as being blue. The multitudinous established vectors allow a much more objective and comprehensive mathematical analysis of the syndesmosis volume, area, and specific coverage.

current data, possibly leading to overtreatment.[75] The review suggested 2.9 mm at the anterior incisura and 3.4 mm at the posterior (tested with a 3 mm probe) as more scientifically sound.[75] Guyton and colleagues had already recommended the use of a 3 mm as able to identify AITFL and interosseous tibiofibular ligament (ITFL) ruptures (**Fig. 5**).[45] The use of distraction to test the syndesmosis was unadvised by Lubberts and colleagues, who found less diastasis when traction was applied.[31]

Calling attention to other instabilities patterns and the limitation when only evaluating the TF relation through a probe placed into the incisura, Massri-Pugin and colleagues[76] showed that only a complete ligament transection was able to produce coronal diastasis, which was better assessed at the posterior incisura margin. They

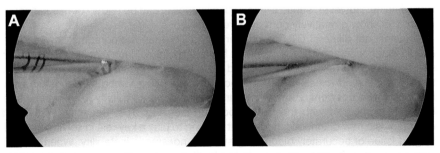

Fig. 5. Intraoperative confirmation of coronal syndesmosis instability is performed arthroscopically by inserting the 3 mm sphere (*A*) at the central aspect of the tibiofibular incisura (*B*).

were followed by Bhimani and colleagues who found higher AUC for instability diagnosis when sagittal stress measurements were combined (AP and posteroanterior [PA]: 0.91) in comparison to coronal stress (anterior and posterior: 0.73).[74] Currently, coronal values above 2.9 mm anteriorly and 3.4 mm posteriorly as well as sagittal values above 2.2 mm in the AP direction and 2.6 mm in the PA direction are considered pathologic.[75] Lubberts and colleagues created a syndesmotic assessment tool using sagittal and coronal translations and found a 3.1 mm threshold for instability diagnosis.[73]

Although presenting a vast 3D view capability, field increase, and dynamic properties, arthroscopy is not free of limitations.[54] Obviously, setting CL parameters for every patient is virtually impossible, what hinders the determination of a normality range in a particular case. Further, longitudinal (and some rotational) instabilities are not fully appreciated through the scope. The lack of good arthroscopy accuracy when assessing syndesmotic reduction from ankle fractures might be a sign that further technical development is necessary.[77]

Quality of Produced Data

The SR performed by Krahenbuhl and colleagues in 2018 on imaging instruments for syndesmotic injury used the Quality Assessment of Diagnostic Accuracy Studies 2 (QUADAS-2) tool found satisfactory methodological quality in the presented studies.[23] Low risk of bias ranged from 50% to 100% and low concerns on applicability from 90% to 100%.[23] The review performed by Raheman and colleagues used the Risk of Bias In Non-randomized Studies (ROBINS-1) tool to evaluate the role of WBCT in identifying unstable injuries and a low risk of bias was observed.[6]

DECISION-MAKING AND TREATMENT OPTION

A review of the studies on the treatment of syndesmotic instability (nonfractured) can be found in **Table 2**. Although general literature is presented in the table, the text focuses on the acute syndesmosis instabilities in the setting of the ankle sprain environment.

The degree of syndesmotic ligament injury—instability parameters—guides the decision-making between operative and nonoperative treatment. Clinical diagnosis has limited evidence, the clinical tests show low accuracy rates for subtle syndesmotic instability; a SR concluded that clinicians could not rely on a single physical examination test to identify syndesmotic injury with certainty.[10] Bilateral comparative mortise and AP conventional radiographic views may be sufficient to demonstrate frank syndesmotic instability, classically defined by a relative widening of the TFCS on the injured ankle. However, subtle syndesmotic instability can be under- or misdiagnosed when CRs show a relatively normal TF relationship.[12]

Conventional bilateral CT has greater sensitivity than radiography; however, the overall diagnostic accuracy is relatively low.[58] The conventional ankle CT scan with stress maneuvers (external rotation and dorsiflexion) in acute isolated syndesmotic instability, showed excellent performance for diagnosing subtle syndesmotic instability, as these positions show a greater accuracy and sensitivity in the ideal cutoff threshold compared with the neutral position (see **Fig. 1**).[51] Recently, WBCT has emerged as a new diagnostic modality. It is going to play a key role in solving the challenging issue of accurately diagnosing subtle syndesmotic instability. When asked if we already have the diagnostic tools to identify and distinguish which syndesmotic injuries are likely to cause clinically relevant instability, many authors state that the answer is still no.[4] The sensitivity and specificity of MRI for detecting syndesmotic

Table 2
Literature review of therapeutic interventions for syndesmosis lesions and instabilities

Study	Sample	Intervention	Results	Complications
Katznelson et al,[162] 1983	5 patients	TF fusion	5/5 good	1 dystrophy
Fritschy,[150] 1989	10 patients	7 Suture + Kwire/screw 3 WB cast 6 wk Direct reduction	9/10 good	1 residual instability (nonop group)
Miller et al,[163] 1995	4 patients	4.5 mm tetracortical screw Direct reduction	3 excellent 1 good	1 calcification
Ogilvie-Harris & Reed,[91] 1994	17 patients	Debridement	17/17 good	Not described
Miller et al,[137] 1999	26 cadavers	Suture construct Tricortical 3.5 mm screw 2 and 5 cm from joint Direct reduction	No differences in load and displacement 5cm stronger than 2 cm	Not assessed
Beumer et al,[151] 2000	9 patients	Chronic: one tetracortical screw and AITFL retensioning Direct reduction	9/9 stable Tegner and Karlsson scores improved	2 dystrophies 1 SPN entrapment
Wolf & Amendola[92] 2002	14 patients	Debridement + screw if unstable	12/14 good or excellent	Not reported
Grass et al,[164] 2003	16 patients	Chronic: PL graft + 1 screw Direct reduction	Karlsson: 88 TCS: 7.0 to 4.8 mm TFO: 3.6 to 6.5 mm CT-TFD: 6.2 to 3.0 mm	1 screw breakage 1 synostosis
Beumer et al,[165] 2005	5 patients	Chronic: one tetracortical screw + AITFL retensioning Direct reduction	Tegner and Karlsson scores improved No pre/postop difference in kinematics	Not assessed
Han et al,[49] 2007	20 patients	Chronic: 10 debridement + screw 10 debridement only Arthroscopic reduction	AOFAS and satisfaction improvement in both groups No difference	None

(continued on next page)

Table 2
(continued)

Study	Sample	Intervention	Results	Complications
Zamzami & Zamzam,[160] 2009	11 patients	Chronic: graft reconstruction + 4.5 mm screw Direct visualization	10/11 good Diastasis: 4.7 to 1.3 mm WPAS: 95.4	2 superficial infections
Schuberth et al,[166] 2008	6 patients	Debridement + 2/3 4.5 mm percutaneous screw Arthroscopic reduction	AOFAS: 32 increase MCS: −3.2 mm	2 synostoses
Morris et al,[167] 2009	8 patients	Chronic: graft reconstruction + 4.5 mm screw Direct visualization	VAS: 73 to 19 AOFAS: 85.4 SF36: 81 MFS: 89.3	1 fusion 1 superficial infection
Teramoto et al,[114] 2011	6 cadavers	One SB vs Two SB vs Anatomic SB vs screw Direct visualization	Single or double: o multidirectional stability. Anatomic: stable. Screw: rigid.	None
Wagener et al,[13] 2011	12 patients	Chronic: one tetracortical screw + AITFL retensioning Direct reduction	11/12 good or excellent 11/12 CR reduction AOFAS: 92	1 superficial infection
Olson et al,[168] 2011	10 patients	Chronic: TF fusion Direct reduction	AOFAS: 37 to 87 10/10 satisfaction	2 prominent implants 1 impingement
Yasui et al,[159] 2011	6 patients	Chronic: Graft reconstruction + 1 3.5 mm screw Direct reduction	AOFAS: 53 to 95 VAS: 95 to 4	None
Valkering et al,[169] 2012	4 patients	Debridement + 4.5 mm screw	3/4 improvement	None
Jain & Kearns,[170] 2014	5 patients	AITFL retensioning + 2 screws with a plate Direct reduction	AOFAS 88.4	1 SPN neuritis
Laver et al,[171] 2015	16 patients	PRP vs control	PRP: shorter RTP; less residual pain	Not reported

Study	N	Intervention	Outcomes	Complications
Ryan & Rodriguez,[172] 2015	19 patients	Chronic: debridement + 2/3 SB Arthroscopic reduction	AOFAS: 48 to 82 VAS: 6 to 1 79% RTP MCS: 5.4 to 4.6 mm TFO: 5.7 to 6.9 mm	1 prominent implant 1 saphenous irritation
Colcuc et al,[158] 2016	32 patients	Chronic 10 Grade I: AITFL suture 12 Grade II: periosteal flap 10 Grade III: plantaris graft All: 1 SB and 1 screw Direct reduction	AOFAS I: 67 to 93 II: 68 to 93 III: 53 to 86	1 superficial infection 2 granulomas
Calder et al,[18] 2016	64 patients	26 grade IIa: nonop 38 grade IIb: 1 SB Arthroscopic reduction	RTP: IIa 45 d; IIb 65 d	2 superficial infections 3 SB removal
LaMothe et al,[118] 2016	11 cadavers	SB vs screw Direct reduction	SB allowed more sagittal motion than screw Both: motion not restored to intact levels	Not reported
Schon et al,[128] 2017	24 cadavers	1 screw vs 1 SB vs 2 SB Direct reduction	All decreased volume from intact state 2 SB decreased more	Not reported
Forschner et al,[138] 2017	19 patients	2 SB Fluoroscopic reduction	AOFAS 100 17 good or excellent	1 failure 9 skin SB irritation 5 SB removal
Li et al,[161] 2019	16 cadavers	1 SB vs graft reconstruction Direct reduction	No differences in displacement, torque, or rotation	Not reported
Kent et al,[157] 2020	138 patients	66 acute vs 43 subacute vs 29 chronic Several fixation types (screws, SB, and graft) Direct reduction	Lower FAOS in chronic patients (−20.7)	Not reported
Kwon et al,[154] 2020	68 patients	1 SB + AITFL tape augmentation Direct reduction	Not reported	1 delayed healing 1 SPN praxia 1 DVT

(continued on next page)

Table 2
(continued)

Study	Sample	Intervention	Results	Complications
Canton et al,[122] 2021	6 patients	2 screws vs 2 SB vs hybrid	DBR No difference in kinematics and ligament elongation All failed to restore the NI parameters FAAM: 95 and 88	Not described
Elghazy et al,[173] 2021	20 patients	1/2 screws vs 1/2 SB	PROMIS: no difference WBCT Screw: area higher than NI SB: area, rotation and anterior higher than NI	Not reported
Schermann et al,[141] 2022	15 cadavers	AITFL tape augmentation vs AITFL tape + 1 SB vs AITFL tape + 2 SB vs 2 SB Direct reduction	1 or 2 SB did not restore stability Tape + 1 SB was similar to intact stage	Not reported
Kingston et al,[174] 2022	70 patients	Chronic: 32 TF fusions vs 38 debridement + 2 SB Direct reduction	AOFAS and Kellgran: no differences No TAR or AA	HWR: 6 fusion vs 1 SB Revision: 2 vs 1 Impingement: 2 vs 1 Infection: 1 vs 0
Altmeppen et al,[175] 2022	41 patients	21 SB vs 20 3.5 mm screw (1) Direct reduction	OMAS and FADI: no difference	20 screw removals 9 SB removals
Takahashi et al,[117] 2022	10 cadavers	1 SB vs 1 SB + AITFL tape augmentation vs 1 SB + PITFL tape augmentation Direct reduction	SB alone did note restore rotation (2.98) SB + augmentation restored NI state	Not reported

Abbreviations: AA, ankle arthrodesis; AITFL, anterior inferior tibiofibular ligament; AOFAS, American Orthopedic Foot and Ankle Society score; CR, conventional radiograph; CT-TFD, compute tomographic tibiofibular distance; DBR, dynamic biplane radiography; DVT, deep vein thrombosis; FAAM, foot and ankle ability measure; FADI, foot and ankle disability index score; FAOS, foot and ankle outcome score; HWR, hardware removal; MFS, maryland foot score; NI, noninjured; Nonop, nonsurgical treatment; OMAS, Olerud-Molander ankle score; PITFL, posterior inferior tibiofibular ligament; PL, peroneal longus; PROMIS, patient-reported outcome measurement information system; PRP, platelet-rich plasma; RTP, return to play; SB, suture buttons; SF36, 36-item short form survey; SPN, superficial peroneal nerve; TAR, total ankle replacement; TCS, total clear space; TF, tibiofibular; TFO, total fibular overlapping; VAS, visual analog score; WB, weight-bearing; WBCT, weight-bearing compute tomography; WPAS, west point ankle score.

injury is virtually 100%. However, because MRI is a static non-weightbearing test, findings do not directly correlate with the presence of syndesmotic instability.[23]

The ESSKA-AFAS consensus on syndesmotic injuries (2016) distinguishes the acute lesions between stable and unstable:[86,87]

- A stable lesion is characterized by an AITFL lesion, with or without IOL lesion, with a competent deltoid ligament.
- An unstable lesion usually combines with a deltoid ligament lesion and is divided into latent or frank diastasis.
  ○ The latent diastasis combines the AITFL rupture with or without IOL and deltoid ligament rupture.
  ○ In frank diastasis all the syndesmotic and deltoid ligaments are ruptured.

Based on this anatomic ligament rupture classification system, there is a consensus that a stable lesion can be treated with conservative measures, which includes a non-WB period followed by protected partial WB and a rehabilitation protocol. Progress through the phases is determined by symptom severity and individual response to treatment.[86,87] However, the controversy in the treatment algorithm remains on how to distinguish especially between on subtle or latent unstable lesions—stable and or unstable lesions.[18]

Surgical Treatment

Arthroscopic assessment
Not only still necessary to confirm the instability, but also to check for associated injuries, clean the joint, and help in the reduction, arthroscopy is a constant step when operating unstable syndesmosis.[88,89] A complete examination, including possible osteochondral lesions, loose bodies, medial and lateral instability should be carried out (please check the Multidirectional chapter on this edition).[89] The TF incisura and the medial gutters need debridement (mild in the acute scenario, more aggressive in the chronic) to optimize reduction and postoperative symptoms.[90] Literature is skeptical when describing debridement as the only treatment for instability, which should not be an option in an unstable joint.[91,92]

Tibiofibular reduction
Research on the reduction capability of different techniques and devices is much focused on the fractured scenario, which might not translate the nuances and particularities of a pure ligamentous instability.[93] However, most of the principles and objectives are the same.[7] Fluoroscopy, used by some authors to check reduction when using percutaneous or arthroscopic-assisted approaches, does not seem to be sufficient.[94,95] Abarca and colleagues used the lateral fluoroscopy of both ankles and found differences in AP fibular distance higher 0.161 having 100% Sn and 97.2% Sp for malreduction.[96] In the work of Koenig and colleagues, surgeons had difficulty in recognizing a 2.5 mm posterior fibular displacement.[94] External rotation was also poorly detected by radiographic indices according to Marmor and colleagues[95] The use of intraoperative 3D imaging might change this perspective in the near future.[97] Cunnningham and colleagues reported a change in 47% of syndemosis reductions after surgeons were presented with 3D fluoroscopic imaging and only 10% malreduction rate in the postoperative CT confrontation.[98] An intraoperative 3D scan was used by Franke and colleagues who observed a 30.7% improvement in TF reductions.[99]

Considering the facts already discussed in this article on the limitations of arthroscopy in diagnosing instability, the same obstacles are present to this technique when used for syndesmosis reduction.[77,100] Overcompression and rotation assessment are challenging throughout the scope.[37] Its use as an adjunctive tool seems more reliable, although this premise still needs to be confirmed.[37] Cassinelli and colleagues evaluated anterior and posterior TF relations and ligament apposition in a cadaveric model to find a 94% of correct reduced or malreduced diagnosis.[101]

Direct reduction presents lower rates of malreduction when compared with other methods according to the literature.[102,103] Visualization and reduction can be achieved through a traditional lateral or anterolateral fibular approach.[7] Few anatomic landmarks have been proposed to guide surgeons, but none became the standard, probably due to individual variabilities.[104] Reb and colleagues proposed the use of a TF line anteriorly to check reduction and found difficulties in the method's reliability.[105] When comparing direct visualization to palpation in cadavers, Pang and colleagues found no differences in the rate of malreduction.[106]

The use of clamps, especially in closed approaches, might lead to malreduction in up to 50% of cases.[107,108] Cosgrove and colleagues and Putnam and colleagues proposed optimal clamp positioning at the anterior medial third of the tibia and 23% of the AP tibia distance, respectively.[107,109] However, a latter study by Cosgrove and colleagues that used CT to determine clamp placement showed a higher risk of malreduction and overcompression when compared with manual digital reduction.[110] A glide-path technique, described Needleman and Harris and colleagues, uses a 1.6 mm wire along the transmalleolar axis to stabilize the fibula in relation to the tibia, allowing a potential more anatomic translation when the construct is fixed.[111,112] The authors found a decrease in malreduction from 44% to 12.5% when using the technique.[111]

Although direct reduction thorough an open approach can be considered the most precise method to reduce the syndesmosis nowadays, it is far from being perfect.[113] No CL templating is available so individual parameters can be respected.[54] Further, rotation and length are still very challenging to be properly corrected and verified even in this scenario.[113] The capability of a flexible implant (or a rigid one when removed) to allow a natural TF relation restauration is debatable. Nonetheless, the range (if any) of an acceptable reduction and the functional impact of potential suboptimal TF interfaces still need more data to clinically support any recommendation. The authors prefer direct reduction assisted by arthroscopy and fluoroscopy. Direct thumb pressure and the glide-path techniques are our preferences. After temporary k-wire stabilization, anatomic landmarks (trifurcation, incisura placement) should be checked as well as lateral and AP views. Not only the relation between tibia and fibula is important, but also the talar position within the mortise in all planes. Ankle range of motion and TF behavior under stress (using the diagnostic tests) might also provide clues if a syndesmosis is not properly reduced.

Screws

The most historical method of syndesmosis stabilization, screw configurations fell into disrepute in the early 2010s when the results of suture button (SB) started to be published.[114–116] Inability of SB to completely restoring TF stability, particularly in the longitudinal and rotational planes, brought the screws back to attention.[117,118] Nowadays, screws constructs have good literature to support their use in severely unstable TF joints, Maisonneuve or high fibula fractures when osseous fixation is not indicated, and other longitudinal patterns where length might be compromised.[93,119–121] These situations also allow the use of hybrid fixation, consisting of a combination of screws and flexible implants.[122,123] Clinical perspective of more recent randomized trials and SRs showed SB superiority over screws although not all studies were not homogenous.[124–127] Screws do not seem to restore TF area, stability, and kinematics in cadaveric models.[122,128] Although it seems more logical that in a nonfracture pure ligamentous instability scenario, flexible implants should be a clear option, this idea is loosely supported by evidence. Lack of specific studies for this condition and contradictory data on the fractured universe are the main issues when making this recommendation.

When using screws, care should be taken when inserting the implants as they were shown to be less forgiving the flexible implants, permitting syndesmotic malreduction while being introduced.[129] The number of screws, its diameter and if they engage three or four cortices do not seem to affect outcomes in a general population.[130,131] Still, for the nonfractured scenario, placement of (at least) two slightly divergent screws must be considered based on the potential highly unstable situation (**Fig. 6**). Screws placed 2 to 5 cm proximal to the tibial plateau and having approximately 30° of anterior angulation seems to respect good parameters.[132] Considering the demographic profile of patients undergoing surgery for syndesmosis instability, hardware removal should always be considered (4 to 6 months after the procedure) to reestablish adequate motion, good kinematics and prevent implant breakage.[88] Once again, literature is controversy when hardware removal is discussed; however, a recent trial showed no superiority on routine screw removal.[133,134] Bioabsorbable and breakable screws might become an option in a near future, but current data are not able to support its use in favor of other implants.[135,136]

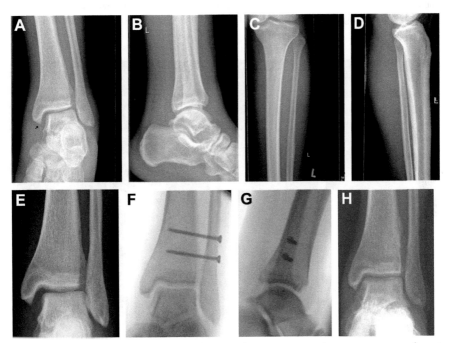

Fig. 6. A 42-year-old male patient who fell with his scooter. Imaging at emergency department without clear fracture of the fibula (*A–D*), a minute avulsion medially and some widening at the medial clear space (MCS). Stress image (*E*) showing frank widening at the MCS. Intraoperative imaging (*E, F*) demonstrates screw placement. Via an anterolateral approach the syndesmosis was cleaned and reduced, temporary wires were placed and two 3.5 mm screws inserted tricortically. One year follow-up image after removal of syndesmotic screws at patient's request (*H*), with a good outcome.

Suture-button

The use of flexible syndesmotic constructions was first attempted by Miller and colleagues in an attempt to offer the TF interface a more physiologic motion while maintaining stability.[137] Since then, the advent of SB constructs completely changed the field and became the standard of care for surgeons.[126,138] Biomechanical studies are contradictory in giving the superiority of SB in relation to screws, particularly the more recent ones.[114,118,128] As discussed above, functionally, SB seems to present better outcomes than the use of screws.[126,139] Lower removal rates (while far from being zero) can support some of the cost-effectiveness' claims in favor of SB over screws.[140] Although not clinically translated yet, recent cadaveric studies showed that SB constructs alone (even when using more than one implant) were not capable of completely restoring TF stability.[117,141] These findings might support the use of SB in conjunction with screws or ligament augmentations considering different circumstances; however, this possibility still needs endorsement.

Notwithstanding the more tolerant characteristic of SB, some of the screw principles for placement should be applied.[5] Placement at 1.5 to 3 cm from the joint in a 20° to 30° anterior inclination has been advocated.[142,143] It is not impossible to malreduce or overcompress the TF with SB.[127,144] The same care, clinical, and imaging meticulous assessment when inserting screws must be replicated in the button scenario (**Fig. 7**).[142] Buttons that rely on the medial tibial cortex for anchorage place the saphenous bundle in risk.[145,146] An approach over the exit point can protect the surrounding structures and allow the local periosteal to be removed and the implant properly seated against the cortex (impeding late reabsorption and potential loss of

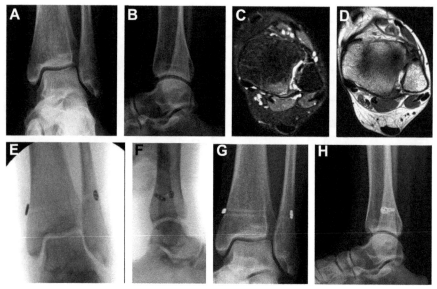

Fig. 7. A 24-year-old female patient who fell and twisted her ankle on the trampoline. Imaging (A, B) obtained at the emergency department showed no fracture distally at the ankle or proximally at the fibula. She was treated conservatively as a sprained ankle. Patient remained symptomatic and an MRI imaging performed at 6 months (C, D) showed anterior and posterior syndesmosis injury. Intraoperative imaging with suture button fixation (E, F) and reefing of the anterior ligaments. Follow-up imaging at 1 year (G, H). The button was removed at the patient's request after 3 years and she had no more complaints.

tension).[143] Although the literature is yet undefined, two slightly divergent SB seem to have a good indication for syndesmotic instability.[147,148] The use of an appropriate lateral plate for the suture-buttons might prevent skiving and fibular stress fractures.[143] As discussed before, longitudinal and severe rotational TF instabilities are not properly stabilized with SB and remain relative contra-indications for its use in isolation.[117,149]

Ligament augmentation

TF ligament repair, tensioning, and reconstruction are also not a novelty in the syndesmosis literature.[13,150,151] Attention has been drawn to the technique over the last few years due to the unsatisfactory biomechanical behavior of SB and screws in TF stability.[117,118,122] Cadaveric studies have been showing superior performance rotationally when an AITFL augmentation is included in an SB construct.[117,141,152,153] Small case series showed good functional results and low complications with the technique.[154,155] Direct repair using suture anchors and synthetic tape or biosynthetic AITFL reconstruction are currently available options.[154,155] Basic concepts of ligament augmentation must be respected, such as the understanding of anatomic footprints and adequate construction tension.[156]

Graft reconstruction

Commonly selected in a chronically unstable scenario, syndesmotic ligament reconstructions using allografts or autografts were presented by few authors.[157–160] Despite the fact good outcomes were reported, no prospective comparative study comparing graft reconstruction with other methods was performed for specific timelines and scenarios. Kent and colleagues were able to demonstrate that chronic patients that underwent graft reconstruction had worse outcomes when compared with SB and screws, but the finding is biased by the nature of the lesion.[157] This is also usually the case when the graft is chosen for more severe cases.[158] A cadaveric study showed similar kinematics.[161] However, there is no proof that native ligaments cannot heal if enough stability and reduction are obtained, even in the chronic situation.

Quality of Produced Data

Many studies combine syndesmosis instabilities in the fracture and the nonfractured scenario to increase the sample number, a characteristic that difficult therapeutic conclusions. The SR performed by Krahenbuhl and colleagues in 2019 on treatment interventions for syndesmotic chronic instabilities used the Coleman score to assess studies' methodology and found the quality to be satisfactory.[139]

Marasco and colleagues, in his overview of SRs, were unreserved in determining the fragility of the produced data regarding the comparison among rigid and flexible fixations.[124] The SRs produced contradicting data in regards of clinical results and complications.[124] Further, the overview stated that a change in outcomes from a very small proportion of the sample could produce completely different conclusions.[124]

AUTHORS' PREFERRED SURGICAL STRATEGY

Much controversy and low quality data inhabit the surgical treatment of nonfractures acute syndesmosis instability.[139] The authors endorse, when syndesmosis instability is questioned and confirmed by arthroscopy (and stress views), a complete joint examination needs to be carried in search of associated injuries, such as medial instability, lateral instability, loose bodies, and osteochondral lesions. When facing such conditions, surgical treatment of all in conjunction with the syndesmosis is needed to prevent late instabilities and osteoarthrosis (please check the Multidirectional

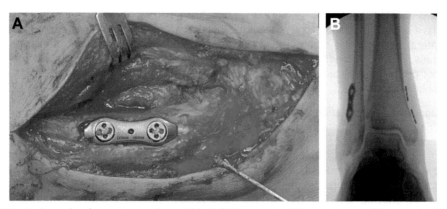

Fig. 8. Example of an acute syndesmotic instability operated through a lateral approach (*A*) for direct visualization of tibiofibular reduction. The syndesmosis was stabilized with two suture buttons (*B*) and an anterior tibiofibular ligament augmentation.

chapter on this edition). It is our preference to reduce and fix the TF articular by direct visualization, after a lateral or anterolateral approach. Arthroscopy can be added, but not used as the only source of reduction as discussed previously. We prefer securing the fibula in a glide-path position with 1 or more k-wires so intraoperative imaging and the scope are used to substantialize the reduction. After good positioning is confirmed, a two- or four-hole lateral plate can be added so two suture-buttons can be placed through it, in a slightly divergent direction in all planes. The authors advocate a medial incision when medial buttons are being used to protect the saphenous nerve and remove the underlying periosteum. To control fibular rotation, an AITFL reconstruction using synthetic tape or biosynthetic graft can be included in the construct (**Fig. 8**).[141]

SUMMARY

Although today we still have more questions than answers, we are undoubtedly much closer of obtaining proper preintervention instability diagnosis. Advancements in clinical assessment and imaging acquisitions are placing providers closer obtaining a correct diagnosis when injury and instability are suspected. Upcoming technological improvement and application are a bright light ahead of us. Better understanding of the extremally intricate syndesmosis anatomy and kinematics also provided much improvement in terms of therapeutic options for TF instability. As in any complex ligament injury, there is a trend toward reconstructions using proper footprints, careful implant placement, and optimal graft tension. The impact of new diagnostic and treatment options on the deleterious effects of a syndesmosis instability is still to be shown. However, the future is very exciting.

CLINICS CARE POINTS

- Clinical suspicion combined with a good physical examination is crucial to identify patients with a potential syndesmosis instability that will require further investigation.
- If available, providers should use all available subsidiary exams to help reaching a decision regarding a possible joint instability that will demand arthroscopic confirmation and

proper treatment. Advanced imaging (MRI and CT) is required since these modalities currently hold the higher accuracies for this condition. Potential adverse consequences of a syndesmotic instability support this profound analysis to obtain the most precise diagnosis.

- Arthroscopic evaluation should contemplate instability in different planes and directions. Associated injuries must also be considered.
- Direct tibiofibular reduction, confirmed by arthroscopy and fluoroscopy, seems to be more reliable than the other methods.
- For most syndesmotic instabilities, suture buttons combined with AITFL augmentation can safely secure the tibiofibular joint and offer a good environment for ligament healing.
- Longitudinal and severe instabilities must be treated with screws, which can be placed in conjunction with flexible implants. Suture buttons do not provide the required stability for these injuries' patterns.

DISCLOSURES

N.S.B. Mansur: American Orthopedic Foot and Ankle Society: Committee Member. Brazilian Orthopedic Foot and Ankle Society: Committee Member. A. L. Godoy-Santos: American Orthopedic Foot and Ankle Society: Committee Member. Brazilian Orthopedic Foot and Ankle Society: Committee Member. Stryker: Paid presenter or speaker, T. Schepers: Nothing to Disclosure. The present study did not receive any grant or funding.

REFERENCES

1. Rammelt S, Zwipp H, Grass R. Injuries to the distal tibiofibular syndesmosis: an evidence-based approach to acute and chronic lesions. Foot Ankle Clin 2008; 13(4):611–33, vii-viii.
2. Williams GN, Jones MH, Amendola A. Syndesmotic ankle sprains in athletes. Am J Sports Med 2007;35(7):1197–207.
3. Zalavras C, Thordarson D. Ankle syndesmotic injury. J Am Acad Orthop Surg 2007;15(6):330–9.
4. de Cesar Netto C, CORR Insights®. Can Weightbearing Cone-beam CT Reliably Differentiate Between Stable and Unstable Syndesmotic Ankle Injuries? A Systematic Review and Meta-Analysis. Clin Orthop Relat Res 2022. https://doi.org/10.1097/corr.0000000000002223.
5. Corte-Real N, Caetano J. Ankle and syndesmosis instability: consensus and controversies. EFORT Open Rev 2021;6(6):420–31.
6. Raheman FJ, Rojoa DM, Hallet C, et al. Can Weightbearing Cone-beam CT Reliably Differentiate Between Stable and Unstable Syndesmotic Ankle Injuries? A Systematic Review and Meta-analysis. Clin Orthop Relat Res 2022;480(8): 1547–62.
7. Tourné Y, Molinier F, Andrieu M, et al. Diagnosis and treatment of tibiofibular syndesmosis lesions. Orthop Traumatol Surg Res 2019;105(8s):S275–86.
8. D'Hooghe P, Grassi A, Alkhelaifi K, et al. Return to play after surgery for isolated unstable syndesmotic ankle injuries (West Point grade IIB and III) in 110 male professional football players: a retrospective cohort study. Br J Sports Med 2020;54(19):1168–73.
9. Schottel PC, Baxter J, Gilbert S, et al. Anatomic Ligament Repair Restores Ankle and Syndesmotic Rotational Stability as Much as Syndesmotic Screw Fixation. J Orthop Trauma 2016;30(2):e36–40.

10. Sman AD, Hiller CE, Rae K, et al. Diagnostic accuracy of clinical tests for ankle syndesmosis injury. Br J Sports Med 2015;49(5):323–9.

11. Kellett JJ. The Clinical Features of Ankle Syndesmosis Injuries: A General Review. Clin J Sport Med 2011;21(6):524–9.

12. Nussbaum ED, Hosea TM, Sieler SD, et al. Prospective evaluation of syndesmotic ankle sprains without diastasis. Am J Sports Med 2001;29(1):31–5.

13. Wagener ML, Beumer A, Swierstra BA. Chronic instability of the anterior tibiofibular syndesmosis of the ankle. Arthroscopic findings and results of anatomical reconstruction. BMC Musculoskelet Disord 2011;12(1):212.

14. Ryan LP, Hills MC, Chang J, et al. The lambda sign: a new radiographic indicator of latent syndesmosis instability. Foot Ankle Int 2014;35(9):903–8.

15. Alonso A, Khoury L, Adams R. Clinical tests for ankle syndesmosis injury: reliability and prediction of return to function. J Orthop Sports Phys Ther 1998; 27(4):276–84.

16. Hopkinson WJ, St Pierre P, Ryan JB, et al. Syndesmosis sprains of the ankle. Foot Ankle 1990;10(6):325–30.

17. de César PC, Ávila EM, de Abreu MR. Comparison of Magnetic Resonance Imaging to Physical Examination for Syndesmotic Injury after Lateral Ankle Sprain. Foot Ankle Int 2011;32(12):1110–4.

18. Calder JD, Bamford R, Petrie A, et al. Stable Versus Unstable Grade II High Ankle Sprains: A Prospective Study Predicting the Need for Surgical Stabilization and Time to Return to Sports. Arthrosc 2016;32(4):634–42.

19. Ogilvie-Harris DJ, Reed SC. Disruption of the ankle syndesmosis: diagnosis and treatment by arthroscopic surgery. Arthroscopy 1994;10(5):561–8.

20. Kiter E, Bozkurt M. The crossed-leg test for examination of ankle syndesmosis injuries. Foot Ankle Int 2005;26(2):187–8.

21. Hunt KJ, Phisitkul P, Pirolo J, et al. High Ankle Sprains and Syndesmotic Injuries in Athletes. J Am Acad Orthopaedic Surgeons 2015;23(11):661–73.

22. Harper MC, Keller TS. A Radiographic Evaluation of the Tibiofibular Syndesmosis. Foot & Ankle 1989;10(3):156–60.

23. Krahenbuhl N, Weinberg MW, Davidson NP, et al. Imaging in syndesmotic injury: a systematic literature review. Skeletal Radiol 2018;47(5):631–48.

24. Ebraheim NA, Lu J, Yang H, et al. Radiographic and CT evaluation of tibiofibular syndesmotic diastasis: a cadaver study. Foot Ankle Int 1997;18(11):693–8.

25. Beumer A, van Hemert WL, Niesing R, et al. Radiographic measurement of the distal tibiofibular syndesmosis has limited use. Clin Orthop Relat Res 2004;423: 227–34.

26. Takao M, Ochi M, Oae K, et al. Diagnosis of a tear of the tibiofibular syndesmosis. J Bone Joint Surg Br 2003;85-B(3):324–9.

27. Schoennagel BP, Karul M, Avanesov M, et al. Isolated syndesmotic injury in acute ankle trauma: comparison of plain film radiography with 3T MRI. Eur J Radiol 2014;83(10):1856–61.

28. Gosselin-Papadopoulos N, Hébert-Davies J, Laflamme GY, et al. A New and More Sensitive View for the Detection of Syndesmotic Instability. J Orthop Trauma 2019;33(9):455–9.

29. Candal-Couto JJ, Burrow D, Bromage S, et al. Instability of the tibio-fibular syndesmosis: have we been pulling in the wrong direction? Injury 2004;35(8): 814–8.

30. Xenos JS, Hopkinson WJ, Mulligan ME, et al. The tibiofibular syndesmosis. Evaluation of the ligamentous structures, methods of fixation, and radiographic assessment. JBJS 1995;77(6):847–56.

31. LaMothe JM, Baxter JR, Karnovsky SC, et al. Syndesmotic Injury Assessment With Lateral Imaging During Stress Testing in a Cadaveric Model. Foot Ankle Int 2018;39(4):479–84.

32. Feller R, Borenstein T, Fantry AJ, et al. Arthroscopic Quantification of Syndesmotic Instability in a Cadaveric Model. Arthrosc 2017;33(2):436–44.

33. Bäcker HC, Vosseller JT, Bonel H, et al. Weightbearing Radiography and MRI Findings in Ankle Fractures. Foot Ankle Spec 2021;14(6):489–95.

34. He JQ, Ma XL, Xin JY, et al. Pathoanatomy and Injury Mechanism of Typical Maisonneuve Fracture. Orthop Surg 2020;12(6):1644–51.

35. Taweel NR, Raikin SM, Karanjia HN, et al. The proximal fibula should be examined in all patients with ankle injury: a case series of missed maisonneuve fractures. J Emerg Med 2013;44(2):e251–5.

36. Beard NM, Gousse RP. Current Ultrasound Application in the Foot and Ankle. Orthop Clin North Am 2018;49(1):109–21.

37. Wake J, Martin KD. Syndesmosis Injury From Diagnosis to Repair: Physical Examination, Diagnosis, and Arthroscopic-assisted Reduction. J Am Acad Orthop Surg 2020;28(13):517–27.

38. Mei-Dan O, Kots E, Barchilon V, et al. A Dynamic Ultrasound Examination for the Diagnosis of Ankle Syndesmotic Injury in Professional Athletes:A Preliminary Study. Am J Sports Med 2009;37(5):1009–16.

39. Hagemeijer NC, Saengsin J, Chang SH, et al. Diagnosing syndesmotic instability with dynamic ultrasound—establishing the natural variations in normal motion. Injury 2020;51(11):2703–9.

40. Shoji H, Teramoto A, Murahashi Y, et al. Syndesmotic instability can be assessed by measuring the distance between the tibia and the fibula using an ultrasound without stress: a cadaver study. BMC Musculoskelet Disord 2022;23(1). https://doi.org/10.1186/s12891-022-05221-z.

41. Hagemeijer NC, Lubberts B, Saengsin J, et al. Portable dynamic ultrasonography is a useful tool for the evaluation of suspected syndesmotic instability: a cadaveric study. Knee Surg Sports Traumatol Arthrosc 2022. https://doi.org/10.1007/s00167-022-07058-4.

42. Cha SW, Bae KJ, Chai JW, et al. Reliable measurements of physiologic ankle syndesmosis widening using dynamic 3D ultrasonography: a preliminary study. Ultrasonography 2019;38(3):236–45.

43. Salat P, Le V, Veljkovic A, et al. Imaging in Foot and Ankle Instability. Foot Ankle Clin 2018;23(4):499–522.e28.

44. Hermans JJ, Beumer A, Hop WCJ, et al. Tibiofibular syndesmosis in acute ankle fractures: additional value of an oblique MR image plane. Skeletal Radiol 2012;41(2):193–202.

45. Guyton GP, DeFontes K 3rd, Barr CR, et al. Arthroscopic Correlates of Subtle Syndesmotic Injury. Foot Ankle Int 2017;38(5):502–6.

46. Oae K, Takao M, Naito K, et al. Injury of the tibiofibular syndesmosis: value of MR imaging for diagnosis. Radiol 2003;227(1):155–61.

47. Clanton TO, Ho CP, Williams BT, et al. Magnetic resonance imaging characterization of individual ankle syndesmosis structures in asymptomatic and surgically treated cohorts. Knee Surg Sports Traumatol Arthrosc 2016;24(7):2089–102.

48. Chun K-Y, Choi YS, Lee SH, et al. Deltoid Ligament and Tibiofibular Syndesmosis Injury in Chronic Lateral Ankle Instability: Magnetic Resonance Imaging Evaluation at 3T and Comparison with Arthroscopy. Korean J Radiol 2015;16(5):1096.

49. Han SH, Lee JW, Kim S, et al. Chronic Tibiofibular Syndesmosis Injury: The Diagnostic Efficiency of Magnetic Resonance Imaging and Comparative Analysis of Operative Treatment. Foot Ankle Int 2007;28(3):336–42.

50. Randell M, Marsland D, Ballard E, et al. MRI for high ankle sprains with an unstable syndesmosis: posterior malleolus bone oedema is common and time to scan matters. Knee Surg Sports Traumatol Arthrosc 2019;27(9):2890–7.

51. Rodrigues JC, Santos ALG, Prado MP, et al. Comparative CT with stress manoeuvres for diagnosing distal isolated tibiofibular syndesmotic injury in acute ankle sprain: a protocol for an accuracy- test prospective study. BMJ Open 2020;10(9):e037239.

52. Spennacchio P, Seil R, Gathen M, et al. Diagnosing instability of ligamentous syndesmotic injuries: A biomechanical perspective. Clin Biomech (Bristol, Avon) 2021;84:105312.

53. Kubik JF, Rollick NC, Bear J, et al. Assessment of malreduction standards for the syndesmosis in bilateral CT scans of uninjured ankles. Bone Joint J 2021; 103-b(1):178–83.

54. Hao KA, Vander Griend RA, Nichols JA, et al. Intraoperative Assessment of Reduction of the Ankle Syndesmosis. Curr Rev Musculoskelet Med 2022; 15(5):344–52.

55. Dikos GD, Heisler J, Choplin RH, et al. Normal tibiofibular relationships at the syndesmosis on axial CT imaging. J Orthop Trauma 2012;26(7):433–8.

56. Taser F, Shafiq Q, Ebraheim NA. Three-dimensional volume rendering of tibiofibular joint space and quantitative analysis of change in volume due to tibiofibular syndesmosis diastases. Skeletal Radiol 2006;35(12):935–41.

57. Malhotra G, Cameron J, Toolan BC. Diagnosing chronic diastasis of the syndesmosis: a novel measurement using computed tomography. Foot Ankle Int 2014; 35(5):483–8.

58. Ahn T-K, Choi S-M, Kim J-Y, et al. Isolated Syndesmosis Diastasis: Computed Tomography Scan Assessment With Arthroscopic Correlation. J Arthroscopic Relat Surg 2017;33(4):828–34.

59. Lepojärvi S, Niinimäki J, Pakarinen H, et al. Rotational Dynamics of the Normal Distal Tibiofibular Joint With Weight-Bearing Computed Tomography. Foot Ankle Int 2016;37(6):627–35.

60. Osgood GM, Shakoor D, Orapin J, et al. Reliability of distal tibio-fibular syndesmotic instability measurements using weightbearing and non-weightbearing cone-beam CT. Foot Ankle Surg 2019;25(6):771–81.

61. Shakoor D, Osgood GM, Brehler M, et al. Cone-beam CT measurements of distal tibio-fibular syndesmosis in asymptomatic uninjured ankles: does weight-bearing matter? Skeletal Radiol 2019;48(4):583–94.

62. Hamard M, Neroladaki A, Bagetakos I, et al. Accuracy of cone-beam computed tomography for syndesmosis injury diagnosis compared to conventional computed tomography. Foot Ankle Surg 2020;26(3):265–72.

63. Burssens A, Krähenbühl N, Weinberg MM, et al. Comparison of External Torque to Axial Loading in Detecting 3-Dimensional Displacement of Syndesmotic Ankle Injuries. Foot Ankle Int 2020;41(10):1256–68.

64. Auch E, Barbachan Mansur NS, Alexandre Alves T, et al. Distal Tibiofibular Syndesmotic Widening in Progressive Collapsing Foot Deformity. Foot Ankle Int 2021;42(6):768–75.

65. Del Rio A, Bewsher SM, Roshan-Zamir S, et al. Weightbearing Cone-Beam Computed Tomography of Acute Ankle Syndesmosis Injuries. J Foot Ankle Surg 2020;59(2):258–63.

66. Bhimani R, Ashkani-Esfahani S, Lubberts B, et al. Utility of Volumetric Measurement via Weight-Bearing Computed Tomography Scan to Diagnose Syndesmotic Instability. Foot Ankle Int 2020;41(7):859–65.
67. Ashkani Esfahani S, Bhimani R, Lubberts B, et al. Volume measurements on weightbearing computed tomography can detect subtle syndesmotic instability. J Orthop Res 2022;40(2):460–7.
68. de Carvalho KAM, Mallavarapu V, Ehret A, et al. The Use of Advanced Semiautomated Bone Segmentation in Hallux Rigidus. Foot Ankle Orthop 2022;7(4). 24730114221137597.
69. Dibbern KN, Li S, Vivtcharenko V, et al. Three-Dimensional Distance and Coverage Maps in the Assessment of Peritalar Subluxation in Progressive Collapsing Foot Deformity. Foot Ankle Int 2021;27. 1071100720983227.
70. Lintz F, Jepsen M, De Cesar Netto C, et al. Distance mapping of the foot and ankle joints using weightbearing CT: The cavovarus configuration. Foot Ankle Surg 2020. https://doi.org/10.1016/j.fas.2020.05.007.
71. Dibbern K, Talaski G, Schmidt E, et al. Ankle syndesmotic instability assessment using a three-dimensional distance mapping algorithm: a cadaveric pilot WBCT study. J Foot Ankle 2022;16(3):190–4.
72. Cohen JF, Korevaar DA, Altman DG, et al. STARD 2015 guidelines for reporting diagnostic accuracy studies: explanation and elaboration. BMJ Open 2016; 6(11):e012799.
73. Lubberts B, Guss D, Vopat BG, et al. The arthroscopic syndesmotic assessment tool can differentiate between stable and unstable ankle syndesmoses. Knee Surg Sports Traumatol Arthrosc 2020;28(1):193–201.
74. Bhimani R, Lubberts B, Sornsakrin P, et al. Do Coronal or Sagittal Plane Measurements Have the Highest Accuracy to Arthroscopically Diagnose Syndesmotic Instability? Foot Ankle Int 2021;42(6):805–9.
75. Hagemeijer NC, Elghazy MA, Waryasz G, et al. Arthroscopic coronal plane syndesmotic instability has been over-diagnosed. Knee Surg Sports Traumatol Arthrosc 2021;29(1):310–23.
76. Massri-Pugin J, Lubberts B, Vopat BG, et al. Effect of Sequential Sectioning of Ligaments on Syndesmotic Instability in the Coronal Plane Evaluated Arthroscopically. Foot Ankle Int 2017;38(12):1387–93.
77. Lucas DE, Watson BC, Simpson GA, et al. Arthroscopic Evaluation of Syndesmotic Instability and Malreduction. Foot Ankle Spec 2016;9(6):500–5.
78. Teitz CC, Harrington RM. A biochemical analysis of the squeeze test for sprains of the syndesmotic ligaments of the ankle. Foot Ankle Int 1998;19(7):489–92.
79. Beumer A, Valstar ER, Garling EH, et al. External rotation stress imaging in syndesmotic injuries of the ankle: Comparison of lateral radiography and radiostereometry in a cadaveric model. Acta Orthop Scand 2003;74(2):201–5.
80. Kim S, Huh YM, Song HT, et al. Chronic tibiofibular syndesmosis injury of ankle: evaluation with contrast-enhanced fat-suppressed 3D fast spoiled gradient-recalled acquisition in the steady state MR imaging. Radiol 2007;242(1):225–35.
81. Femino JE, Vaseenon T, Phisitkul P, et al. Varus external rotation stress test for radiographic detection of deep deltoid ligament disruption with and without syndesmotic disruption: a cadaveric study. Foot Ankle Int 2013;34(2):251–60.
82. Lubberts B, Guss D, Vopat BG, et al. The effect of ankle distraction on arthroscopic evaluation of syndesmotic instability: A cadaveric study. Clin Biomech (Bristol, Avon) 2017;50:16–20.

83. Gosselin-Papadopoulos N, Hébert-Davies J, Laflamme GY, et al. Intraoperative Torque Test to Assess Syndesmosis Instability. Foot Ankle Int 2019;40(4): 408–13.

84. Mousavian A, Shakoor D, Hafezi-Nejad N, et al. Tibiofibular syndesmosis in asymptomatic ankles: initial kinematic analysis using four-dimensional CT. Clin Radiol 2019;74(7):571.e1–8.

85. Hagemeijer NC, Chang SH, Abdelaziz ME, et al. Range of Normal and Abnormal Syndesmotic Measurements Using Weightbearing CT. Foot Ankle Int 2019;40(12):1430–7.

86. van Dijk CN, Longo UG, Loppini M, et al. Classification and diagnosis of acute isolated syndesmotic injuries: ESSKA-AFAS consensus and guidelines. Knee Surg Sports Traumatol Arthrosc 2016;24(4):1200–16.

87. van Dijk CN, Longo UG, Loppini M, et al. Conservative and surgical management of acute isolated syndesmotic injuries: ESSKA-AFAS consensus and guidelines. Knee Surg Sports Traumatol Arthrosc 2016;24(4):1217–27.

88. Stenquist DS, Ye MY, Kwon JY. Acute and Chronic Syndesmotic Instability: Role of Surgical Stabilization. Clin Sports Med Oct 2020;39(4):745–71.

89. Rellensmann K, Behzadi C, Usseglio J, et al. Acute, isolated and unstable syndesmotic injuries are frequently associated with intra-articular pathologies. Knee Surg Sports Traumatol Arthrosc 2021;29(5):1516–22.

90. Kurokawa H, Li H, Angthong C, et al. APKASS Consensus Statement on Chronic Syndesmosis Injury, Part 2: Indications for Surgical Treatment, Arthroscopic or Open Debridement, and Reconstruction Techniques of Suture Button and Screw Fixation. Orthop J Sports Med Jun 2021;9(6). 23259671211021063.

91. Ogilvie-Harris DJ, Reed SC. Disruption of the ankle syndesmosis: Diagnosis and treatment by arthroscopic surgery. J Arthroscopic Relat Surg 1994;10(5):561–8. https://doi.org/10.1016/S0749-8063(05)80015-5.

92. Wolf BR, Amendola A. Syndesmosis injuries in the athlete: when and how to operate. Curr Opin Orthopaedics 2002;13(2):151–4.

93. Regauer M, Mackay G, Nelson O, et al. Evidence-Based Surgical Treatment Algorithm for Unstable Syndesmotic Injuries. J Clin Med 2022;11(2):331.

94. Koenig SJ, Tornetta P 3rd, Merlin G, et al. Can We Tell if the Syndesmosis Is Reduced Using Fluoroscopy? J Orthop Trauma 2015;29(9):e326–30.

95. Marmor M, Hansen E, Han HK, et al. Limitations of standard fluoroscopy in detecting rotational malreduction of the syndesmosis in an ankle fracture model. Foot Ankle Int 2011;32(6):616–22.

96. Abarca M, Besa P, Mora E, et al. The use of intraoperative comparative fluoroscopy allows for assessing sagittal reduction and predicting syndesmosis reduction in ankle fractures. Foot Ankle Surg 2022;28(6):750–5.

97. Beisemann N, Tilk AM, Gierse J, et al. Detection of fibular rotational changes in cone beam CT: experimental study in a specimen model. BMC Med Imaging Oct 19 2022;22(1):181.

98. Cunningham BA, Warner S, Berkes M, et al. Effect of Intraoperative Multidimensional Fluoroscopy Versus Conventional Fluoroscopy on Syndesmotic Reduction. Foot Ankle Int 2021;42(2):132–6.

99. Franke J, von Recum J, Suda AJ, et al. Intraoperative three-dimensional imaging in the treatment of acute unstable syndesmotic injuries. J Bone Joint Surg Am Aug 1 2012;94(15):1386–90.

100. Watson BC, Lucas DE, Simpson GA, et al. Arthroscopic Evaluation of Syndesmotic Instability in a Cadaveric Model. Foot Ankle Int 2015;36(11):1362–8.

101. Cassinelli SJ, Harris TG, Giza E, et al. Use of Anatomical Landmarks in Ankle Arthroscopy to Determine Accuracy of Syndesmotic Reduction: A Cadaveric Study. Foot Ankle Spec 2020;13(3):219–27.

102. Stenquist DS, Kwon JY. Strategies to Avoid Syndesmosis Malreduction in Ankle Fractures. Foot Ankle Clin 2020;25(4):613–30.

103. Miller AN, Carroll EA, Parker RJ, et al. Direct Visualization for Syndesmotic Stabilization of Ankle Fractures. Foot Ankle Int 2009;30(5):419–26.

104. Acevedo JI, Busch MT, Ganey TM, et al. Coaxial portals for posterior ankle arthroscopy. J Arthroscopic Relat Surg 2000;16(8):836–42.

105. Reb CW, Hyer CF, Collins CL, et al. Clinical Adaptation of the "Tibiofibular Line" for Intraoperative Evaluation of Open Syndesmosis Reduction Accuracy:A Cadaveric Study. Foot Ankle Int 2016;37(11):1243–8.

106. Pang EQ, Coughlan M, Bonaretti S, et al. Assessment of Open Syndesmosis Reduction Techniques in an Unbroken Fibula Model: Visualization Versus Palpation. J Orthop Trauma 2019;33(1):e14–8.

107. Cosgrove CT, Putnam SM, Cherney SM, et al. Medial Clamp Tine Positioning Affects Ankle Syndesmosis Malreduction. J Orthop Trauma 2017;31(8):440–6.

108. Miller AN, Barei DP, Iaquinto JM, et al. Iatrogenic syndesmosis malreduction via clamp and screw placement. J Orthop Trauma 2013;27(2):100–6.

109. Putnam SM, Linn MS, Spraggs-Hughes A, et al. Simulating clamp placement across the trans-syndesmotic angle of the ankle to minimize malreduction: A radiological study. Injury 2017;48(3):770–5.

110. Cosgrove CT, Spraggs-Hughes AG, Putnam SM, et al. A Novel Indirect Reduction Technique in Ankle Syndesmotic Injuries: A Cadaveric Study. J Orthop Trauma 2018;32(7):361–7.

111. Harris MC, Lause G, Unangst A, et al. Prospective Results of the Modified Glide Path Technique for Improved Syndesmotic Reduction During Ankle Fracture Fixation. Foot Ankle Int 2022;43(7):923–7.

112. Needleman RL. Accurate Reduction of an Ankle Syndesmosis With the "Glide Path" Technique. Foot Ankle Int 2013;34(9):1308–11.

113. Shaner AC, Sirisreetreerux N, Shafiq B, et al. Open versus minimally invasive fixation of a simulated syndesmotic injury in a cadaver model. J Orthopaedic Surg Res 2017;12(1). https://doi.org/10.1186/s13018-017-0658-0.

114. Teramoto A, Suzuki D, Kamiya T, et al. Comparison of different fixation methods of the suture-button implant for tibiofibular syndesmosis injuries. Am J Sports Med 2011;39(10):2226–32.

115. Schepers T. Acute distal tibiofibular syndesmosis injury: a systematic review of suture-button versus syndesmotic screw repair. Int Orthopaedics 2012;36(6):1199–206.

116. Inge SY, Pull Ter Gunne AF, Aarts CAM, et al. A systematic review on dynamic versus static distal tibiofibular fixation. Injury Dec 2016;47(12):2627–34.

117. Takahashi K, Teramoto A, Murahashi Y, et al. Comparison of Treatment Methods for Syndesmotic Injuries With Posterior Tibiofibular Ligament Ruptures: A Cadaveric Biomechanical Study. Orthop J Sports Med 2022;10(9). 23259671221122811.

118. LaMothe JM, Baxter JR, Murphy C, et al. Three-Dimensional Analysis of Fibular Motion After Fixation of Syndesmotic Injuries With a Screw or Suture-Button Construct. Foot Ankle Int 2016;37(12):1350–6.

119. Solan MC, Davies MS, Sakellariou A. Syndesmosis Stabilisation: Screws Versus Flexible Fixation. Foot Ankle Clin 2017;22(1):35–63.

120. Kortekangas T, Savola O, Flinkkila T, et al. A prospective randomised study comparing TightRope and syndesmotic screw fixation for accuracy and maintenance of syndesmotic reduction assessed with bilateral computed tomography. Injury 2015;46(6):1119–26.
121. Kortekangas TH, Pakarinen HJ, Savola O, et al. Syndesmotic fixation in supination-external rotation ankle fractures: a prospective randomized study. Foot Ankle Int 2014;35(10):988–95.
122. Canton SP, Gale T, Onyeukwu C, et al. Syndesmosis Repair Affects in Vivo Distal Interosseous Tibiofibular Ligament Elongation Under Static Loads and During Dynamic Activities. J Bone Joint Surg Am 2021;103(20):1927–36.
123. Kim GB, Park CH. Hybrid Fixation for Danis-Weber Type C Fractures With Syndesmosis Injury. Foot Ankle Int 2021;42(2):137–44.
124. Marasco D, Russo J, Izzo A, et al. Static versus dynamic fixation of distal tibiofibular syndesmosis: a systematic review of overlapping meta-analyses. Knee Surg Sports Traumatol Arthrosc 2021;29(11):3534–42.
125. Ræder BW, Stake IK, Madsen JE, et al. Randomized trial comparing suture button with single 3.5 mm syndesmotic screw for ankle syndesmosis injury: similar results at 2 years. Acta Orthopaedica 2020;91(6):770–5.
126. Ræder BW, Figved W, Madsen JE, et al. Better outcome for suture button compared with single syndesmotic screw for syndesmosis injury: five-year results of a randomized controlled trial. Bone Joint J 2020;102-b(2):212–9.
127. Lehtola R, Leskelä H-V, Flinkkilä T, et al. Suture button versus syndesmosis screw fixation in pronation-external rotation ankle fractures: A minimum 6-year follow-up of a randomised controlled trial. Injury 2021;52(10):3143–9.
128. Schon JM, Williams BT, Venderley MB, et al. A 3-D CT Analysis of Screw and Suture-Button Fixation of the Syndesmosis. Foot Ankle Int 2017;38(2):208–14.
129. Chen CY, Lin KC. Iatrogenic syndesmosis malreduction via clamp and screw placement. J Orthop Trauma 2013;27(10):e248–9.
130. Peek AC, Fitzgerald CE, Charalambides C. Syndesmosis screws: How many, what diameter, where and should they be removed? A literature review. Injury 2014/08/01/2014;45(8):1262–7. https://doi.org/10.1016/j.injury.2014.05.003.
131. Schepers T, van der Linden H, van Lieshout EM, et al. Technical aspects of the syndesmotic screw and their effect on functional outcome following acute distal tibiofibular syndesmosis injury. Injury Apr 2014;45(4):775–9.
132. McBryde A, Chiasson B, Wilhelm A, et al. Syndesmotic Screw Placement: A Biomechanical Analysis. Foot Ankle Int 1997;18(5):262–6.
133. Dingemans SA, Rammelt S, White TO, et al. Should syndesmotic screws be removed after surgical fixation of unstable ankle fractures? a systematic review. Bone Joint J 2016;98-b(11):1497–504.
134. Sanders FRK, Birnie MF, Dingemans SA, et al. Functional outcome of routine versus on-demand removal of the syndesmotic screw: a multicentre randomized controlled trial. Bone Joint J 2021;103-b(11):1709–16.
135. Ahmad J, Raikin SM, Pour AE, et al. Bioabsorbable screw fixation of the syndesmosis in unstable ankle injuries. Foot Ankle Int 2009;30(2):99–105.
136. van der Eng DM, Schep NW, Schepers T. Bioabsorbable Versus Metallic Screw Fixation for Tibiofibular Syndesmotic Ruptures: A Meta-Analysis. J Foot Ankle Surg Jul-Aug 2015;54(4):657–62.
137. Miller RS, Weinhold PS, Dahners LE. Comparison of tricortical screw fixation versus a modified suture construct for fixation of ankle syndesmosis injury: a biomechanical study. J Orthop Trauma 1999;13(1):39–42.

138. Förschner PF, Beitzel K, Imhoff AB, et al. Five-Year Outcomes After Treatment for Acute Instability of the Tibiofibular Syndesmosis Using a Suture-Button Fixation System. Orthopaedic J Sports Med 2017;5(4). 232596711770285.
139. Krähenbühl N, Weinberg MW, Hintermann B, et al. Surgical outcome in chronic syndesmotic injury: A systematic literature review. Foot Ankle Surg Oct 2019; 25(5):691–7.
140. Weber AC, Hull MG, Johnson AJ, et al. Cost analysis of ankle syndesmosis internal fixation. J Clin Orthopaedics Trauma 2019/01/01/2019;10(1):173–7. https://doi.org/10.1016/j.jcot.2017.08.008.
141. Schermann H, Ogawa T, Lubberts B, et al. Comparison of Several Combinations of Suture Tape Reinforcement and Suture Button Constructs for Fixation of Unstable Syndesmosis. J Am Acad Orthop Surg 2022;30(10):e769–78.
142. Andersen MR, Figved W. Use of Suture Button in the Treatment of Syndesmosis Injuries. JBJS Essent Surg Tech 2018;8(2):e13.
143. Güvercin Y, Abdioğlu AA, Dizdar A, et al. Suture button fixation method used in the treatment of syndesmosis injury: A biomechanical analysis of the effect of the placement of the button on the distal tibiofibular joint in the mid-stance phase with finite elements method. Injury 2022;53(7):2437–45.
144. Gonzalez T, Egan J, Ghorbanhoseini M, et al. Overtightening of the syndesmosis revisited and the effect of syndesmotic malreduction on ankle dorsiflexion. Injury 2017/06/01/2017;48(6):1253–7. https://doi.org/10.1016/j.injury.2017.03.029.
145. Reb CW, Brandão RA, Watson BC, et al. Medial Structure Injury During Suture Button Insertion Using the Center-Center Technique for Syndesmotic Stabilization. Foot Ankle Int 2018;39(8):984–9.
146. Lehtonen EJ, Pinto MC, Patel HA, et al. Syndesmotic Fixation With Suture Button: Neurovascular Structures at Risk: A Cadaver Study. Foot Ankle Spec 2020; 13(1):12–7.
147. Parker AS, Beason DP, Slowik JS, et al. Biomechanical Comparison of 3 Syndesmosis Repair Techniques With Suture Button Implants. Orthop J Sports Med Oct 2018;6(10). 2325967118804204.
148. Clanton TO, Whitlow SR, Williams BT, et al. Biomechanical Comparison of 3 Current Ankle Syndesmosis Repair Techniques. Foot Ankle Int 2017;38(2):200–7.
149. Ebramzadeh E, Knutsen AR, Sangiorgio SN, et al. Biomechanical Comparison of Syndesmotic Injury Fixation Methods Using a Cadaveric Model. Foot Ankle Int 2013;34(12):1710–7.
150. Fritschy D. An unusual ankle injury in top skiers. Am J Sports Med 1989;17(2): 282–5 [discussion: 285–6].
151. Beumer A, Heijboer RP, WPJ Fontijne, et al. Late reconstruction of the anterior distal tibiofibular syndesmosis: Good outcome in 9 patients. Acta Orthop Scand 2000;71(5):519–21.
152. Shoji H, Teramoto A, Suzuki D, et al. Suture-button fixation and anterior inferior tibiofibular ligament augmentation with suture-tape for syndesmosis injury: A biomechanical cadaveric study. Clin Biomech 2018/12/01/2018;60:121–6
153. Jamieson MD, Stake IK, Brady AW, et al. Anterior Inferior Tibiofibular Ligament Suture Tape Augmentation for Isolated Syndesmotic Injuries. Foot Ankle Int 2022;43(7):994–1003.
154. Kwon JY, Stenquist D, Ye M, et al. Anterior Syndesmotic Augmentation Technique Using Nonabsorbable Suture-Tape for Acute and Chronic Syndesmotic Instability. Foot Ankle Int 2020;41(10):1307–15.

155. Kim JS, Shin HS. Suture Anchor Augmentation for Acute Unstable Isolated Ankle Syndesmosis Disruption in Athletes. Foot Ankle Int 2021;42(9):1130–7.

156. Lan R, Piatt ET, Bolia IK, et al. Suture Tape Augmentation in Lateral Ankle Ligament Surgery: Current Concepts Review. Foot Ankle Orthop Oct 2021;6(4). 24730114211045978.

157. Kent S, Yeo G, Marsland D, et al. Delayed stabilisation of dynamically unstable syndesmotic injuries results in worse functional outcomes. Knee Surg Sports Traumatol Arthrosc 2020;28(10):3347–53.

158. Colcuc C, Fischer S, Colcuc S, et al. Treatment strategies for partial chronic instability of the distal syndesmosis: an arthroscopic grading scale and operative staging concept. Arch Orthop Trauma Surg 2016;136(2):157–63.

159. Yasui Y, Takao M, Miyamoto W, et al. Anatomical reconstruction of the anterior inferior tibiofibular ligament for chronic disruption of the distal tibiofibular syndesmosis. Knee Surg Sports Traumatol Arthrosc 2011;19(4):691–5.

160. Zamzami MM, Zamzam MM. Chronic isolated distal tibiofibular syndesmotic disruption: diagnosis and management. Foot Ankle Surg 2009;15(1):14–9.

161. Li H-Y, Zhou R-S, Wu Z-Y, et al. Strength of suture-button fixation versus ligament reconstruction in syndesmotic injury: a biomechanical study. Int Orthopaedics 2019;43(3):705–11.

162. Katznelson A, Lin E, Militiano J. Ruptures of the ligaments about the tibio-fibular syndesmosis. Injury 1983;15(3):170–2.

163. Miller CD, Shelton WR, Barrett GR, et al. Deltoid and syndesmosis ligament injury of the ankle without fracture. Am J Sports Med 1995;23(6):746–50.

164. Grass R, Rammelt S, Biewener A, et al. Peroneus Longus Ligamentoplasty for Chronic Instability of the Distal Tibiofibular Syndesmosis. Foot Ankle Int 2003; 24(5):392–7.

165. Beumer A, Valstar ER, Garling EH, et al. Kinematics before and after reconstruction of the anterior syndesmosis of the ankle. Acta Orthopaedica 2005;76(5): 713–20.

166. Schuberth JM, Jennings MM, Lau AC. Arthroscopy-Assisted Repair of Latent Syndesmotic Instability of the Ankle. J Arthroscopic Relat Surg 2008;24(8): 868–74. https://doi.org/10.1016/j.arthro.2008.02.013.

167. Morris MW, Rice P, Schneider TE. Distal tibiofibular syndesmosis reconstruction using a free hamstring autograft. Foot Ankle Int 2009;30(6):506–11.

168. Olson KM, Dairyko GH Jr, Toolan BC. Salvage of chronic instability of the syndesmosis with distal tibiofibular arthrodesis: functional and radiographic results. J Bone Joint Surg Am 2011;93(1):66–72.

169. Valkering KP, Vergroesen DA, Nolte PA. Isolated syndesmosis ankle injury. Orthopedics 2012;35(12):e1705–10.

170. Jain SK, Kearns SR. Ligamentous advancement for the treatment of subacute syndesmotic injuries. Report of a new technique in 5 cases. Foot Ankle Surg 2014;20(4):281–4.

171. Laver L, Carmont MR, McConkey MO, et al. Plasma rich in growth factors (PRGF) as a treatment for high ankle sprain in elite athletes: a randomized control trial. Knee Surg Sports Traumatol Arthrosc 2015;23(11):3383–92.

172. Ryan PM, Rodriguez RM. Outcomes and Return to Activity After Operative Repair of Chronic Latent Syndesmotic Instability. Foot Ankle Int 2015;37(2): 192–7.

173. Elghazy MA, Hagemeijer NC, Guss D, et al. Screw versus suture button in treatment of syndesmosis instability: Comparison using weightbearing CT scan. Foot Ankle Surg 2021;27(3):285–90.

174. Kingston KA, Lin Y, Bradley AT, et al. Salvage of Chronic Syndesmosis Instability: A Retrospective Review With Mid-Term Follow-Up. J Foot Ankle Surg
2022. S1067-2516(22)00205-00208.
175. Altmeppen JN, Colcuc C, Balser C, et al. A 10-Year Follow-Up of Ankle Syndesmotic Injuries: Prospective Comparison of Knotless Suture-Button Fixation and
Syndesmotic Screw Fixation. J Clin Med 2022;11(9):2524.

Multidirectional Chronic Ankle Instability: What Is It?

Cesar de Cesar Netto, MD, PhD[a,b,*], Victor Valderrabano, MD, PhD[c],
Nacime Salomão Barbachan Mansur, MD, PhD[a,d]

KEYWORDS

- Ankle • Lateral • Syndesmosis • Multidirectional • Combined • Rotational
- Instability • Sprain

KEY POINTS

- The high incidence of ankle sprains creates the perfect environment for the development of associated chronic ankle instabilities.
- Combined medial with lateral (rotational), lateral with syndesmosis, and medial with syndesmosis have been described in different clinical scenarios.
- Multidirectional chronic ankle instability can be defined by the association of lateral chronic ankle instability, medial chronic ankle instability (MCAI), and chronic syndesmotic instability.
- A high suspicion index for combined and multidirectional instabilities should be raised when evaluating simple sprains or presumed isolated ankle instability.
- Reconstruction of all ligament complexes in MCAI aims to restore global stability, improving pain and function.

BACKGROUND

The fact that chronic ankle instability (CAI) can occur in more than one plane is not something recently described.[1,2] As new patterns of ankle lesions, sprains, and mechanical behaviors were described by researchers, the topographical name was attributed to the instability (please check the distinct instabilities' articles in this same Foot and Ankle Clinics edition). Therefore, lateral complex ligament injuries producing recurrent inversion sprains were termed lateral chronic ankle instabilities (LCAI).[3–5] Deltoid ligament lesions causing medial giving away sensation or pain received the medial chronic ankle instability (MCAI) nomenclature.[6–8] Valderrabano

[a] University of Iowa, Carver College of Medicine, 200 Hawkins Drive, John PappaJohn Pavillion (JPP), Room 01066, Lower Level, Iowa City, IA 52242, USA; [b] Duke University Medical Center, USA; [c] Swiss Ortho Center & University of Basel, Schmerzklinik Basel, Swiss Medical Network, Hirschgässlein 15, 4010 Basel, Switzerland; [d] Escola Paulista de Medicina – Universidade Federal de São Paulo, 740 Botucatu Street, Sao Paulo, SP, Brazil 04023-062
* Corresponding author.
E-mail address: cesar-netto@uiowa.edu

Foot Ankle Clin N Am 28 (2023) 405–426
https://doi.org/10.1016/j.fcl.2023.01.012
1083-7515/23/© 2023 Elsevier Inc. All rights reserved.

and colleagues[9] described the rotational (rotational CAI) as the combination of LCAI and MCAI. Finally, chronic syndesmosis instability (CSI) was characterized as injuries occurring at the distal tibiofibular syndesmosis generating diastasis, pain, or abnormal fibular motion.[10,11]

Nowadays, we know these specific instabilities do not occur in a single direction and they usually extend beyond the coronal plane.[12–14] Lateral and medial ligaments also restrain the talar bone inside the mortise anteriorly and posteriorly.[15,16] Specific ligament bands in all complexes are responsible to stabilize the talus or fibula in the rotational plane.[17–19] When considering these concepts, the combination of chronic lateral, medial, or syndesmotic instabilities can happen and produce considerable clinical symptoms.[20–22] Some attention has been given to the combination of LCAI, MCAI, or SI, which have been called multidirectional CAI by some authors.[6,21,22] However, instabilities in all three "complexes" were recently described, challenging the proposed nomenclature, and potentially confusing the health care population. Attempts in defining some of these episodes as "rotational instabilities" brought more misunderstanding to the whole scenario.[23,24]

With that in mind, our objective in this review article was to assess the current literature on the combined CAI and multidirectional CAI. The analyses were performed in the chronic instability scenario while taking some of the acute concepts into consideration. We also proposed new definitions for the current nomenclature of chronic ankle instabilities.

COMBINED INSTABILITY

Associations among two topographical instabilities are common in the literature, having a longstanding background. Objectivating a more precise understanding, we recommend that combined CAI be used only for combinations of two of the three ligament complexes. **Table 1** summarizes the current literature on associated ankle instabilities.

Rotational Chronic Ankle Instability: Lateral Chronic Ankle Instability with Medial Chronic Ankle Instability

Studies explored the association between lateral chronic ankle instability (LCAI)and MCAI (**Fig. 1**) in the last decades. Valderrabano and colleagues[9] defined rotational CAI as the combined CAI of LCAI and MCAI. Hintermann and colleagues,[25] while describing adjunctive lesions in LCAI arthroscopies, found MCAI in 36% of their sample. The same authors repeated the arthroscopic evaluation in MCAI patients, finding a 77% of LCAI occurrence.[26] A medial and lateral ankle ligament repair was proposed by Buchorn and colleagues[27] to 81 patients having what he called "rotational" instability. They found 83% correlation between clinical presentation and arthroscopy findings for the instabilities.[27] Yasuda and colleagues performed a medial repair and a lateral reconstruction in patients having both LCAI and MCAI with good clinical results. Interestingly, preoperative MR imaging did not show deep deltoid striation in 29 of the 30 ankles.[16] Medial and lateral arthroscopic ligament repair was proposed by Vega and colleagues[24] when treating combined LCAI and MCAI with good results.

A few theories tried to elucidate why the medial ankle ligament complex (deltoid ligament and spring ligament) might become unstable in an LCAI condition.[22,28] The fact that some patients may not recall an eversion/external rotation moment occurring in isolation or within an inversion trauma can explain some of these occurrences.[24] The anterolateral talar dislocation in common sprains could also place continuous stress on the superficial and deep deltoid ligament.[29–31] Impingement between the

Table 1
Literature review on combined chronic ankle instabilities

Study	Type	Sample	Definition	Results
Hintermann et al,[25] 2002	Case Series	148 ankles Lateral	Physical examination and Arthroscopy	26% clinical LCAI and MCAI 36% arthroscopic LCAI and MCAI
Hintermann et al,[26] 2004	Case Series	52 ankles Medial	Arthroscopy	77% arthroscopic MCAI and LCAI Medial and lateral open repair 90% good results
Han et al,[87] 2007	Diagnostic Study	20 ankles Syndesmosis	MR imaging and Arthroscopy	25% associated CSI and LCAI
Teramoto et al,[39] 2008	Cadaveric	7 cadavers	Tracking system	Syndesmosis injury produced talar internal rotation
Choi et al,[20] 2008	Case Series	65 ankles Lateral	Physical examination, CR, MR imaging, and Arthroscopy	Lateral open repair 29.2% of combined LCAI and CSI 11.1 OR for unfavorable outcomes with CSI
Yoo[88] 2009	Case Report	1 ankle Lateral + Medial	Physical examination and Radiographs	Medial and lateral graft reconstruction Good result
Hua et al,[35] 2010	Case Series	81 ankles Lateral	Physical examination, CR, MR imaging, and Arthroscopy	Lateral open repair 6.9% of combined LCAI and CSI
Buchorn et al,[27] 2011	Case Series	81 ankles Lateral + Medial	Physical examination and Arthroscopy	Medial and lateral open repair AOFAS: 63–94 VAS: 4–2 Compl: 4%
Kim et al,[21] 2015	Comparative	276 ankles Lateral + Medial + Syndesmosis CLAI + CMAI + CSI: 5% CLAI + CMAI: 7% CLAI + CSI: 4%	Physical examination, MR imaging, and Arthroscopy	Medial and lateral open repair, syndesmosis fixation Unfavorable: LCAI + MCAI: 3.8 OR LCAI + CSI: 4 OR LCAI + MCAI + CSI: 11.7 OR

(continued on next page)

Table 1
(continued)

Study	Type	Sample	Definition	Results
Yasuda et al,[16] 2017	Case Series	30 ankles Lateral + Medial	Physical examination, Stress CR, MR imaging, and Arthroscopy	Open medial repair and lateral reconstruction Karlsson: 69–96 JSSF: 69–94 Varus: 16 –4° Valgus: 4–1° Anterior: 20–10 mm
Vega et al,[24] 2020	Case Series	13 ankles Lateral + Medial	Physical examination and Arthroscopy	Medial and lateral arthroscopic repair AOFAS: 77–100
Mansur et al,[22] 2021	Case Series	30 ankles Lateral + Medial	Physical examination and Arthroscopy	Medial and lateral arthroscopic repair AOFAS: 49–92 VAS: 7–1 Compl: 16%

Abbreviations: AOFAS, American Orthopaedic Foot and Ankle Society; Compl, complications; CR, conventional radiographs; CSI, chronic syndemosis instability; JSSF, Japanese Society for Surgery of the Foot score; LCAI, lateral chronic ankle instability; MCAI, medial chronic ankle instability; mm, millimeters; OR, odds-ratio; VAS, visual analog score.

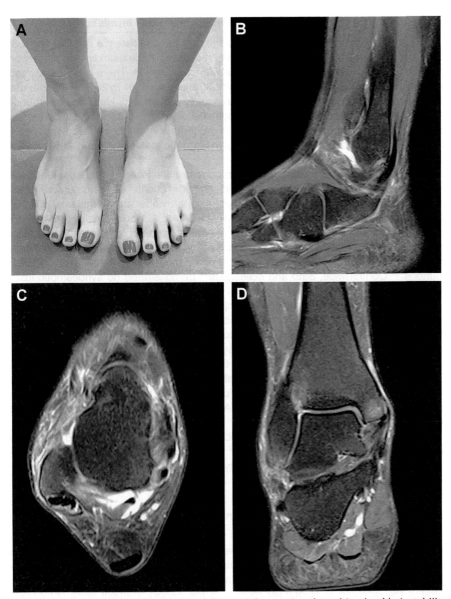

Fig. 1. Example of combined ankle instability, a right rotational combined ankle instability consisting of MCAI and lateral CAI. The patient is a ballet dancer (A) with a longstanding history of ankle sprains and failure with non-surgical treatments. MR imaging (T2 ponderation) demonstrates the lateral ligament injury in the sagittal (B) and axial (C) views. Deltoid superficial lesion can be noted in the axial cut (C), whereas the anterior layer of the deep deltoid is found incompetent in the coronal view (D).

talus and medial malleolus might also weaken the deep deltoid bands according to previous authors.[8] Although the notion that a lateral chronic unstable ankle (not only multiple sprains) should place more lasting tension on the medial ligaments (as a medial chronic instability also would place on the lateral ligaments) makes sense, this was never fully substantiated by biomechanical or clinical data.[31]

Lateral Chronic Ankle Instability with Chronic Syndesmosis Instability

There is a paucity of available studies addressing the coexistence of LCAI and CSI. Kim and colleagues,[21] whose study is further discussed in the multidirectional section, found a 4% lateral and syndesmosis instability combination. There is a classic association between ankle sprains and syndesmotic injuries in 10% to 20% of the traumas, but they do not translate into any definite instability pattern.[32–34] Hua and colleagues[35] described 6.9% syndesmotic injuries (not specified) in 81 ankles that underwent arthroscopic evaluation before a Bröstrom procedure. A diagnostic study assessing the MR imaging capability in predicting syndesmotic instability found 25% of LCAI in the studied cohort.[36]

An unstable lateral complex produces recurrent ankle inversion traumas that might predispose a patient to sprains in different directions as commented above (**Fig. 2**).[24,37] This can place the syndesmosis in jeopardy after an external rotation force. Superior translation of the talus as demonstrated in LCAI could employ stress at the tibiofibular joint.[29] Patel and colleagues[36] demonstrated fibular posterior translation when applying inversion stress to normal ankles, which increased when the syndesmosis was injured. Curiously, the motion was restored by screw fixation, but not by suture buttons.[36] Contrariwise, Sato and colleagues[38] demonstrated no syndesmotic instability in cadavers after the lateral ligaments were resected. When the interosseous ligament was transected, even partial lateral injuries produced an unstable syndesmosis.[38]

A hypermobile fibula in a CSI scenario could dispose the lateral ligament complex to injuries or persistent stretching. Teramoto and colleagues[39] showed an increase in cadaveric talar internal rotation when the syndesmosis was injured. However, Bhimani and colleagues[40] did not find instability at the lateral ligaments in cadavers with an unstable syndesmosis. When the anterior talofibular ligament (ATFL) was cut, progressive lateral instability was observed.[40] Further studies are still necessary to better understand the correlations between LCAI and CSI while establishing any potential etiological relation among them.

A varus hindfoot alignment can be observed in this population and should be considered during clinical evaluation.[41,42] This mechanical predisposition or associated condition contributes to the instability picture and could require a different strategy when present.[42,43]

Medial Chronic Ankle Instability with Chronic Syndesmosis Instability

Despite the fact that syndesmosis injuries are directly correlated to medial ankle ligament complex lesions in the ankle fracture scenario (**Fig. 3**), a concept still underestimated and forgotten by many orthopedic surgeons, this assumption in the "pure ligament" scenario is not completely substantiated.[44–47] Few cadaveric studies demonstrated the increase in tibiofibular motion as the deltoid ligament were combinedly sectioned with the syndesmotic structures.[48–50] Equivalently, medial instability was found to increase in the presence of an unstable syndesmosis.[30,50] In the clinical scenario, the deltoid injury was correlated to good accuracies when diagnosing CSI through MR imaging (please consult the article Nacime Salomão Barbachan Mansur and colleagues "High-Ankle Sprain and Syndesmotic Instability: How Far Have We Come with Diagnosis and Treatment?" for further details).[51,52] Further, clinical guidelines suggest medial assessment and treatment when treating CSI.[53,54] In MCAI patients, the syndesmosis should also be evaluated in search for latent CSI.[6,7]

Loss in the medial constraints could change the syndesmotic kinematic as the talus increases lateral translation, valgus, and external rotation in this situation.[23,30,55,56] This idea was only corroborated by limited articles that demonstrated syndesmosis

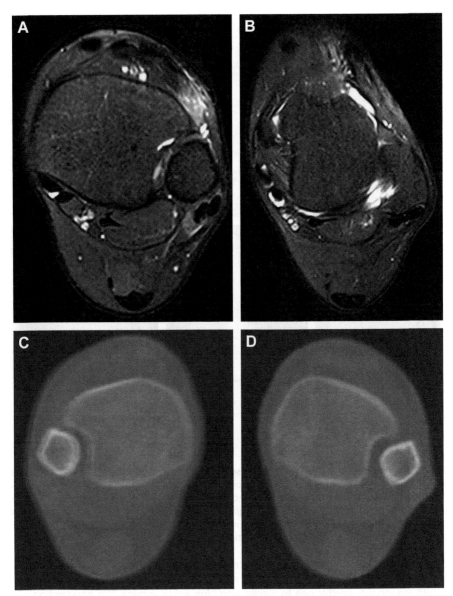

Fig. 2. A professional dancer with a confirmed left combined ankle instability, lateral CAI, and CSI. Axial views from the MR imaging (T2 ponderation) display prior injury to the AITFL and the interosseus (*A*) as well as undefinition of the ATFL (*B*). Bilateral comparative WBCT axial cuts demonstrate tibiofibular relations in the non-injured (*C*) and injured (*D*) sides.

instability after isolated deltoid ligament transection.[30,57] Other studies found an adjunctive syndesmotic ligament lesion, anterior inferior tibiofibular ligament (AITFL) for instance, necessary for the establishment of tibiofibular instability.[58–60]

Combined MCAI and CSI might occasionally be clinically identified through a hind-foot valgus or an asymmetrical progressive collapsing foot deformity.[26,61,62] Delayed

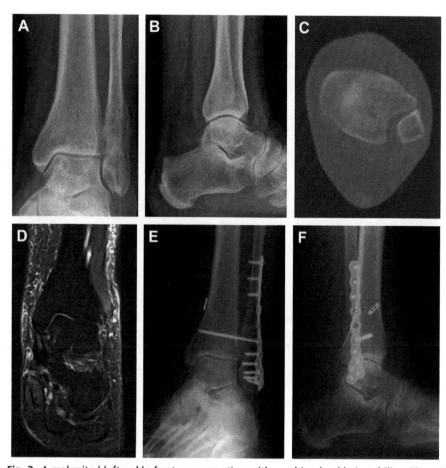

Fig. 3. A malunited left ankle fracture presenting with combined ankle instability, CSI and MCAI. Conventional radiographs (*A, B*) depict the shortened and rotated lateral malleolus. WBCT axial view (*C*) shows a malpositioned syndesmosis, with diastasis, anterior displacement, and rotation of the fibula. R imaging (T2 ponderation) exhibits chronic injury to the superficial and deep layers of the deltoid ligament (*D*). Fibular, medial, and syndesmosis reconstructions were performed in this patient (*E, F*).

presentations can produce or deteriorate malignment in patients with chronic medial and syndesmotic injuries.[6,7,26] Although a collapsed arch and a valgus of the hindfoot could reasonably predispose to medial and high ankle sprains, this assumption was never substantiated.

MULTIDIRECTIONAL CHRONIC ANKLE INSTABILITY

The term has been used by four studies, three clinical and one cadaveric. Teramoto and colleagues[39] hypothesized that syndesmosis injuries could cause MD-CAI. The authors tested motion between the tibia, fibula, and talus after syndesmotic lesions and found an increase in the talar internal rotation (7.1° to 9.4°) after the AITFL.[39] Kim and colleagues[21] used the nomenclature to describe associations between two or more types of instabilities. The authors found this pattern in 16.3% of their 231 patients, whereas 5% had the three instabilities altogether.[21] By fixing the syndesmosis with a button and repairing medial and lateral ligaments, they found that patients with combined MCAI and CSI had higher chances of negative outcomes.[21] Mansur and colleagues[22] named as multidirectional his sample of 29 patients (30 ankles) with lateral and medial instabilities. The conditions were determined by a combination of clinical and arthroscopic evaluation.[22] The authors proposed an arthroscopic repair of the ATFL and superficial deltoid with good results and a low complication rate.[22]

Although these three studies used multidirectional to quote their findings, they all defined instabilities and presented results by dealing with two of the three ligament complexes.[22,39] In a diagnostic study, Schafer and colleagues[63] proposed that the available tests would be able to detect a multidirectional pattern of instability. However, the authors never clearly defined what this would be.[63] We believe that the name MD-CAI should be used only for cases where a complete association of LCAI, MCAI, and CSI is found.

Only one study reported the presentation of LCAI, MCAI, and CSI in conjunction so far (Kim and colleagues[21]), but few tried to correlate ligament injuries. When assessing the time to return to play in 147 patients undergoing acute grade III lateral ligament repair, Hong and colleagues[64] observed 7% of deltoid injuries and 4% of syndesmosis instabilities. In the MR imaging performed after ankle sprains, Debieux and colleagues[65] described the coexistence between lateral and medial lesions as being 45% and among lateral and syndesmosis as 11%. Chun and colleagues[52] retrospectively reviewed MR imaging from 50 patients undergoing surgical LCAI treatment. They found deltoid injuries in 36% and syndesmotic injuries in 42% of the cohort, with a high accuracy for arthroscopic confirmation. Athletes (n = 261) having an MR imaging after an ankle sprain were reviewed by Roemer and colleagues,[34] who described 20.3% injuries to the syndesmosis and 49% to the deltoid. Jeong and colleagues[66] studied MR imagings from 36 patients with acute deltoid injury finding concomitant syndesmosis tear in 55% and lateral ligament rupture in 44%. Schafer and colleagues,[1] when evaluating adjunctive findings in 110 LCAI arthroscopies, found 32% of deltoid and 7% of syndesmosis lesions. The same authors repeated the evaluation in 148 patients when deltoid and syndesmosis lesions were seen in 40% and 9%, respectively.[25]

None of these studies directly reported the number of patients having structural injuries in the three topographies concurrently. Nevertheless, based on the presented numbers, it would be fair to conclude that multifilamentary injuries are present in a substantial portion of ankle sprains, which could be a potential source for CMAI. Further, the deleterious effect of isolated LCAI, MCAI, or CSI in its neighboring structures might also take some of the blame for MCAI development as explained above.[21,29]

AUTHORS' PREFERRED MANAGEMENT
Preoperative Assessment

Any patient having an established or suspected diagnosis of isolated LCAI, MCAI, or CSI should be considered and investigated for potential MD-CAI. A full clinical evaluation (please also check the articles of the correspondent instabilities), starting with a complete anamnesis inquiring about prior traumas to ankle, injury mechanisms, and sprain directions should be carried out. Questioning regarding anteromedial and syndesmotic pain as well as the instability pattern (inversion, medial giving away, dynamic collapse) is important to raise suspicion on the different presentations.[5,67]

Gutters and syndesmosis (distal to proximal) palpations might indicate pain that could be correlated to impingement and chronic regional instability.[26,68,69] The lateral complex is evaluated through the anterolateral drawer test and the varus stress test.[67,70] Although potentially negative in the chronic scenario, the syndesmosis is addressed with the Pillings test, the external rotational test, and the fibula drawer test.[11] Medial instability is tested using the eversion stress test, eversion-external rotation test, Kleiger test, and anteromedial drawer test.[5,6] An actual full anterior drawer should raise suspicion of combined medial and lateral instabilities due to the loss of both restraints (**Fig. 4**).[70]

Weight-bearing comparative (bilateral) conventional foot, ankle, and hindfoot radiographs, although very unspecific, can demonstrate syndesmotic diastasis, anteroposterior fibular displacement, talar tilting, bone impingement, and peritalar subluxation, suggesting the aforementioned instabilities.[51,71] More subtle changes in the syndesmotic interaction (**Fig. 5**) and overall alignment can be noted with a weight-bearing computed tomography (WBCT).[28,72] Stress acquisitions can be added to increase the diagnostic capability of radiographs and WBCT.[72,73] In our opinion, MR imaging is crucial when assessing any ankle instability or the possibility of MCAI due to its plethora of potential findings, including chronic ligament injuries and associated lesions that might increase clinical suspicions (**Fig. 6**).[51,74,75]

Even with negative clinical and imaging results, the multidirectional suspicion must be carried to the operating room. The surgeon should be prepared to perform a full reconstruction if intraoperative and arthroscopic tests are found to be positive. In our opinion, this must also be planned when performing "simple" and "straightforward" LCAI cases. As stated before, the prevalence of MCAI could be much higher than what is described.[21]

Arthroscopic Evaluation

Arthroscopic evaluation of the complete cavity is mandatory (**Fig. 7**), which includes intraoperative assessment of specific instabilities and evaluation of other potential conditions. The lateral instability is confirmed by arthroscopic varus and anterior drawer tests in conjunction with the low ATFL quality as described by Vega and colleagues and talar excursion by Hintermann and colleagues[25,76,77] The syndesmosis is tested for instability using the spheres as described by Guyton and colleagues[78] The capability of inserting a 3 mm sphere at the tibiofibular (TF) incisura, 5 mm posterior to the anterior fibular margin, is considered positive.[78] Using the parameters

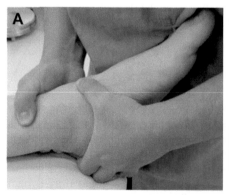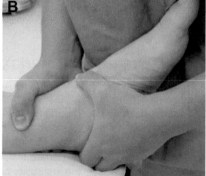

Fig. 4. A "full" anterior drawer (*A, B*) test should raise suspicion for combined and multidirectional ankle instabilities. Only when both medial and lateral constraints are lost, the talus can move freely anteriorly out of the mortise.

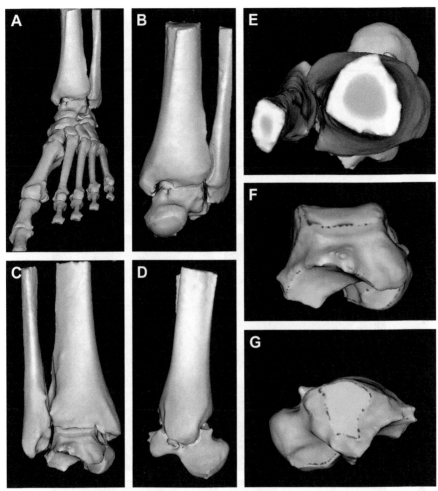

Fig. 5. Bone segmentation from WBCT (*A–G*) imaging allows the creation of distance and coverage maps between structures. When applied to the multidirectional scenario, the technology can help identify subtle changes in bone interactions. Color mapping can be used to show distances (*B–E*; *red* and *yellow* closer relations; *green* and *blue* increase in distance) or coverage (*F, G*; *green* covered; *blue* less covered; *no color* not covered).

described by Femino and colleagues and Hintermman and colleagues, medial instability is established by either a positive drive-through sign at the anteromedial corner or medial gutters (5-mm probe) or a varus-external rotation test with medial space opening.[6,19,26]

Reduction and Reconstruction

Arthroscopic debridement of gutters and syndesmotic space is carried out to allow proper reduction and treat pain sites. Possible associated injuries, such as osteochondral lesions and impingements, are treated accordingly. In a supine position, a lateral approach is directed to the distal fibula and the fourth ray is carried (**Figs. 8** and **9**). The remaining scar tissue at the syndesmosis is removed with care to the peroneal artery.

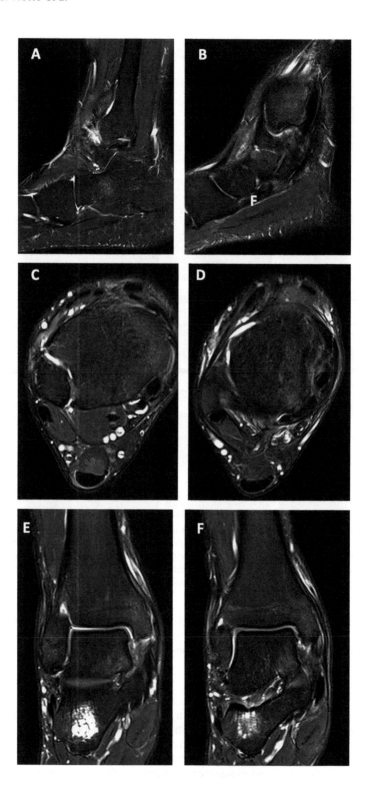

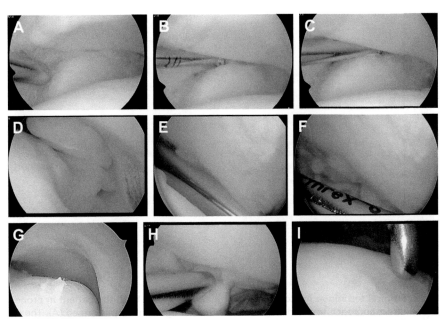

Fig. 7. A full arthroscopic evaluation is necessary not only to confirm the instabilities but also to check for potential associated injuries and to debride the joint. Lateral ligament insufficiency is observed (*A*). The syndesmosis is assessed for instability in the sagittal plane, by provoking a posterior fibular translation (*A*), and in the coronal plane, by inserting a 3 mm sphere (*B*) at the anterior aspect of the incisura (*C*). The medial compartment is exanimated for signs of MCAI, such as deltoid ligament ruptures (*D*), drive-through sign (*E*), or lateral talar translation (*F*). By applying a varus-external rotation test, an anteromedial (*G*) or medial gutter opening can also indicate an unstable medial ankle. Synovial and fibrotic scar tissues (*H*) are removed in conjunction with any loose body. Presence of adjunctive lesions, such as talar osteochondral lesions (*I*), must also be inspected and properly treated.

The lateral ligaments (ATFL and CFL) should not be incised at this moment as this would produce severe talar instability and loss of many reduction parameters. A medial approach, at the medial malleolus midline and directed to the navicular, is then performed.[6,62] The superficial deltoid band (mainly tibionavicular and tibiospring), often curiously spared in the MCAI scenario, is opened in a "t" shape fashion to allow its proper tensioned closure. The deep deltoid is inspected and any exuberant scar is removed. In case of severe MCAI or if both anterior and posterior deep deltoid ligaments are insufficient, reconstruction of the two components is advised. The medial body talar fossa is prepared to receive a 4.5 mm eyelet anchor with a synthetic

Fig. 6. MR imaging (T2 ponderation) assessment in a patient with confirmed right multidirectional CAI after a single ankle sprain 10 months before the clinical visit. Sagittal views display signs of prior injury at the lateral (*A*) and medial (*B*) ligament complexes. Axial cuts demonstrate lesion to the syndesmosis (*C*), AITFL, interosseus ligament, and posterior inferior tibiofibular ligaments, and to the ATFL (*D*). Finally, coronal views can portray injury to the posterior (*E*) and anterior (*F*) fascicules of the deep deltoid ligament.

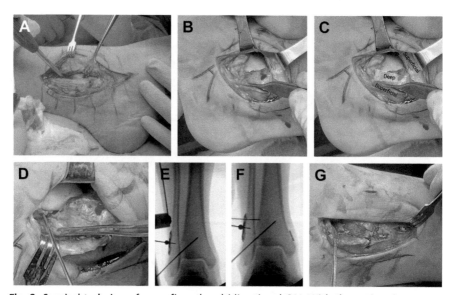

Fig. 8. Surgical technique for confirmed multidirectional CAI. With the patient in prone, a lateral direct approach to the distal fibula and lateral ligaments is performed (A). The syndesmosis is cleaned but the lateral ligaments are not incised (A). A midline approach to the medial malleolus is carried (B) and the superficial deltoid is opened to expose the deep component (C). In this case, only the anterior layer of the deep deltoid was affected and, therefore, reconstructed. The talar footprint for the anterior deep deltoid is prepared and a 3.75/4.5 mm eyelet anchor positioned (D). Attention is brought back laterally, where the syndesmosis is directly reduced with thumb pressure and secured with a k-wire (E). After arthroscopic, fluoroscopic, and clinical confirmation, two endo-buttons are placed throughout the fibular plate (F) while medially checking for any potential entrapment or periosteal interposition (G).

tape/biosynthetic graft/allograft/autograft and the posterior band of the reconstruction. Before proceeding with the medial construct, attention is brought back to the syndesmosis.

The fibula is directly reduced to the incisura and secured with two 1.5-mm k-wires.[79] Fluoroscopy, the medial approach, and arthroscopy are used to check syndesmotic and medial space reduction. A lateral two- hole or four-hole plate is positioned posterolaterally at the fibula. The guidewire for the most distal suture buttons is placed through the plate, 1.5 cm proximal to the tibial plafond, and followed by a second more proximal. Positions are checked and the medial incision is used to observe medial button exits. The two buttons are tightened after the reduction k-wires are receded and the ankle is placed in a neutral position. One of the reduction k-wires is advanced again to secure the TF position until the end of the whole syndesmotic procedure. Augmentation of the syndesmosis reconstruction is obtained with an AITFL tape/graft placement using the ligament footprints and 3.75/4.5 mm eyelet anchors.[80–82] The ankle is positioned in neutral for this step.

The medial reconstruction is then resumed by preparing the intercollicular groove to receive another 4.5 mm eyelet anchor.[6] When inserting the tensioned tape/graft, the ankle is positioned in 15° plantarflexion. Another tunnel, for the anterior deep deltoid band, is placed 5 to 10 mm anterior at the body–neck transition. For this band, the ankle is placed at neutral, internally rotated, and the hindfoot is positioned in valgus to maximize tension.[6] The syndesmotic reduction k-wire is finally removed. A formal

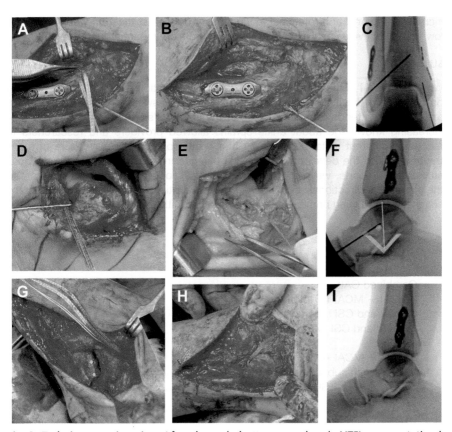

Fig. 9. Technique continuation. After the endo-buttons are placed, AITFL augmentation is performed respecting tibial (*A*) and fibular (*B*) footprints. The surgery returns to the medial side, where the tibial tunnel for the deep deltoid reconstruction is made at the intercollicular notch (*C, D*). Another eyelet anchor is placed with the proper construct tension and a superficial deltoid repair is performed (*E*). Back again laterally, the ATFL augmentation is prepared using the talar footprint (*F*), the anterior aspect of the lateral process proximal end. A Bröstrom procedure (*G*) is then carried out using one or two intraosseous anchors (*yellow dots*) and the augmentation is finalized through fibular anchor placement (*H*). Fluoroscopy confirms final overall positioning and proper tunnel placement (*I*).

Bröstrom-Gould procedure is then carried out using one and two anchors.[3] An ATFL lateral augmentation with tape/graft and 3.75/4.5 mm eyelet anchors (while observing proper tension and placement) concludes the whole surgical intervention.[83,84]

Postoperative Protocol

Patients are placed in a splint for 1 week and a short leg cast for another 2 weeks.[6] They are kept non-weight-bearing for 3 weeks. When sutures are removed in the third postoperative week, they are transitioned to a pneumatic postoperative boot and progressive load is initiated. Range of motion (ROM) is also allowed at this time, mainly active and limited to about 10° of plantarflexion and 20° of dorsiflexion. No eversion, inversion, or rotations are permitted. At 6 weeks, patients are placed in a rigid ankle brace and referred to physical therapy, where ankle sagittal ROM is progressively increased. Coronal and rotational motion are introduced at the 10th week. Return to low-impact activities might begin at 8 weeks and high-impact around the 12th.

SUMMARY

What is MD-CAI of the ankle? Does it exist? What situations does that apply to? Is it proper to call it that? Although there are no definitive answers to these questions, this review article intends to present some of the literature's explanations to them. The increasing knowledge about ankle sprains allowed providers and researchers to recognize different instability patterns that might contribute to the failure of many treatments and the development of ankle osteoarthrosis.[21,85,86] Based on previous studies and reports, we presented the current associated instabilities picture and the actual multidirectional scenario. As proper definitions are still lacking, we hereby suggest the following nomenclature when dealing with ankle instabilities.

- Isolated CAI:
  - ○ LCAI
  - ○ MCAI
  - ○ CSI
- Combined CAI:
  - ○ LCAI + MCAI = Rotational CAI
  - ○ LCAI and CSI (often with varus hindfoot)
  - ○ MCAI and CSI (often with valgus hindfoot)
- MD-CAI:
  - ○ LCAI + MCAI + CSI = MD-CAI
- MD-CAI with subtalar instability
  - ○ LCAI, MCAI, CSI, and STI

CLINICS CARE POINTS

- Any clinical assessment of simple or severe ankle sprain should consider combined CAI or MD-CAI as possible diagnoses. Isolated ankle instabilities must also be approached with this possibility in mind, devoting attention to all ligament complexes.

- Even when the preoperative clinical and imaging evaluation is negative for associated conditions, surgeons must be prepared to arthroscopically evaluate all complexes and approach potential instabilities that might be found. Surgical planning should consider these possibilities.

- Although always considering health care limitations and proper clinical guidance, subsidiary exams are necessary to present the provider and patient with the best possible data for treatment decisions. Ankle instabilities' deleterious effect and the high incidence of ankle arthritis secondary to these conditions support a more meticulous investigation.

- When facing MD-CAI, all ligament complexes will require reconstruction. Arthroscopy is not only necessary to confirm the diagnosis but also to clean the joint. Consider open approaches that allow a direct reduction of the syndesmosis and the medial gutter. Ligament augmentations and tendon grafts are good options for poor local tissues while also providing higher structural stability.

DISCLOSURES

N.S.B. Mansur: American Orthopaedic Foot and Ankle Society: Committee Member. Brazilian Orthopaedic Foot and Ankle Society: Committee Member. V. Valderrabano:

European Foot & Ankle Society: EFAS Research Foundation President. Exactech, Inc: IP royalties; Paid consultant; Paid presenter or speaker, Geistlich Surgery: Paid presenter or speaker. German-Austrian-Swiss Sports Orthopaedics Society: Board or committee member. Medartis: IP royalties; Paid consultant; Paid presenter or speaker. Swiss Foot & Ankle Society: Board member, Past President. C. de Cesar Netto: American Orthopaedic Foot and Ankle Society: Committee Member. Brazilian Orthopaedic Foot and Ankle Society: Committee Member. C. De Cesar Netto, MD, PhD (Iowa City, IA). American Orthopaedic Foot and Ankle Society: Board or committee member. CurveBeam: Paid consultant; Stock or stock options. Foot and Ankle International: Editorial or governing board. Nextremity: Paid consultant; Ossio: Paid consultant; Paragon 28: IP royalties; Paid consultant. Weightbearing CT International Study Group: Board or committee member. Zimmer: Paid consultant. This study did not receive any grants or funding.

REFERENCES

1. Schäfer D, Hintermann B. Arthroscopic assessment of the chronic unstable ankle joint. Knee Surg Sports Traumatol Arthrosc 1996;4(1):48–52.
2. Hopkinson WJ, St Pierre P, Ryan JB, et al. Syndesmosis sprains of the ankle. Foot Ankle 1990;10(6):325–30.
3. Porter DA, Kamman KA. Chronic Lateral Ankle Instability: Open Surgical Management. Foot Ankle Clin 2018;23(4):539–54.
4. Gribble PA, Bleakley CM, Caulfield BM, et al. Evidence review for the 2016 International Ankle Consortium consensus statement on the prevalence, impact and long-term consequences of lateral ankle sprains. Br J Sports Med 2016;50(24):1496–505.
5. Knupp M, Lang TH, Zwicky L, et al. Chronic ankle instability (medial and lateral). Clin Sports Med 2015;34(4):679–88.
6. de Cesar Netto C, Femino JE. State of the art in treatment of chronic medial ankle instability. Foot Ankle Clin 2021;26(2):329–44.
7. Alshalawi S, Galhoum AE, Alrashidi Y, et al. Medial ankle instability: the deltoid dilemma. Foot Ankle Clin 2018;23(4):639–57.
8. Ferran NA, Oliva F, Maffulli N. Ankle instability. Sports Med Arthrosc Rev 2009;17(2):139–45.
9. Valderrabano V, Wiewiorski M, Frigg A, et al. [Chronic ankle instability]. Unfallchirurg 2007;110(8):691–9. https://doi.org/10.1007/s00113-007-1310-y [quiz: 700]. Chronische Instabilität des oberen Sprunggelenks.
10. Stenquist DS, Ye MY, Kwon JY. Acute and chronic syndesmotic instability: role of surgical stabilization. Clin Sports Med 2020;39(4):745–71.
11. Tourné Y, Molinier F, Andrieu M, et al. Diagnosis and treatment of tibiofibular syndesmosis lesions. Orthop Traumatol Surg Res 2019;105(8s):S275–86.
12. Doherty C, Bleakley C, Hertel J, et al. Dynamic balance deficits in individuals with chronic ankle instability compared to ankle sprain copers 1 year after a first-time lateral ankle sprain Injury. Knee Surg Sports Traumatol Arthrosc 2016;24(4):1086–95.
13. Koshino Y, Ishida T, Yamanaka M, et al. Kinematics and muscle activities of the lower limb during a side-cutting task in subjects with chronic ankle instability. Knee Surg Sports Traumatol Arthrosc 2016;24(4):1071–80.
14. Hashimoto T, Inokuchi S. A kinematic study of ankle joint instability due to rupture of the lateral ligaments. Foot Ankle Int 1997;18(11):729–34.

15. Dalmau-Pastor M, Malagelada F, Calder J, et al. The lateral ankle ligaments are interconnected: the medial connecting fibres between the anterior talofibular, calcaneofibular and posterior talofibular ligaments. Knee Surg Sports Traumatol Arthrosc 2020;28(1):34–9.

16. Yasuda T, Shima H, Mori K, et al. Simultaneous reconstruction of the medial and lateral collateral ligaments for chronic combined ligament injuries of the ankle. Am J Sports Med 2017;45(9):2052–60.

17. Mococain P, Bejarano-Pineda L, Glisson R, et al. Biomechanical effect on joint stability of including deltoid ligament repair in an ankle fracture soft tissue injury model with deltoid and syndesmotic disruption. Foot Ankle Int 2020;41(9):1158–64.

18. Lepojärvi S, Niinimäki J, Pakarinen H, et al. Rotational dynamics of the normal distal tibiofibular joint with weight-bearing computed tomography. Foot Ankle Int 2016;37(6):627–35.

19. Femino JE, Vaseenon T, Phisitkul P, et al. Varus external rotation stress test for radiographic detection of deep deltoid ligament disruption with and without syndesmotic disruption: a cadaveric study. Foot Ankle Int 2013;34(2):251–60.

20. Choi WJ, Lee JW, Han SH, et al. Chronic lateral ankle instability:the effect of intra-articular lesions on clinical outcome. Am J Sports Med 2008;36(11):2167–72.

21. Kim JS, Young KW, Cho HK, et al. Concomitant syndesmotic instability and medial ankle instability are risk factors for unsatisfactory outcomes in patients with chronic ankle instability. Arthroscopy 2015;31(8):1548–56.

22. Mansur NSB, Lemos AVKC, Baumfeld DS, et al. Medial and lateral combined ligament arthroscopic repair for multidirectional ankle instability. Foot & Ankle Orthopaedics 2021;6(1). 247301142098615.

23. Longo UG, Loppini M, Fumo C, et al. Deep deltoid ligament injury is related to rotational instability of the ankle joint: a biomechanical study. Knee Surg Sports Traumatol Arthrosc 2021;29(5):1577–83.

24. Vega J, Allmendinger J, Malagelada F, et al. Combined arthroscopic all-inside repair of lateral and medial ankle ligaments is an effective treatment for rotational ankle instability. Knee Surg Sports Traumatol Arthrosc 2020;28(1):132–40.

25. Hintermann B, Boss A, Schäfer D. Arthroscopic findings in patients with chronic ankle instability. Am J Sports Med 2002;30(3):402–9.

26. Hintermann B, Valderrabano V, Boss A, et al. Medial ankle instability: an exploratory, prospective study of fifty-two cases. Am J Sports Med 2004;32(1):183–90.

27. Buchhorn T, Sabeti-Aschraf M, Dlaska CE, et al. Combined medial and lateral anatomic ligament reconstruction for chronic rotational instability of the ankle. Foot Ankle Int 2011;32(12):1122–6.

28. Ikuta Y, Nakasa T, Sumii J, et al. Quantitative analysis of deltoid ligament degradation in patients with chronic ankle instability using computed tomographic images. Foot Ankle Int 2021;42(7):952–8.

29. Caputo AM, Lee JY, Spritzer CE, et al. In vivo kinematics of the tibiotalar joint after lateral ankle instability. Am J Sports Med 2009;37(11):2241–8.

30. Goetz JE, Vaseenon T, Tochigi Y, et al. 3D talar kinematics during external rotation stress testing in hindfoot varus and valgus using a model of syndesmotic and deep deltoid instability. Foot Ankle Int 2019;40(7):826–35.

31. Ziai P, Benca E, Skrbensky GV, et al. The role of the medial ligaments in lateral stabilization of the ankle joint: an in vitro study. Knee Surg Sports Traumatol Arthrosc 2015;23(7):1900–6.

32. Corte-Real N, Caetano J. Ankle and syndesmosis instability: consensus and controversies. EFORT Open Reviews 2021;6(6):420–31.

33. McCollum GA, van den Bekerom MP, Kerkhoffs GM, et al. Syndesmosis and del-toid ligament injuries in the athlete. Knee Surg Sports Traumatol Arthrosc 2013; 21(6):1328–37.

34. Roemer FW, Jomaah N, Niu J, et al. Ligamentous injuries and the risk of associ-ated tissue damage in acute ankle sprains in athletes: a cross-sectional MRI study. Am J Sports Med 2014;42(7):1549–57.

35. Hua Y, Chen S, Li Y, et al. Combination of modified Broström procedure with ankle arthroscopy for chronic ankle instability accompanied by intra-articular symp-toms. Arthroscopy 2010;26(4):524–8.

36. Patel NK, Murphy CI, Pfeiffer TR, et al. Sagittal instability with inversion is impor-tant to evaluate after syndesmosis injury and repair: a cadaveric robotic study. Journal of Experimental Orthopaedics 2020;7(1). https://doi.org/10.1186/ s40634-020-00234-w.

37. Doherty C, Bleakley C, Delahunt E, et al. Treatment and prevention of acute and recurrent ankle sprain: an overview of systematic reviews with meta-analysis. Br J Sports Med 2017;51(2):113–25.

38. Sato G, Saengsin J, Bhimani R, et al. Isolated injuries to the lateral ankle liga-ments have no direct effect on syndesmotic stability. Knee Surg Sports Traumatol Arthrosc 2022;30(11):3881–7.

39. Teramoto A, Kura H, Uchiyama E, et al. Three-dimensional analysis of ankle insta-bility after tibiofibular syndesmosis injuries. Am J Sports Med 2008;36(2):348–52.

40. Bhimani R, Sato G, Saengsin J, et al. Fluoroscopic evaluation of the role of syn-desmotic injury in lateral ankle instability in a cadaver model. Foot Ankle Int 2022; 43(11):1482–92.

41. Lalevée M, Anderson DD, Wilken JM. Current challenges in chronic ankle insta-bility: review and perspective. Foot Ankle Clin. doi:10.1016/j.fcl.2022.11.003.

42. Kisamori K, Kimura T, Saito M, et al. Lateralizing calcaneal osteotomy and first metatarsal dorsiflexion osteotomy for cavovarus foot and peroneal sheath release with peroneus brevis repair for peroneal tendinopathy in chronic ankle instability and sprain. Cureus 2022. https://doi.org/10.7759/cureus.32235.

43. Lintz F, Bernasconi A, Baschet L, et al. Relationship between chronic lateral ankle instability and hindfoot varus using weight-bearing cone beam computed tomog-raphy. Foot Ankle Int 2019;40(10):1175–81.

44. Whitlock KG, LaRose M, Barber H, et al. Deltoid ligament repair versus trans-syndesmotic fixation for bimalleolar equivalent ankle fractures. Injury 2022; 53(6):2292–6.

45. Doty JF, Dunlap BD, Panchbhavi VK, et al. Deltoid ligament injuries associated with ankle fractures: arguments for and against direct repair. J Am Acad Orthop Surg 2021;29(8):e388–95.

46. Barbachan Mansur NS, Raduan FC, Lemos AVKC, et al. Deltoid ligament arthro-scopic repair in ankle fractures: case series. Injury 2021;52(10):3156–60.

47. Butler BA, Hempen EC, Barbosa M, et al. Deltoid ligament repair reduces and stabilizes the talus in unstable ankle fractures. J Orthop 2020;17:87–90.

48. Massri-Pugin J, Lubberts B, Vopat BG, et al. Effect of sequential sectioning of lig-aments on syndesmotic instability in the coronal plane evaluated arthroscopically. Foot Ankle Int 2017;38(12):1387–93.

49. Feller R, Borenstein T, Fantry AJ, et al. Arthroscopic quantification of syndesmotic instability in a cadaveric model. Arthroscopy 2017;33(2):436–44.

50. LaMothe JM, Baxter JR, Karnovsky SC, et al. Syndesmotic injury assessment with lateral imaging during stress testing in a cadaveric model. Foot Ankle Int 2018; 39(4):479–84.

51. Krähenbühl N, Weinberg MW, Davidson NP, et al. Imaging in syndesmotic injury: a systematic literature review. Skeletal Radiol 2018;47(5):631–48.

52. Chun K-Y, Choi YS, Lee SH, et al. Deltoid ligament and tibiofibular syndesmosis injury in chronic lateral ankle instability: magnetic resonance imaging evaluation at 3T and comparison with arthroscopy. Korean J Radiol 2015;16(5):1096.

53. van Dijk CN, Longo UG, Loppini M, et al. Classification and diagnosis of acute isolated syndesmotic injuries: ESSKA-AFAS consensus and guidelines. Knee Surg Sports Traumatol Arthrosc 2016;24(4):1200–16.

54. van Dijk CN, Longo UG, Loppini M, et al. Conservative and surgical management of acute isolated syndesmotic injuries: ESSKA-AFAS consensus and guidelines. Knee Surg Sports Traumatol Arthrosc 2016;24(4):1217–27.

55. Campbell KJ, Michalski MP, Wilson KJ, et al. The ligament anatomy of the deltoid complex of the ankle: a qualitative and quantitative anatomical study. J Bone Joint Surg Am 2014;96(8):e62.

56. Xenos JS, Hopkinson WJ, Mulligan ME, et al. The tibiofibular syndesmosis. Evaluation of the ligamentous structures, methods of fixation, and radiographic assessment. JBJS 1995;77(6):847–56.

57. Krähenbühl N, Bailey TL, Weinberg MW, et al. Impact of torque on assessment of syndesmotic injuries using weightbearing computed tomography scans. Foot Ankle Int 2019;40(6):710–9.

58. Beumer A, Valstar ER, Garling EH, et al. External rotation stress imaging in syndesmotic injuries of the ankle: comparison of lateral radiography and radiostereometry in a cadaveric model. Acta Orthop Scand 2003;74(2):201–5.

59. Hunt KJ, Goeb Y, Behn AW, et al. Ankle joint contact loads and displacement with progressive syndesmotic injury. Foot Ankle Int 2015;36(9):1095–103.

60. Krähenbühl N, Bailey TL, Weinberg MW, et al. Is load application necessary when using computed tomography scans to diagnose syndesmotic injuries? A cadaver study. Foot Ankle Surg 2020;26(2):198–204.

61. Auch E, Barbachan Mansur NS, Alexandre Alves T, et al. Distal tibiofibular syndesmotic widening in progressive collapsing foot deformity. Foot Ankle Int 2021;42(6):768–75.

62. Fonseca LF, Baumfeld D, Mansur N, et al. Deltoid Insufficiency and Flatfoot—Oh Gosh, I'm Losing the Ankle! What Now? Techniques in Foot & Ankle Surgery 2019;18(4):202–7.

63. Schäfer D, Hintermann B. [Diagnostic imaging of ankle joint instability]. Sportverletz Sportschaden 1996;10(3):55–7. https://doi.org/10.1055/s-2007-993399. Bildgebende Diagnostik der Sprunggelenksinstabilität.

64. Hong CC, Calder J. Ability to return to sports after early lateral ligament repair of the ankle in 147 elite athletes. Knee Surg Sports Traumatol Arthrosc 2022. https://doi.org/10.1007/s00167-022-07270-2.

65. Debieux P, Wajnsztejn A, Mansur NSB. Epidemiology of injuries due to ankle sprain diagnosed in an orthopedic emergency room. Einstein (Sao Paulo). 2020;18:eAO4739.

66. Jeong MS, Choi YS, Kim YJ, et al. Deltoid ligament in acute ankle injury: MR imaging analysis. Skeletal Radiol 2014;43(5):655–63.

67. Tourne Y, Besse JL, Mabit C, et al. Chronic ankle instability. Which tests to assess the lesions? Which therapeutic options? Orthop Traumatol Surg Res 2010;96(4):433–46.

68. Stenquist DS, Miller C, Velasco B, et al. Medial tenderness revisited: is medial ankle tenderness predictive of instability in isolated lateral malleolus fractures? Injury 2020;51(6):1392–6.

69. Williams BT, Ahrberg AB, Goldsmith MT, et al. Ankle syndesmosis: a qualitative and quantitative anatomic analysis. Am J Sports Med 2015;43(1):88–97.
70. Miller AG, Myers SH, Parks BG, et al. Anterolateral drawer versus anterior drawer test for ankle instability: a biomechanical model. Foot Ankle Int 2016;37(4): 407–10.
71. Spennacchio P, Seil R, Gathen M, et al. Diagnosing instability of ligamentous syndesmotic injuries: A biomechanical perspective. Clin Biomech 2021;84:105312.
72. Ashkani Esfahani S, Bhimani R, Lubberts B, et al. Volume measurements on weightbearing computed tomography can detect subtle syndesmotic instability. J Orthop Res 2022;40(2):460–7.
73. Rodrigues JC, Santos ALG, Prado MP, et al. Comparative CT with stress manoeuvres for diagnosing distal isolated tibiofibular syndesmotic injury in acute ankle sprain: a protocol for an accuracy- test prospective study. BMJ Open 2020; 10(9):e037239.
74. Chun DI, Cho JH, Min TH, et al. Diagnostic accuracy of radiologic methods for ankle syndesmosis injury: a systematic review and meta-analysis. J Clin Med 2019;8(7). https://doi.org/10.3390/jcm8070968.
75. Salat P, Le V, Veljkovic A, et al. Imaging in foot and ankle instability. Foot Ankle Clin Dec 2018;23(4):499–522 e28.
76. Wiebking U, Pacha TO, Jagodzinski M. An accuracy evaluation of clinical, arthrometric, and stress-sonographic acute ankle instability examinations. Foot Ankle Surg 2015;21(1):42–8.
77. Vega J, Malagelada F, Dalmau-Pastor M. Arthroscopic all-inside ATFL and CFL repair is feasible and provides excellent results in patients with chronic ankle instability. Knee Surg Sports Traumatol Arthrosc 2020;28(1):116–23.
78. Guyton GP, DeFontes K 3rd, Barr CR, et al. Arthroscopic correlates of subtle syndesmotic injury. Foot Ankle Int 2017;38(5):502–6.
79. Harris MC, Lause G, Unangst A, et al. Prospective results of the modified glide path technique for improved syndesmotic reduction during ankle fracture fixation. Foot Ankle Int 2022;43(7):923–7.
80. Schermann H, Ogawa T, Lubberts B, et al. Comparison of several combinations of suture tape reinforcement and suture button constructs for fixation of unstable syndesmosis. J Am Acad Orthop Surg 2022;30(10):e769–78.
81. Takahashi K, Teramoto A, Murahashi Y, et al. Comparison of treatment methods for syndesmotic injuries with posterior tibiofibular ligament ruptures: a cadaveric biomechanical study. Orthop J Sports Med 2022;10(9). https://doi.org/10.1177/ 23259671221122811. 23259671221122811.
82. Jamieson MD, Stake IK, Brady AW, et al. Anterior inferior tibiofibular ligament suture tape augmentation for isolated syndesmotic injuries. Foot Ankle Int 2022; 43(7):994–1003.
83. Lan R, Piatt ET, Bolia IK, et al. Suture Tape Augmentation in Lateral Ankle Ligament Surgery: Current Concepts Review. Foot Ankle Orthop 2021;6(4). https:// doi.org/10.1177/24730114211045978. 24730114211045978.
84. Porter M, Shadbolt R, Ye X, et al. Ankle lateral ligament augmentation versus the modified brostrom-gould procedure: a 5-year randomized controlled trial Am J Sports Med 2019;47(3):659–66.
85. Saltzman CL, Salamon ML, Blanchard GM, et al. Epidemiology of ankle arthritis: report of a consecutive series of 639 patients from a tertiary orthopaedic center. Iowa Orthop J 2005;25:44–6.
86. Valderrabano V, Horisberger M, Russell I, et al. Etiology of ankle osteoarthritis. Clin Orthop Relat Res 2009;467(7):1800–6.

87. Han SH, Lee JW, Kim S, et al. Chronic tibiofibular syndesmosis injury: the diagnostic efficiency of magnetic resonance imaging and comparative analysis of operative treatment. Foot Ankle Int 2007;28(3):336–42.
88. Yoo JH, Lee WC, Moon JS. Simultaneous reconstruction of the medial and lateral ligament complexes of the ankle joint with semitendinosus tendon allograft. A case report. J Bone Joint Surg Am 2009;91(6):1491–6.

Acute and Chronic Subtalar Joint Instability

Does It Really Exist?

Kerri Lynne Bell, MD[a], Brandon William King, MD[a,*],
Bruce J. Sangeorzan, MD[b]

KEYWORDS

- Subtalar • Instability • Cervical ligament • Calcaneofibular ligament
- Interosseous ligament

KEY POINTS

- Ten to twenty-five percent of patients with ankle instability have concurrent subtalar instability.
- There is no current consensus to the evaluation of subtalar instability. Current imaging techniques have poor reliability for the diagnosis of subtalar instability.
- The initial non operative management of subtalar instability is similar to ankle instability.
- Operative treatment can be considered after 3 to 6 months of failed nonoperative treatment. Lateral ligament repair, anatomic, and nonanatomic reconstruction techniques exist and have limited data supporting their use.

INTRODUCTION

Subtalar instability remains an uncertain (controversial) topic in orthopaedics. The clinical presentation of subtalar instability is often vague. Given the clinical and radiographic overlap between lateral ankle instability and subtalar instability, the diagnosis remains challenging and may be commonly missed. It has been suggested that subtalar instability can occur in isolation but is much more common concomitant with lateral ankle instability.[1] Undiagnosed subtalar joint instability over time can lead to pain, functional impairment and may lead to degenerative changes and subsequent disability.[2]

Drs B W. King and B. Sangeorzan have no conflicts of interest.
No funding was received in support of this article.
[a] Orthopaedic Surgery, Henry Ford Health, 2799 West Grand Boulevard K12, Detroit, MI 48202, USA; [b] Orthopaedic Surgery, Harborview Medical Center, University of Washington, Seattle, WA 98104, USA
* Corresponding author. 2799 West Grand Boulevard K12, Detroit, MI 48202.
E-mail address: Bking13@hfhs.org

Foot Ankle Clin N Am 28 (2023) 427–444
https://doi.org/10.1016/j.fcl.2022.12.008
1083-7515/23/© 2023 Elsevier Inc. All rights reserved.

ANATOMY

The subtalar joint is a complex synovial joint, composed of the articulations of the anterior, middle, and posterior facets of the talus and calcaneus. The subtalar joint allows for accommodation when walking over uneven ground.[3]

The anterior subtalar joint, also known as the talocalcaneonavicular joint or acetabulum pedis, is composed of convex anterior and middle talar facets, the concave anterior and middle calcaneal facets, the head of the talus, and the concave proximal surface of the navicular.[2,4–6] This articulation is most similar to a ball-and-socket joint.[4] Viladot and colleagues[7] found that the anterior and middle facets of the anterior subtalar joint have great individual variation and can be subclassified by type into an ovoid, bean, or two-part morphology.

The posterior subtalar joint is a saddle-shaped joint formed from the concave inferior posterior facet of the talus and the convex superior posterior facet of the calcaneus.[2,4,5] The anterior and posterior subtalar joints are separated by the sinus tarsi and the canalis tarsi. They also have separate ligamentous joint capsules.[4] The posterior subtalar joint has a 45° oblique axis in relation to the longitudinal axis of the foot.[2,5,7] The posterior facet is the largest articulation and is separated from the anterior and middle facets by the interosseous talocalcaneal ligament (ITCL).[2] The dorsal surface of the middle calcaneal facet contributes to the sustentaculum tali, under which the flexor hallucis longus tendon glides.[8]

In addition to the bony stability provided by the convex and concave facets, several ligaments provide additional support. The ligaments surrounding the subtalar joint are primary stabilizers. The cervical ligament (CL) and ITCL are the intrinsic ligaments of the subtalar joint and provide anterior and medial support[2,5] (**Fig. 1**). Within the tarsal sinus, some cadaver studies have demonstrated two ligaments with unique insertions and running patterns.[9,10] As a result, some authors suggest that the anterior capsular ligament (also known as the interosseous ligament vertical segment) should be considered unique and distinct from the ITCL (also known as interosseous ligament oblique segment), as it runs more lateral and posterior to the ITCL.[1,5,11] Yoon and colleagues[12] reported that an absence or complete tear of the anterior capsular ligament occurs with much higher frequency in patients with subtalar instability compared with those with lateral ankle instability (60% vs 13%). The three roots of the inferior extensor retinaculum, the ITCL, and the anterior capsular ligament are located in the small area between the tarsal canal and the posterior aspect of the tarsal sinus.[11]

The extrinsic ligaments of the subtalar joint include the calcaneofibular ligament (CFL), the tibiocalcaneal portion of the deltoid ligament, and the superomedial aspect of the spring ligament (also known as the plantar calcaneonavicular ligament).[2,5] The CFL provides the majority of stabilization when the ankle is in neutral position; during plantarflexion, it is assisted by the anterior talofibular ligament.

The specific functions of each ligament have been elucidated through the use of several cadaver studies involving the isolated sectioning of individual ligaments.[13] Stormont and colleagues[14] found that the CFL is the primary restraint for external rotation. Cahill[15], Smith,[16] and Kjaersgaard-Andersen and colleagues[17] reported that the CL prevents talar inversion, talar rotation, and excessive motion within the subtalar joint. Tochigi and colleagues[18] described the role of the ITCL as primarily maintaining talus–calcaneus apposition and stabilizing the joint against inversion forces.

Some authors have also divided the lateral talocalcaneal ligaments into superficial and deep compartments. The superficial compartment is composed of the CL, the sinus tarsi ligaments, and the superficial and intermediate layers of the inferior extensor

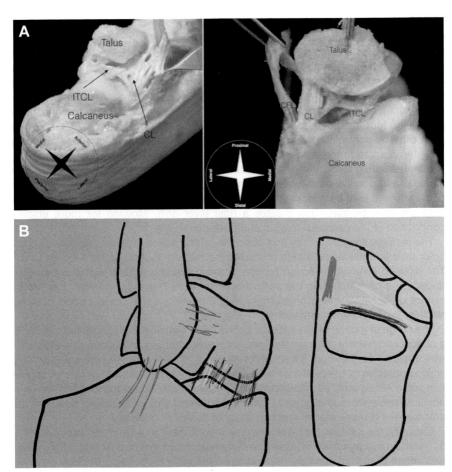

Fig. 1. Subtalar joint anatomy. ACL, anterior capsular ligament; ATFL, anterior talofibular ligament; CFL, calcaneofibular ligament; CL, cervical ligament; ITCL, interosseous talocalcaneal ligament. Top image from CreativeCommons. No further licensing necessary. (*From* Pereira BS, Andrade R, Espregueira-Mendes J, Marano RPC, Oliva XM, Karlsson J. Current Concepts on Subtalar Instability. Orthop J Sports Med. 2021 Aug 19;9(8):23259671211021352. https://doi.org/10.1177/23259671211021352. PMID: 34435065; PMCID: PMC8381447.)

retinaculum. The deep compartment includes the canalis tarsi ligaments in addition to the ITCL and the deep layer of the inferior extensor retinaculum.[5]

The medial subtalar ligament complex is composed of the tibiosubtalar portion of the deltoid ligament and the superomedial aspect of the spring ligament. The medial complex provides stability during sliding, rolling, and torsion.[5]

HINDFOOT BIOMECHANICS

The functional weight-bearing subtalar joint is complex and has a multiplanar range of motion. The transition from swing to stance phase is the most unstable stage of the gait cycle for the subtalar joint.[13,19] With normal gait, pronation begins during the heel strike and continues through toe strike. Pronation of the hindfoot initiates with internal rotation of the tibia, causing internal rotation of the talus–navicular, which then rotates medially (plantar flexes and adducts) on calcaneus which moves in a valgus (lateral) direction. This positioning allows for shock absorption, equilibrium, and accommodation on uneven terrain, as the talonavicular and calcaneocuboid joints are divergent, thus dissipating the vertical compressive force in addition to the anterior and medial shearing forces. With this unlocking of the midfoot, the forefoot can more easily adapt to uneven terrain, thus improving equilibrium. As the gait cycle continues, the foot moves from stance phase into swing phase. During the midstance phase, the foot transitions into a supinated position to allow for a rigid lever arm for push off. The contralateral leg swings past the weight-bearing leg, which promotes an external rotation force on the weight-bearing leg. The external rotation produces a lateral shearing force, instigating supination. The calcaneus is inverted which then abducts and dorsiflexes the talus via the sustentaculum tali. This supination motion of the subtalar joint thus locks the midtarsal joints; the talonavicular and calcaneocuboid are now parallel. This creates a rigid lever arm, allowing for more efficient contraction of the peroneus longus and posterior tibialis.[20,21]

The reciprocating convexity and concavity of the paired anterior, middle, and posterior talar and calcaneal facets produces the rotatory motion at the subtalar joint.[21] The isolated inversion/eversion motion of the posterior subtalar joint can be reproduced by a clinician when the patient is non-weight-bearing. However, this motion cannot be isolated during physiologic weight-bearing, as the anterior and posterior subtalar joints move simultaneously.[21]

The range of motion of the subtalar joint is often simplified for clinical purposes. For a clinical perspective, the subtalar joint is assumed to have an oblique axis of rotation which allows for hindfoot inversion/eversion.[3,22–24] On average, the subtalar axis, which originates at the posterior talocalcaneal articulation, has 23° of medial angulation and a 42° upward tilt in relation to the perpendicular axis at the foot.[4,25] The anterior and posterior subtalar joints share a common axis of rotation; however, the anterior joint is more medial and has a higher center of rotation.[4]

Clinically, the subtalar joint has been reported to have a range of motion from 39° to 54°, with an average of 46°. Studies have demonstrated that clinical evaluation of subtalar range of motion can vary depending on the technique used.[5] Buckley and Hunt found poor inter-examiner and intra-examiner reliability when assessing subtalar motion in orthopedic surgeons.[26] Computed tomography (CT) 3D motion analysis demonstrated a smaller range of motion, from 5° to 16°; the threefold increase in clinical subtalar motion was attributed to soft tissue and talocrural motion and not true subtalar motion.[25]

Etiology/Epidemiology

Chronic ankle instability is attributed to either mechanical insufficiency, function insufficiency, or a combination. Mechanical instability can be due to pathologic laxity, restrictions in arthrokinematics, degenerative changes, or synovial changes. These can occur either together or in isolation. Functional instability can be an impaired proprioception, impaired neuromuscular control, impaired postural control, or deficits in strength.[4]

It has been reported that approximately 10% to 25% of patients with ankle instability have subtalar instability.[27] Subtalar injury can occur through a variety of injury patterns.[28] Subtalar injury occurs most often when the ankle is in a dorsiflexed or neutral position and experiences forced inversion/supination, which can lead to injury to the CFL, CL, and ITCL.[5,28] Taillard and colleagues[29] demonstrated that when a constant inversion stress is applied across the foot and ankle, the CFL is the first ligament to fail, followed by the CL and then finally the ITCL. The failure of the CFL versus the CL or the ITCL as the primary cause of subtalar instability remains controversial.[5,28,30–35] A systematic review by Michels and colleagues found that no single ligament was the primary cause for failure, and it is likely a combination of injury to several ligaments.[36]

Clinical Evaluation

Good history taking can aid in the diagnosis of subtalar instability. With acute injuries, many patients will report an inversion injury and may report hearing a "pop" when the injury occurred.[6] The acute presentation may appear as a severe ankle sprain.[28] However, most of the patients present with chronic symptoms. Kato noted that many of his patients with subtalar instability did not report any history of injury.[37] Patients may report recurrent swelling, a sense of the ankle "giving way," diffuse heel and hind foot pain, difficulty wearing high-heeled shoes, and stiffness of the subtalar joint; these symptoms are often aggravated when ambulating on uneven terrain or when playing sports.[5,6,34] Careful history taking can help differentiate true patient instability from apprehension by clarifying when and how the symptoms present.

The physical examination should include a general overview of the foot and ankle in all planes. The foot should be assessed for any flexible or rigid deformities including cavus, equinus, varus, or valgus. Several examination maneuvers can be used to isolate concomitant or confounding pathologies. A Silfverskiold test can gauge for gastrocnemius contracture. A Malloy impingement test can identify synovial impingement.

Acutely, patients may have ecchymosis, swelling, and tenderness diffusely throughout the ankle.[28] They may demonstrate increased inversion with varus ankle stress. With chronic presentations, there may be swelling located laterally and sinus tarsi tenderness. Owing to pain, there may be ankle and hindfoot stiffness from disuse; however, the subtalar joint will still demonstrate increased inversion.[5,28]

Several authors hypothesize that the subtalar instability has both a tilt and rotational component.[28] Subtle examination findings of these include an increase in internal rotation of the subtalar joint and an increase in forward translation of the calcaneus underneath the talus.[28,38] Thermann and colleagues proposed an examination for subtalar instability on which the heel and forefoot were held fixed with the foot in 10° of dorsiflexion, with an inversion and external rotation stress applied through the heel, and adduction stress was then applied through the forefoot. Subtalar instability was reported when the examiner could feel a medial shift of the calcaneus beneath the talus and an opening of the talocalcaneal angle. They confirmed these findings with radiographs.[38] The anterior lateral drawer test is commonly used to assess the laxity of the subtalar joint; a positive test results in an increased anteromedial shift and varus tilt to the hind foot.[5,22,24] A talar tilt stress test can identify laxity or disruption of the CFL, but a negative test did not rule out subtalar instability.[39] A medial subtalar glide test can also be used to test for subtalar instability.[4,40] A systematic review by Netterström-Wedin reported that only the anterior talofibular ligament had reliable and accurate clinical diagnostic testing for injury to the ligament. Tenderness to palpation of the anterior talofibular ligament was highly sensitive, whereas the anterior drawer test was highly specific. The talar tilt test was found to be highly specific for calcaneofibular injury.[41] Vaseenon and colleagues[42] and Miller and colleagues[43] reported that the anterolateral drawer test was more reliable and sensitive compared with the anterior drawer test in cadaver models. There remains no examination test for the intrinsic ligaments of the subtalar joint, which contributes to the difficulty in diagnosing subtalar instability.

There is no current consensus on the optimal method to evaluate for subtalar instability.[5] A set of five clinical criteria to help diagnose subtalar instability was proposed.[5,11,12,27] Per this guideline, the patient must have four of the five following criteria to receive a diagnosis of subtalar instability: (1) recurrent ankle sprains, (2) sinus tarsi pain and tenderness, (3) hindfoot looseness or giving way, (4) hindfoot instability on physical examination, and (5) radiographic subtalar instability on ankle and Broden varus stress views, defined as ipsilateral subtalar tilt greater than 10° or contralateral subtalar tilt difference greater than 5°.

LATERAL ANKLE INSTABILITY VERSUS SUBTALAR INSTABILITY

Lateral ankle instability and subtalar instability can have similar presentations. Williams and colleagues[44] suggest that localized, selective injections of a local anesthetic could help to distinguish between pain originating from the subtalar joint and the lateral gutter of the ankle.

IMAGING

Several different imaging modalities can be used in the diagnosis of subtalar instability including radiographs, CT, ultrasound, arthrography, and MRI.

Stress radiographs were initially used to evaluate subtalar instability (**Fig. 2**). Stress radiography can be performed manually or with an arthrometer. It was first described by Ruben and Witten in 1962 for ankle instability, when inversion stress was applied through the hindfoot in a Broden's view tomogram.[28,45] Subsequent authors continued to use stress radiographs to determine diagnostic criteria to define subtalar instability.[5,28] However, radiographic parameters did not consistently correlate with symptoms. Louwerens and colleagues[46] followed by Harper and colleagues[47] found no correlation between subtalar tilt and symptoms. Stress radiographs also did not correlate with CT findings. The talar tilt seen in all patients during stress radiographs was not found in any of the patients by either author in the CT imaging.[48,49]

The use of anterior stress has been suggested as a method of stress radiography. First pioneered by Kato[37] and later supported by Ishii and colleagues,[50] increased translation of the subtalar joint was found to correlate with clinical instability. A systematic review by Michels and colleagues[36] concluded that Broden's stress radiographs should not be used, and instead, anterior drawer-supination radiographs should be used to diagnose subtalar instability.

Ultrasound has also been used for subtalar instability. Waldecker and Blatter described a ratio between the sonographic neutral and stress-inverted fibula-trochlear angle. A ratio greater than 1.6 correlated with a radiographically measured subtalar instability, whereas a ratio less than 1.2 was correlated with a stable subtalar joint.[51] Wenning and colleagues[52] described a method of using a stress sonography for the diagnosis of subtalar instability in a controlled observational study. Ultrasound usage is limited as a widespread diagnostic tool, however, as it relies on the operator experience and expertise.[5]

CT permits more precise and in-depth analysis of osseous deformities of the hindfoot. However, CT alone does not provide much additional information regarding subtalar instability, as this etiology is largely soft tissue related. CT arthrography has been used to demonstrate injury to subtalar structures.[53] Pisani described a loss of the synovial recess at the sinus tarsi, which he attributed to reparative processes of the talocalcaneal ligaments following major inversion sprains.[34] Meyer and Lagier reported dye leakage from the sinus tarsi correlated with an ITCL tear, whereas dye from the lateral posterior capsule was associated with a tear of the lateral calcaneal ligament.[54]

MRI is the gold standard for evaluating soft tissues. Identifying which ligaments may be involved is important, as patients with both CL and intraosseous talocalcaneal

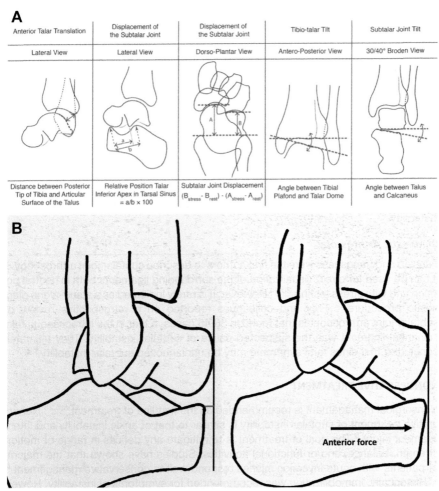

Fig. 2. (*A*) Stress imaging assessing anterior talar translation, displacement of subtalar joint and lateral and AP views, tibio-talar tilt and subtalar tilt with permission. (*B*) Stress maneuver for radiographs used for imaging in suspected subtalar instability. Stress imaging with permission. (*From* Krähenbühl N, Weinberg MW, Davidson NP, Mills MK, Hintermann B, Saltzman CL, et al. Currently used imaging options cannot accurately predict subtalar joint instability. Knee Surg Sports Traumatol Arthrosc Off J ESSKA 2019;27:2818–30. https://doi.org/10.1007/s00167-018-5232-8.)

ligament injuries have been shown to have worse clinical outcomes.[5] Partial or complete tears of the ligaments that support the subtalar joint can be seen in addition to increased intensity suggestive of bone marrow edema on T2-weighted sequences. Yuki and colleagues found a relationship between an ITCL lesion found on MRI with symptoms of giving way, pain, and limitation of ankle motion. They also found a statistically significant relationship between CL lesion found on MRI and the symptoms of giving way and pain.[55] Kim and colleagues reported that patients diagnosed with subtalar instability had significantly small anterior capsular ligament thickness and width and that the significantly higher rates of complete tears or absence of this ligament. They also noted higher rates of tears of the calcaneofibular and anterior talofibular ligament in patients with subtalar instability, but this trend was not statistically significant.[11] However, other investigators report poor correlation between MRI findings and severity of clinical instability.[22,30] Jung and colleagues[27] also found poor correlation between MRI reported chronic tears in the intraosseous talocalcaneal ligament (30%) and observed tears (100%) during surgical reconstruction for subtalar instability.

A method for better MRI diagnostic accuracy for ankle soft tissue injury was proposed by Ringleb and colleagues.[56] They described a 3D stress MRI technique using cadaver tissue and reported improved detection using this method. Wenning and colleagues[52] found similar value in using stress MRI in diagnosing ankle instability in a cross-sectional study. Seebauer and colleagues[57] found that increased subtalar tilt and anterior and medial talocalcaneal displacement were seen on stress MRIs in patients with subjective subtalar instability.

A recent systemic review by Krahenbuhl and colleagues[58] found that current imaging modalities cannot reliably differentiate subtalar instability from lateral ankle instability.

Diagnostic Arthroscopy

Parisien and Vangsness were the first authors to describe subtalar joint arthroscopy.[59] It can be used for direct visualization of the surrounding ligaments both in neutral position and with stress testing.[30,44] However, it is rarely indicated as a stand-alone diagnostic procedure.[22] Frey and colleagues reported on a retrospective review on subtalar joint arthroscopies that found in 36/45 cases, a tear in the intraosseous talocalcaneal ligament was the suspected cause of subtalar instability. They ultimately concluded that sinus tarsi syndrome may be undiagnosed subtalar instability.[60]

NONOPERATIVE TREATMENT

Nonsurgical management is recommended as the first line of treatment.[5,6,28] Nonoperative treatment of subtalar instability is similar to that of ankle instability and lateral ligament injury.[5] The goal of treatment is to mitigate any deficits in range of motion, strength, balance, and/or functional activities. Studies have shown that the majority of patients with acute inversion injuries respond well to conservative management.[6]

Historically, immobilization was recommended for symptoms of instability. However, functional treatment is now thought to be the optimal nonsurgical management.[61]

A tailored physical therapy regimen is a key for improving range of motion, strength, and proprioception. The ankle and hip work simultaneously for postural control; ankle injuries therefore can drastically impact balance and equilibrium.[62] Therapy has been shown to improve patient-reported outcomes and prevent recurrence of episodes of instability.[5] A recent meta-analysis by Luan and colleagues[62] found that strength training did not provide any improvement in clinical outcomes in activities of daily living or sport performance in patients with chronic ankle instability. However, in the same study, Luan and colleagues found benefit in neuromuscular control training. Neuromuscular control training improves deficits by increasingly challenging the sensorimotor system to adapt to varying tasks and environments. It has been shown to improve subjective symptoms of instability and prevent recurrence.[5,62,63]

Maharaj and colleagues suggested that alteration of gait can decrease subtalar moments and energy cost while walking. They found that a stride greater than the preferred step width reduced both the positive and negative work at the subtalar joint, which they hypothesized would be helpful in rehabilitation of subtalar injuries.[64]

Ankle bracing can be another effective component of nonoperative treatment. Ankle orthotics are reusable, cost-effective, easy to use, cause no skin irritation, and have no or minimal effects on performance.[65] The use of ankle braces has been shown to reduce subsequent ankle injuries.[5,66,67]

Ankle braces restrict inversion of both the talocrural and subtalar joints.[5,68,69] Braces also have been shown to preload the ankle and guide it in a more anatomically and mechanically favorable position before heel strike.[65] Ankle braces are generally one of two types: semirigid or soft lace up. Controversy exists as to which type of brace is ideal.[5,61,65,70,71]

A biomechanical study by Kamiya and colleagues[13] found that an ankle brace limited inversion of the subtalar joint with pure inversion and eversion forces. It did not offer support, however, with inversion and eversion torque. Although ankle braces help reduce talar inversion, studies have shown there continues to be increased subtalar anterior translation despite the brace in patients with chronic ankle instability.[72] Ankle braces have been shown to be more effective than elastic bandages or tape.[5,65,73–75]

It is recommended that bracing should be a supplemental component and not used alone.[5] A meta-analysis by Raymond and colleagues reported that neither the use of an ankle brace nor of taping the ankle was shown to affect the proprioceptive acuity of patients with chronic ankle instability. The investigators attributed that the reducing in ankle reinjury was likely due to restriction of joint range-of-motion, reduced mechanical instability, or improved confidence with the task, rather than increased proprioception.[66]

Foot insoles can also be considered. A cadaveric study by Tochigi demonstrated reduced abnormal maximal internal rotation of the ankle following sectioning of the anterior talofibular ligament and ITCL with the use of an insole designed to support the medial longitudinal and transverse arches. The investigator suggests that the use of an insole can be considered for patients who continue have subjective instability with walking or running despite the use of an ankle brace.[76]

A systematic review by Kerkhoffs and colleagues investigating outcomes following operative and nonoperative treatments for lateral ligament injuries of the ankle found inconclusive and heterogenous evidence and were unable to provide any strong conclusions. However, they reported that based on the included studies, surgical treatments were associated with improved stability, fewer recurrence, and less residual pain. Surgical management, however, was also associated with higher complication rates, longer duration of time off from work, higher costs, and no significant benefits in clinical outcomes.[77]

Operative Treatment

Operative treatment can be considered if there is no improvement in symptoms following 3 to 6 months of conservative management.[5,78] Many surgical techniques have been described in the literature and can broadly be classified as nonanatomic or anatomic. Schon and colleagues[79] found that in most cases of subtalar instability, reconstruction procedures are more reliable than imbrication or repair.

The Brostrom-Gould procedure is an effective surgical option for lateral ankle instability. The Brostrom procedure, initially described in 1966, is based on the direct midsubstance repair of the anterior talofibular ligament and the CFL. The original technique was reported to have a successful outcome in 80% of patients.[80] Gould and colleagues[81] later modified the technique by augmenting the repair with the lateral aspect of the inferior extensor retinaculum. This provided additional subtalar and talocrural joint stability. Outcomes following the Brostrom-Gould procedure have reported 85% to 95% success rates.[82]

Nonanatomic reconstruction can be performed when the ligaments cannot be directly repaired. These procedures usually involve tendon transfer or tenodesis techniques using the peripheral tendons to provide stability. A variety of graft types and placement can be used. The most commonly cited techniques include the Elmslie (**Fig. 3**), Watson-Jones (**Fig. 4**), Evans tenodesis (**Fig. 5**), Chrisman–Snook (**Fig. 6**), and Larsen techniques.[5,6] Most of these techniques involve using the peroneus brevis, peroneus longus, or plantaris tendon to reconstruct the anterior talofibular ligament.[5,6,79]

The Elmslie procedure (see **Fig 3**), originally described in 1934, involves routing a strip of autograft fascia lata through tunnels in the fibula, talus, and calcaneus to compensate for calcaneofibular and talofibular ligament injury.[83] The Chrisman–Snook technique, a modification from the Elmslie procedure, described reconstructing both the anterior talofibular ligament and the CFL. This technically demanding procedure uses half of the longitudinally split peroneus brevis which is rerouted through tunnels in the calcaneus and fibula. Chrisman and Snook reported on outcomes following their eponymous procedure; long-term follow (4–24 years) was found to have excellent or good function in 45/48 ankles, with two ankles still reporting improved but persistent instability and one ankle with no improvement.[84] Various modifications of this method continued to report good outcomes.[6,37,85–87] However, it has been noted that this procedure can inhibit inversion, which can lead to pain due to constrained range of motion.[88]

The Larsen technique uses the peroneus brevis to reconstruct the CFL. The peroneus brevis tendon is released as proximally as possible. The proximal end is then tenodesed to the peroneus longus. The free distal tendon is then rerouted starting at the insertion at the base of the fifth metatarsal proximal through an oblique tunnel in the distal fibula. It is then passed through a second more vertical tunnel in the distal fibula and anchored into the calcaneus.[89] Although all 25 patients at mid-term follow-up following this method of stabilization had satisfactory return to activity, the complication rate was high (11%).[90]

The nonanatomic reconstruction techniques are effective in reducing subtalar motion. However, they do not restore the normal arthrokinematics of the ankle. As a result, they are associated with a higher risk of developing subtalar stiffness and osteoarthritis.[28]

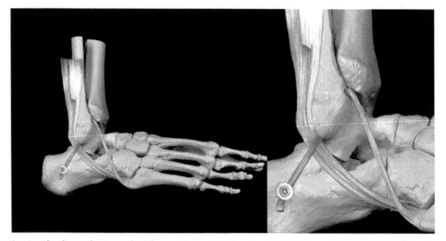

Fig. 3. Elmslie technique. (*With permission* Mittlmeier T, Wichelhaus A. Subtalar joint instability. Eur J Trauma Emerg Surg. 2015 Dec;41(6):623-9. https://doi.org/10.1007/s00068-015-0588-7. Epub 2015 Oct 28. PMID: 26510942.)

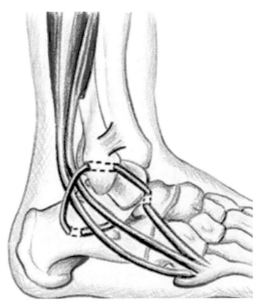

Fig. 4. Watson-Jones technique. (*With permission* granted by CreativeCommons license from Al-Mohrej OA, Al-Kenani NS. Chronic ankle instability: Current perspectives. Avicenna J Med. 2016 Oct-Dec;6(4):103-108. https://doi.org/10.4103/2231-0770.191446. PMID: 27843798; PMCID: PMC5054646.)

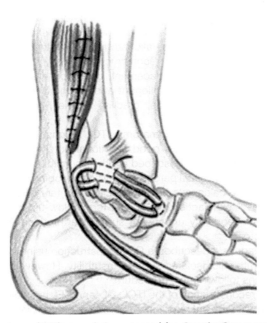

Fig. 5. Evans technique. (*With permission* granted by CreativeCommone license from Al-Mohrej OA, Al-Kenani NS. Chronicans ankle instability: Current perspectives. Avicenna J Med. 2016 Oct-Dec;6(4):103-108. https://doi.org/10.4103/2231-0770.191446. PMID: 27843798; PMCID: PMC5054646.)

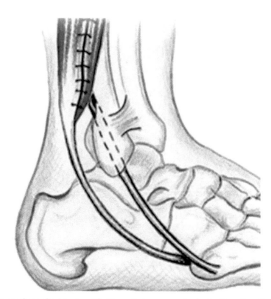

Fig. 6. Crissman–Snook technique with Permission granted via CreativeCommons. (*From* Al-Mohrej OA, Al-Kenani NS. Chronicans ankle instability: Current perspectives. Avicenna J Med. 2016 Oct-Dec;6(4):103-108. https://doi.org/10.4103/2231-0770.191446. PMID: 27843798; PMCID: PMC5054646.)

Anatomic reconstruction seeks to restore the major subtalar ligaments, including the CFL, ITCL, and CL, in order to restore normal arthrokinematics. Anatomic reconstruction is considered superior to the older nonanatomic techniques, especially in cases with isolated subtalar laxity.[5] This can be accomplished either through direct repair, with or without autologous, allographic, or synthetic supplementation or through autologous or synthetic reconstruction. Many techniques have been described, with variations in tunnel placement, graft type, graft positioning, and fixation techniques.[5,6] Several different allograft and autograft tendons have been proposed including the semitendinosus, gracilis, Achilles, plantaris, and peroneus brevis.[5]

Kato was the first to describe an anatomic ITCL reconstruction; he used a partial Achilles tendon graft. He reported good functional outcomes with low complications.[37] Pasini and colleagues[34] described another technique for ITCL reconstruction using the anterior half of the distal peroneus brevis and looping it through tunnels in the anterior process of the calcaneus into the neck of the talus. For his original article, Pisani reported a 91% satisfaction rate at long-term follow-up; however, it was noted that six patients subsequently underwent subtalar arthrodesis for residual pain or insufficiency symptoms.[34]

Schon and colleagues[79] described a CL reconstruction using half of the peroneus brevis in patients with mild, isolated subtalar instability. However, they did not report on patient outcomes following this procedure.

Tri-ligamentous reconstruction of the ITCL, CL, and CFL has been well described. It can be performed with the entire or half of peroneus brevis, plantaris, or the Achilles tendon.[6,28,79,91] Schon and colleagues[79] noted that using the plantaris in this procedure avoids sacrificing tendons around the ankle that contribute to proprioceptive stability; they do acknowledge, however, difficulties using the plantaris including locating the tendon, additional incisions, and the occasional fragility of the tendon.

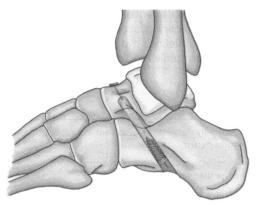

Fig. 7. Anatomic cervical ligament reconstruction with graft. (*With permission* granted via CreativeCommons license From Iglesias-Durán E, Guerra-Pinto F, García-Esteo F, Vilá-Rico J. Anatomic Arthroscopic Graft Reconstruction of the Interosseous Talocalcaneal Ligament for Subtalar Instability. Arthrosc Tech. 2020 Nov 25;9(12):e1903-e1906. https://doi.org/10.1016/j.eats.2020.08.020. PMID: 33381399; PMCID: PMC7768199.)

Karlsson and colleagues described a technique for anatomic repair/reconstruction of the calcaneofibular, lateral talocalcaneal, and CL. With the ankle in neutral position, the CFL was cut, the ends imbricated with appropriate tension and sutured to the distal fibula and the inferior extensor retinaculum. The lateral talocalcaneal and CLs were tightened, imbricated, and sutured to the distal fibula. The investigators reported satisfactory outcomes in 18/22 patients. Of the two patients with poor results, both continued to have symptoms of functional instability.[88]

Coughlin and colleagues used an ipsilateral gracilis autograft in a case series of 28 patients with chronic instability. They used the free gracilis tendon to anatomically reconstruct the anterior talofibular ligament and CFL. Following the reconstruction, the remnants of the anterior talofibular ligament were directly repaired via the Brostrom procedure. They reported all patients had excellent or good outcomes at long-term follow-up (12–52 months).[92]

Arthroscopic reconstruction or endoscopy-assisted approaches have recently been reported in the literature. So and colleagues[93] described an accurate, reproducible, percutaneous method for placing a tunnel at the footprint of the ITCL, using a fluoroscopic-guided technique in cadaver feet. Liu and colleagues[94] described a case report using ankle arthroscopy to assist in a reconstruction of the ITCL using a gracilis autograft. They believed that using ankle arthroscopy allowed for improved accuracy in the placement of anchor tunnels. More recently, Iglesias-Duran and colleagues[95] published a new "all inside" arthroscopic technique for ITCL reconstruction (**Fig. 7**).

Subtalar arthrodesis can be considered in patients with persistent subtalar instability following failure of ligament reconstruction.[96]

SUMMARY

Isolated subtalar instability continues to be a difficult entity to define, detect, and treat. Current imaging modalities continue to lack the specificity and sensitivity for this condition and much of the treatment for subtalar instability overlaps lateral ankle instability. Isolated subtalar instability seems to continue to be a diagnosis of exclusion.

Patients who fail nonoperative intervention are candidates for operative intervention and the risks and benefits of surgery must be carefully balanced. The ideal reconstruction technique is currently not defined owing to the rarity of this condition with little literature besides small cohort studies and case reports with significant heterogeneity.

CLINICS CARE POINTS

- Inital treatment is essentially the same as lateral ankle sprains, but a high suspicion should be maintained if symptoms persist.
- Imaging is not always reliable and multiple modalities including stress imaging and MRI may be required tomake the diagnosis.
- Multiple procedures have been described but few have strong support in the literature. Procedure selection should be based on surgeon comfort level and patient symptoms.

REFERENCES

1. Jung H-G, Moon SG, Yoon DY, et al. Feasibility of MRI for the evaluation of interosseous ligament vertical segment via subtalar arthroscopy correlation: comparison of 2D and 3D MR images. BMC Musculoskelet Disord 2021;22:869.
2. Krähenbühl N, Horn-Lang T, Hintermann B, et al. The subtalar joint: a complex mechanism. EFORT Open Rev 2017;2:309–16.
3. Maceira E, Monteagudo M. Subtalar anatomy and mechanics. Foot Ankle Clin 2015;20:195–221.
4. Hertel J. Functional anatomy, pathomechanics, and pathophysiology of lateral ankle instability. J Athl Train 2002;37:364–75.
5. Pereira BS, Andrade R, Espregueira-Mendes J, et al. Current Concepts on Subtalar Instability. Orthop J Sports Med 2021;9. 23259671211021350.
6. Karlsson J, Eriksson BI, Renström PA. Subtalar ankle instability. A review. Sports Med Auckl NZ 1997;24:337–46.
7. Viladot A, Lorenzo JC, Salazar J, et al. The subtalar joint: embryology and morphology. Foot Ankle 1984;5:54–66.
8. Olexa TA, Ebraheim NA, Haman SP. The sustentaculum tali: anatomic, radiographic, and surgical considerations. Foot Ankle Int 2000;21:400–3.
9. Jotoku T, Kinoshita M, Okuda R, et al. Anatomy of ligamentous structures in the tarsal sinus and canal. Foot Ankle Int 2006;27:533–8. ⟍.
10. Li S-Y, Hou Z-D, Zhang P, et al. Ligament structures in the tarsal sinus and canal. Foot Ankle Int 2013;34:1729–36.
11. Kim TH, Moon SG, Jung H-G, et al. Subtalar instability: imaging features of subtalar ligaments on 3D isotropic ankle MRI. BMC Musculoskelet Disord 2017;18:475.
12. Yoon DY, Moon SG, Jung H-G, et al. Differences between subtalar instability and lateral ankle instability focusing on subtalar ligaments based on three dimensional isotropic magnetic resonance imaging. J Comput Assist Tomogr 2018;42:566–73.
13. Kamiya T, Kura H, Suzuki D, et al. Mechanical stability of the subtalar joint after lateral ligament sectioning and ankle brace application: a biomechanical experimental study. Am J Sports Med 2009;37:2451–8.
14. Stormont DM, Morrey BF, An KN, et al. Stability of the loaded ankle. Relation between articular restraint and primary and secondary static restraints. Am J Sports Med 1985;13:295–300.

15. Cahill DR. The anatomy and function of the contents of the human tarsal sinus and canal. Anat Rec 1965;153:1–17.
16. Smith JW. The ligamentous structures in the canalis and sinus tarsi. J Anat 1958; 92:616–20.
17. Kjaersgaard-Andersen P, Wethelund JO, Helmig P, et al. The stabilizing effect of the ligamentous structures in the sinus and canalis tarsi on movements in the hindfoot. An experimental study. Am J Sports Med 1988;16:512–6.
18. Tochigi Y, Amendola A, Rudert MJ, et al. The role of the interosseous talocalcaneal ligament in subtalar joint stability. Foot Ankle Int 2004;25:588–96.
19. Wright DG, Desai SM, Henderson WH. Action of the subtalar and ankle-joint complex during the stance phase of walking. J Bone Joint Surg Am 1964;46:361–82.
20. Donatelli RA. Normal biomechanics of the foot and ankle. J Orthop Sports Phys Ther 1985;7:91–5.
21. Medina McKeon JM, Hoch MC. The ankle-joint complex: a kinesiologic approach to lateral ankle sprains. J Athl Train 2019;54:589–602.
22. Mittlmeier T, Wichelhaus A. Subtalar joint instability. Eur J Trauma Emerg Surg 2015;41:623–9.
23. Bartoníček J, Rammelt S, Naňka O. Anatomy of the subtalar joint. Foot Ankle Clin 2018;23:315–40.
24. Mittlmeier T, Rammelt S. Update on subtalar joint instability. Foot Ankle Clin 2018; 23:397–413.
25. Pearce TJ, Buckley RE. Subtalar joint movement: clinical and computed tomography scan correlation. Foot Ankle Int 1999;20:428–32.
26. Buckley RE, Hunt DV. Reliability of clinical measurement of subtalar joint movement. Foot Ankle Int 1997;18:229–32.
27. Jung H-G, Park J-T, Shin M-H, et al. Outcome of subtalar instability reconstruction using the semitendinosus allograft tendon and biotenodesis screws. Knee Surg Sports Traumatol Arthrosc 2015;23:2376–83.
28. Keefe DT, Haddad SL. Subtalar instability. Etiology, diagnosis, and management. Foot Ankle Clin 2002;7:577–609.
29. Taillard W, Meyer JM, Garcia J, et al. The sinus tarsi syndrome. Int Orthop 1981;5: 117–30.
30. Barg A, Tochigi Y, Amendola A, et al. Subtalar instability: diagnosis and treatment. Foot Ankle Int 2012;33:151–60.
31. Bonnel F, Toullec E, Mabit C, et al. Chronic ankle instability: biomechanics and pathomechanics of ligaments injury and associated lesions. Orthop Traumatol Surg Res OTSR 2010;96:424–32.
32. Ringleb SI, Dhakal A, Anderson CD, et al. Effects of lateral ligament sectioning on the stability of the ankle and subtalar joint. J Orthop Res 2011;29:1459–64.
33. Heilman AE, Braly WG, Bishop JO, et al. An anatomic study of subtalar instability. Foot Ankle 1990;10:224–8.
34. Pisani G. Chronic laxity of the subtalar joint. Orthopedics 1996;19:431–7.
35. Pisani G, Pisani PC, Parino E. Sinus tarsi syndrome and subtalar joint instability. Clin Podiatr Med Surg 2005;22:63–77, vii.
36. Michels F, Clockaerts S, Van Der Bauwhede J, et al. Does subtalar instability really exist? A systematic review. Foot Ankle Surg 2020;26:119–27.
37. Kato T. The diagnosis and treatment of instability of the subtalar joint. J Bone Joint Surg Br 1995;77:400–6.
38. Thermann H, Zwipp H, Tscherne H. Treatment algorithm of chronic ankle and subtalar instability. Foot Ankle Int 1997;18:163–9.

39. Usuelli FG, Mason L, Grassi M, et al. Lateral ankle and hindfoot instability: a new clinical based classification. Foot Ankle Surg Off J Eur Soc Foot Ankle Surg 2014; 20:231–6.

40. Hertel J, Denegar CR, Monroe MM, et al. Talocrural and subtalar joint instability after lateral ankle sprain. Med Sci Sports Exerc 1999;31:1501–8.

41. Netterström-Wedin F, Matthews M, Bleakley C. Diagnostic accuracy of clinical tests assessing ligamentous injury of the talocrural and subtalar joints: a systematic review with meta-analysis. Sports Health 2022;14:336–47.

42. Vaseenon T, Gao Y, Phisitkul P. Comparison of two manual tests for ankle laxity due to rupture of the lateral ankle ligaments. Iowa Orthop J 2012;32:9–16.

43. Miller AG, Myers SH, Parks BG, et al. Anterolateral drawer versus anterior drawer test for ankle instability: a biomechanical model. Foot Ankle Int 2016;37:407–10.

44. Williams M, Ferkel R. Subtalar arthroscopy: indications, technique, and results. Arthrosc J Arthrosc Relat Surg 1998;14:373–81.

45. Rubin G, Wittin M. The subtalar joint and the symptom of turning overr on the ankle: a new method of evaluation utilizing tomography. Am J Orthop 1962; 4:16–9.

46. Louwerens JW, Ginai AZ, van Linge B, et al. Stress radiography of the talocrural and subtalar joints. Foot Ankle Int 1995;16:148–55.

47. Harper MC. Stress radiographs in the diagnosis of lateral instability of the ankle and hindfoot. Foot Ankle 1992;13:435–8.

48. van Hellemondt FJ, Louwerens JWK, Sijbrandij ES, et al. Stress Radiography and Stress Examination of the Talocrural and Subtalar Joint on Helical Computed Tomography. Foot Ankle Int 1997;18:482–8.

49. Sijbrandij ES, van Gils APG, van Hellemondt FJ, et al. Assessing the subtalar joint: the brodén view revisited. Foot Ankle Int 2001;22:329–34.

50. Ishii T, Miyagawa S, Fukubayashi T, et al. Subtalar stress radiography using forced dorsiflexion and supination. J Bone Joint Surg Br 1996;78:56–60.

51. Waldecker U, Blatter G. Sonographic measurement of instability of the subtalar joint. Foot Ankle Int 2001;22:42–6.

52. Wenning M, Gehring D, Lange T, et al. Clinical evaluation of manual stress testing, stress ultrasound and 3D stress MRI in chronic mechanical ankle instability. BMC Musculoskelet Disord 2021;22:198.

53. Goossens M, De Stoop N, Claessens H, et al. Posterior subtalar joint arthrography. A useful tool in the diagnosis of hindfoot disorders. Clin Orthop 1989;249: 248–55.

54. Meyer JM, Lagier R. Post-traumatic sinus tarsi syndrome. An anatomical and radiological study. Acta Orthop Scand 1977;48:121–8.

55. Tochigi Y, Yoshinaga K, Wada Y, et al. Acute inversion injury of the ankle: magnetic resonance imaging and clinical outcomes. Foot Ankle Int 1998;19:730–4.

56. Ringleb SI, Udupa JK, Siegler S, et al. The effect of ankle ligament damage and surgical reconstructions on the mechanics of the ankle and subtalar joints revealed by three-dimensional stress MRI. J Orthop Res 2005;23:743–9.

57. Seebauer CJ, Bail HJ, Rump JC, et al. Ankle laxity: stress investigation under MRI control. AJR Am J Roentgenol 2013;201:496–504.

58. Krähenbühl N, Weinberg MW, Davidson NP, et al. Currently used imaging options cannot accurately predict subtalar joint instability. Knee Surg Sports Traumatol Arthrosc Off J ESSKA 2019;27:2818–30.

59. Parisien JS, Vangsness T. Arthroscopy of the subtalar joint: an experimental approach. Arthrosc J Arthrosc Relat Surg 1985;1:53–7.

60. Frey C, Feder KS, DiGiovanni C. Arthroscopic evaluation of the subtalar joint: does sinus tarsi syndrome exist? Foot Ankle Int 1999;20:185–91.

61. van den Bekerom MPJ, van Kimmenade R, Sierevelt IN, et al. Randomized comparison of tape versus semi-rigid and versus lace-up ankle support in the treatment of acute lateral ankle ligament injury. Knee Surg Sports Traumatol Arthrosc 2016;24:978–84.

62. Luan L, Adams R, Witchalls J, et al. Does strength training for chronic ankle instability improve balance and patient-reported outcomes and by clinically detectable amounts? A systematic review and meta-analysis. Phys Ther 2021;101: pzab046.

63. de Vries JS, Krips R, Sierevelt IN, et al. Interventions for treating chronic ankle instability. Cochrane Database Syst Rev 2011;CD004124. https://doi.org/10.1002/14651858.CD004124.pub3.

64. Maharaj JN, Murry LE, Cresswell AG, et al. Increasing step width reduces the requirements for subtalar joint moments and powers. J Biomech 2019;92:29–34.

65. Zhang S, Wortley M, Chen Q, et al. Efficacy of an ankle brace with a subtalar locking system in inversion control in dynamic movements. J Orthop Sports Phys Ther 2009;39:875–83.

66. Raymond J, Nicholson LL, Hiller CE, et al. The effect of ankle taping or bracing on proprioception in functional ankle instability: a systematic review and meta-analysis. J Sci Med Sport 2012;15:386–92.

67. Barlow G, Donovan L, Hart JM, et al. Effect of lace-up ankle braces on electromyography measures during walking in adults with chronic ankle instability. Phys Ther Sport 2015;16:16–21.

68. Choisne J, McNally A, Hoch MC, et al. Effect of simulated joint instability and bracing on ankle and subtalar joint flexibility. J Biomech 2019;82:234–43.

69. Choisne J, Hoch MC, Bawab S, et al. The effects of a semi-rigid ankle brace on a simulated isolated subtalar joint instability. J Orthop Res 2013;31:1869–75.

70. Cordova ML, Dorrough JL, Kious K, et al. Prophylactic ankle bracing reduces rearfoot motion during sudden inversion. Scand J Med Sci Sports 2007;17: 216–22.

71. Simpson KJ, Cravens S, Higbie E, et al. A comparison of the Sport Stirrup, Malleoloc, and Swede-O ankle orthoses for the foot-ankle kinematics of a rapid lateral movement. Int J Sports Med 1999;20:396–402.

72. Cao S, Wang C, Zhang G, et al. Effects of an ankle brace on the in vivo kinematics of patients with chronic ankle instability during walking on an inversion platform. Gait Posture 2019;72:228–33.

73. Kobayashi T, Saka M, Suzuki E, et al. The effects of a semi-rigid brace or taping on talocrural and subtalar kinematics in chronic ankle instability. Foot Ankle Spec 2014;7:471–7.

74. Paris DL, Kokkaliaris J, Vardaxis V. Ankle ranges of motion during extended activity periods while taped and braced. J Athl Train 1995;30:223–8.

75. Vorhagen FA, van der Beek AJ, van Mechelen W. The effect of tape, braces and shoes on ankle range of motion. Sports Med Auckl NZ 2001;31:667–77.

76. Tochigi Y. Effect of arch supports on ankle-subtalar complex instability: a biomechanical experimental study. Foot Ankle Int 2003;24:634–9.

77. Kerkhoffs GMMJ, Handoll HHG, de Bie R, et al. Surgical versus conservative treatment for acute injuries of the lateral ligament complex of the ankle in adults. Cochrane Database Syst Rev 2007;CD000380. https://doi.org/10.1002/14651858.CD000380.pub2.

78. Michels F, Pereira H, Calder J, et al. Searching for consensus in the approach to patients with chronic lateral ankle instability: ask the expert. Knee Surg Sports Traumatol Arthrosc 2018;26:2095–102.

79. Schon LC, Clanton TO, Baxter DE. Reconstruction for subtalar instability: a review. Foot Ankle 1991;11:319–25.

80. Broström L. Sprained ankles. VI. Surgical treatment of "chronic" ligament ruptures. Acta Chir Scand 1966;132:551–65.

81. Gould N, Seligson D, Gassman J. Early and late repair of lateral ligament of the ankle. Foot Ankle 1980;1:84–9.

82. So E, Preston N, Holmes T. Intermediate- to long-term longevity and incidence of revision of the modified broström-gould procedure for lateral ankle ligament repair: a systematic review. Sports Med 2017;56:1076–80.

83. Elmslie RC. Recurrent subluxation of the ankle-joint. Ann Surg 1934;100:364–7.

84. Snook GA, Chrisman OD, Wilson TC. Long-term results of the Chrisman-Snook operation for reconstruction of the lateral ligaments of the ankle. J Bone Joint Surg Am 1985;67:1–7.

85. Marsh JS, Daigneault JP, Polzhofer GK. Treatment of ankle instability in children and adolescents with a modified Chrisman-Snook repair: a clinical and patient-based outcome study. J Pediatr Orthop 2006;26:94–9.

86. Bernhard JA, Burckhardt A. [Long-term results following fibulo-tarsal ligament reconstruction. Comparison of the Watson-Jones and the (modified) Chrisman-Snook techniques]. Swiss Surg Schweiz Chir Chir Suisse Chir Svizzera 1996;2: 274–9.

87. Noyez JF, Martens MA. Secondary reconstruction of the lateral ligaments of the ankle by the Chrisman-Snook technique. Arch Orthop Trauma Surg Arch Orthopadische Unf-Chir 1986;106:52–6.

88. Karlsson J, Eriksson BI, Renström P. Subtalar instability of the foot. A review and results after surgical treatment. Scand J Med Sci Sports 1998;8:191–7.

89. Larsen E. Tendon transfer for lateral ankle and subtalar joint instability. Acta Orthop Scand 1988;59:168–72.

90. Larsen E. Static or dynamic repair of chronic lateral ankle instability. A prospective randomized study. Clin Orthop 1990;257:184–92.

91. Solheim LF, Denstad TF, Roaas A. Chronic lateral instability of the ankle. A method of reconstruction using the Achilles tendon. Acta Orthop Scand 1980;51:193–6.

92. Coughlin MJ, Schenck RC, Grebing BR, et al. Comprehensive reconstruction of the lateral ankle for chronic instability using a free gracilis graft. Foot Ankle Int 2004;25:231–41.

93. So E, Weber J, Berlet G, Bull P. Surgical treatment of subtalar joint instability: safety and accuracy of a new technique in a cadaver model. J Foot Ankle Surg 2020;59(1):38–43.

94. Liu C, Jiao C, Hu Y, et al. Interosseous talocalcaneal ligament reconstruction with hamstring autograft under subtalar arthroscopy: case report. Foot Ankle Int 2011; 32:1089–94.

95. Iglesias-Durán E, Guerra-Pinto F, García-Esteo F, et al. Anatomic arthroscopic graft reconstruction of the interosseous talocalcaneal ligament for subtalar instability. Arthrosc Tech 2020;9:e1903–6.

96. Mann RA, Beaman DN, Horton GA. Isolated subtalar arthrodesis. Foot Ankle Int 1998;19:511–9.

Ligament Ruptures in Ankle Fractures—Was Lauge-Hansen Right?

Stefan Rammelt, MD, PhD[a],*, Andrzej Boszczyk, MD, PhD[b]

KEYWORDS

- Ankle • Malleolar • Fracture • Lateral ligaments • Syndesmosis
- Interosseous ligament

KEY POINTS

- The contribution of Lauge-Hansen to the understanding and treatment of ankle fractures cannot be underestimated, an unquestionable merit being the analysis of the ligamentous component of these injuries that are considered as equivalent to the respective malleolar fractures.
- When revisiting the Lauge-Hansen experiments, biomechanical and observational studies suggest that a substantial amount of fracture patterns regarded as supination-external rotation injuries were, in fact, produced by a pronation force.
- In numerous clinical and biomechanical studies, the lateral ankle ligaments are ruptured either together with or instead of the syndesmotic ligaments, as predicted by the Lauge-Hansen stages.
- The differences between the Lauge-Hansen and current experiments as well as the variable patterns of purely ligamentous and bony components in ankle factures may be explained partly by the individual bone quality resulting in a variable morphology of malleolar fractures through a similar mechanism of injury.
- A ligament-based view on malleolar fractures may deepen the understanding of the mechanism of injury and lead to a stability-based evaluation and treatment of the 4 osteoligamentous pillars (malleoli) at the ankle.

INTRODUCTION

The notable variability of ankle fracture morphology and associated ligamentous injuries has been fascinating surgeons and researchers alike since the advent of modern orthopedics and traumatology. Early researchers solved the task of categorizing ankle fractures by grouping similar fractures together and assigning them an eponym like,

[a] University Center for Orthopaedic, Trauma and Plastic Surgery, University Hospital Carl Gustav Carus at the TU Dresden, Fetscherstrasse 74, Dresden 01307, Germany; [b] Idea Ortopedia, Piękna 15 Str, Warsaw 00-549, Poland
* Corresponding author.
E-mail address: stefan.rammelt@uniklinikum-dresden.de

Foot Ankle Clin N Am 28 (2023) 445–461
https://doi.org/10.1016/j.fcl.2023.01.007
1083-7515/23/© 2023 Elsevier Inc. All rights reserved.

foot.theclinics.com

for example, Pott, Dupuytren, Maisonneuve, and Volkmann fracture.[1–3] These morphology-based classifications added little, however, to the understanding of the injury and planning of treatment. The question of the exact mechanism, that is, which positions and forces explain these highly different patterns of ankle fracture morphology, has been keeping surgeons and researchers busy for at least 150 years now. The landmark Lauge-Hansen studies from the late 1940s associated fracture morphology with the position of the foot and the direction of deforming force acting on the joint at the time of injury.[2,4–6] If this association was as strong as suggested by Lauge-Hansen, then the defined set of positions (supination/pronation) and forces (adduction/abduction/external rotation) would consistently produce fractures belonging to a defined family (**Fig. 1**). In the reverse analysis, recognition of fracture patterns belonging to a defined family would enable the researcher to deduct the forces having produced them.

Lauge-Hansen's studies, however, despite their logic appeal, in fact produced more questions than they solved. There is a growing body of literature supporting doubts about the mechanistic explanation offered by them. Studies questioning the Lauge-Hansen "laws" can be categorized in 2 groups. A first group of studies were those attempting to reproduce the Lauge-Hansen experiments either exactly or with various modifications. A second group of studies used observational methods in order to correlate fracture morphology and the mechanism of injury. Independent of these findings, an unquestionable merit of Lauge-Hansen was the analysis of the ligamentous component of these injuries that were considered as equivalent to the malleolar fractures.[5]

THE LAUGE-HANSEN EXPERIMENTS REVISITED

Reproducing the original Lauge-Hansen experiments is not trivial because he did not place the extremity in a constant position and applied the forces (mainly external rotation) manually. Numerous researchers attempting to recreate the Lauge-Hansen experiments achieved variable results.

Stiehl and colleagues[7] loaded 26 cadaveric ankles at a fixed degree of pronation/supination or dorsiflexion/plantar flexion or both in external rotation and found only a weak correlation between foot position (pronation/supination) and injury pattern.

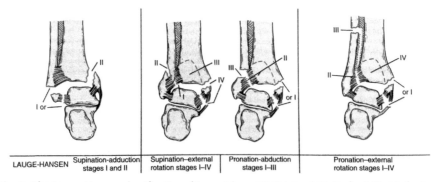

| LAUGE-HANSEN | Supination-adduction stages I and II | Supination–external rotation stages I–IV | Pronation-abduction stages I–III | Pronation–external rotation stages I–IV |

Fig. 1. The Lauge-Hansen classification. (*From* Adams SB, Tainter DM, Taylor MA: Malleolar fractures and soft-tissue injuries to the ankle. In: Browner BD, Jupiter JB, Krettek C, Anderson PA (eds.): Skeletal Trauma, 6th Edition, Philadelphia, Elsevier Saunders, 2019, pp. 2446-2496.)

Overall, only 67% of male and 40% of female specimens had an oblique fibular fracture, torn anterior tibiofibular ligament, and torn deltoid ligament corresponding to a supination-external rotation (SER) stage 2 (4) fracture. In female specimens, 45% had a transverse fibular fracture without any syndesmotic or deltoid injury. The angle of supination or pronation did not correlate with a specific injury pattern.

Michelson and colleagues[8] observed, that axial loading and external rotation did not result in the typical Lauge-Hansen SER type fractures in 32 cadaver ankles placed in neutral position on a foot plate with 25° of supination. This was not altered when the ankle specimens initially were placed in plantar flexion or dorsiflexion. The authors concluded that pure supination and external rotation do not lead to the predicted SER fracture pattern. The addition of a valgus load, which pushes the talus laterally against the fibula (ie, an abduction force), resulted in the classic Lauge-Hansen SER type fracture pattern. All specimens either had an isolated lateral injury or a lateral injury that preceded medial injury.

Haraguchi and Arminger[9] produced the typical oblique distal fibular fracture that was thought to be characteristic of a SER-injury with a pronation-external rotation (PER) mechanism. Adding an additional momentum of external lateral force (abduction) produced a high fibular fracture with a reversed fracture line or comminuted fracture. The authors concluded that most malleolar fractures except for supination-adduction (SAD) injuries are produced with the foot in pronation.

Zahn and colleagues[10] applied SER forces together with axial load and ankle dorsiflexion to 29 osteoporotic cadaveric ankles. They reproduced SER injury patterns according to Lauge-Hansen in 45% of specimens without and 65% of specimens with additional application of a lateral force. A SER4 injury was induced in 25% only. A lower bone density correlated with the angle of the fibular fracture. The obligatory lesion of the anterior inferior tibiofibular (syndesmotic) ligament (AITFL) at stage 2 of SER according to Lauge-Hansen was observed in 50% only, whereas half of the specimens had an intact syndesmosis. Lateral ligament injuries (bony avulsions of the anterior talofibular ligament, ATFL) were only seen without lateral force application.

In an attempt to recreate the original Lauge-Hansen experiments, Kwon and colleagues[11] loaded 10 feet axially in neutral position (plantarflexion/dorsiflexion) and supination manually with external rotation until osseous and ligamentous injuries occurred. Although several specimens exhibited findings consistent with certain SER stages, no specimen demonstrated the complete sequence of osseous and soft-tissue injuries as predicted by the Lauge-Hansen stages. Interestingly, 3 of 10 specimens displayed a rupture of the lateral collateral ligaments, that is, the ATFL and calcaneofibular ligament (CFL). One of them also had an AITFL rupture and fibular avulsion fracture, one had an additional deltoid ligament rupture, and the third one had no other injuries. Only 4 specimens had a short oblique fibular fracture and 2 of them had an additional AITFL rupture corresponding to the SER stage 2 pattern. The posterior inferior tibiofibular ligament (PITFL) was disrupted in 1 specimen, and there was no posterior malleolar fracture.

CLINICAL OBSERVATIONS OF THE INJURY MECHANISM

Another set of studies attempted on searching for real-life observations of forces producing discriminate types of fracture.

In a remarkable study, Rodriguez and colleagues[12] analyzed 30 YouTube videos—mostly of skateboarding injuries—and managed to obtain the corresponding postinjury radiographs. Due to the selective patient age group and injury patterns captured on YouTube videos, the authors observed 16 SAD mechanisms and 14 PER mechanisms. Although they found no video evidence of an SER injury mechanism, there were 8 SER fracture patterns on radiographs that were actually caused by a pronation fracture mechanism. The accuracy of the Lauge-Hansen classification of radiographs in predicting the mechanism of injury was calculated with 65%. This concordance may still be relatively high because of the atypical population studied. Due to the specific sports and age groups present at the Internet platform at the time of the study, SAD fractures, that typically account for around 1% of fractures, comprised 60% of the whole study group. The concordance between fracture mechanism on video and radiographic pattern of injury was 75% for the SAD mechanism and only 36% for the PER mechanism.[12]

Recent studies based on patient-reported mechanisms of injury were able to recruit a more representative population with ankle fractures.[13,14] In the study by Boszczyk and colleagues,[13] 110 patients slated for ankle fracture surgery were interviewed and 71% of them were able to provide the circumstances of their injury. The group included 43 women and 35 men aged from 19.5 to 88.4 years. Both pronation (45%) and supination (35%) were reported by patients as an injury mechanism, followed by hyperplantarflexion in 20% of cases. The concordance between the mechanism described by the patient and the fracture pattern according to the Lauge-Hansen classification was 45% only. When the Lauge-Hansen classification was used to predict the mechanism reported by the patients, the concordance reached 48%. This translates to a concordance below random statistical distribution.

In a sequel of this study using the same group of patients,[14] radiological features useful in predicting mechanism of injury have been identified. It has been confirmed that absolute determination of the mechanism of injury based on radiograph features in not possible. Some correlations, however, were identified. Pure ligamentous or chip-avulsion medial side injury was correlated with supination, while anterior colliculus fractures at the medial malleolus were correlated with pronation. Posterior malleolar fractures were significantly correlated with pronation. The lateral side injury was not able to predict mechanism of injury, except for infrasyndesmotic fractures pointing to supination, which is in line with observations by Rodriguez and colleagues.[12]

Considered together, the biomechanical studies by Haraguchi and Arminger[9] and the observational studies of Rodriguez and colleagues[12] and Boszczyk and colleagues[13,14] suggest that a substantial amount of fracture patterns regarded as SER injuries were in fact produced by a pronation force. In a recent clinical study of 153 patients, Patton and colleagues[15] did not find any significant association between the Lauge-Hansen injury mechanism and posterior malleolar fracture morphology as expressed by the Bartoníček/Rammelt and Haraguchi classifications.[16]

Questioning the association between mechanism of fracture and its resulting morphology offered by Lauge-Hansen leads to reopening of the search for a theory explaining the existence of so many different patterns of ankle fractures. This question is especially interesting as each scientist and clinician inherently feels that the fractures form discrete patterns.

LIGAMENTOUS INJURIES IN MALLEOLAR FRACTURES
Equivalence of Ligament Ruptures, Avulsions, and Malleolar Fractures

Ankle fractures are osteoligamentous injuries affecting the system formed by the tibiofibular mortise, the talus, and numerous ligaments interconnecting these bones.[1–6] The sheer term "ankle fracture" as well as x-ray-based imaging techniques as primary modalities focus attention on the bony part of the injury. It should be, however, noted that the ligamentous complex is at least equally important to stability. Applying a ligament-centered analysis to ankle fractures can lead to new insights. With this approach, the majority of osseous injuries in the wake of ankle fractures can be interpreted as ligamentous avulsion fractures. A similar biomechanical effect can be expected from purely ligamentous injuries without bone involvement and bony avulsions of the ligaments presenting as fractures. Beginning–again–with Lauge-Hansen,[5] these former injuries are being termed the soft tissue equivalent of the fracture.[16]

This type of analysis has been exemplarily well illustrated for the deltoid ligament and medial malleolus complex by Pankovich and colleagues[17,18] as early as 1979. Pankovich pointed out that the medial malleolus comprises an anterior and posterior colliculus separated by intercollicular groove. The deep posterior tibiotalar portion of the deltoid ligament that is crucial for talar stability in the ankle mortise inserts to the posterior colliculus and intercollicular groove. The anterior colliculus receives insertion of deep anterior tibiotalar portion at its apex and the superficial layer of the deltoid ligament on its body.[19] In his classification, Pankovich interpreted medial malleolar fractures as avulsions of certain parts of the deltoid ligament. Accordingly, the medial injury may take a form of.

1. Rupture of deep and superficial portions of the deltoid ligament, representing the soft-tissue equivalent of a fracture
2. Fracture of the anterior colliculus, representing avulsion of the deep anterior tibiotalar ligament while the deep posterior part of tibiotalar ligament remains intact, offering stability to the joint
3. Fracture of anterior colliculus and tear of the deep posterior tibiotalar ligament rendering the talus unstable in the mortise
4. Fracture of the posterior colliculus of medial malleolus
5. Supracollicular fractures of the medial malleolus representing avulsion of whole deltoid ligament, which remains intact
6. Chip-avulsion fractures representing avulsion of the superficial deltoid.

This latter was considered by Pankovich as benign. Recently, however, observation of a "medial malleolar fleck sign," corresponding to this type 6 injury, has been linked to deltoid incompetence.[20] Contrary to Pankovich's observations, the authors intraoperatively observed the deep layer of the deltoid ligament partially attached to the avulsed fragment (fleck).[20]

Similar analysis can be applied to the other ankle ligaments. Injuries to AITFL, for example, may take a form of ligamentous avulsion, that is, a Chaput and/or Wagstaffe fracture—all leading to similar mechanical effects (**Fig. 2**). According to the classification of the anterolateral distal tibia (anterior malleolus) fractures, type 1 represents a small bony avulsion of the AITFL, type 2 represents a fracture of the anterolateral distal tibia extending into the tibial incisura and joint surface, whereas type 3 fractures represent anterolateral tibial plafond impaction, most likely resulting from an abduction mechanism.[21] Failure to treat acute, displaced avulsion fractures may result in chronic instability necessitating secondary surgery (**Fig. 3**). Similarly, a Bartoníček/Rammelt type 1 posterior malleolus fracture represents a shell-like avulsion of the PITFL and types 2 to 4 would represent various avulsion fractures of the PITFL (and probably interosseous tibiofibular ligament [ITFL]) involving the tibial incisura.[16] Additional forces such as axial impaction may produce intercalary fragments and impaction of the tibial plafond in both anterior (type 3) and posterior (types 2–4) malleolar fractures.[16,21] Finally, an SA1 type lateral malleolus fracture according to Lauge-Hansen represents an avulsion of the ATFL and CFL.

It follows from the above that ligamentous injuries and their corresponding avulsion fractures represent 2 forms of the same injury because they likely result from the same

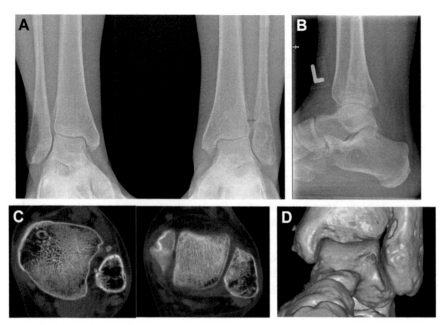

Fig. 2. (*A, B*) Standing radiographs of a 55-year-old female patient presenting with persisting pain 18 months after trimalleolar fracture fixation and 1 year after implant removal. Note the slightly increased tibiofibular clear space (*double arrow* in *A*) and obvious incongruence between the distal fibula and lateral talar facet. (*C*) CT imaging including (*D*) 3D-reconstruction reveal an untreated, displaced avulsion of the anterolateral distal tibia (tubercule de Tillaux-Chaput) corresponding to a type 1 anterior malleolar fracture,[21] resulting in external rotation of the distal fibula.

forces. Once the excessive force has been applied to the bone-ligament-bone system, it fails. The point of failure is the least resistant point (**Fig. 4**). This *locus minoris resistentiae* is located within the bone in some cases (above all with poor bone quality) and within the ligament in other cases. Thus, the same energy and direction of force is able to produce different fracture patterns. In this way, the injury indirectly tests the relative resistance of ligaments and their bony attachments. This concept is well understood in wrist traumatology, that is, in the analysis of perilunate injuries. These injuries may take a form of pure ligamentous rupture, may also take a transscaphoid, transradial, and transcapitate routes.[22]

The point of lowest resistance
The notion that in ankle injury the energy dissipates through the path of least resistance is supported by several observations that can be grouped in 3 categories.

1. Studies identifying anatomical predispositions to certain forms of ankle injury
2. Studies observing the correlation between lateral malleolar fracture morphology and syndesmotic injury
3. Studies observing the correlation between injury pattern and bone quality

A first set of studies looked at anatomical predispositions to sustaining certain forms of ankle injury. Boszczyk and colleagues[23] identified features of syndesmotic anatomy that predispose to pure ligamentous syndesmotic injury in ankle fractures. Computed

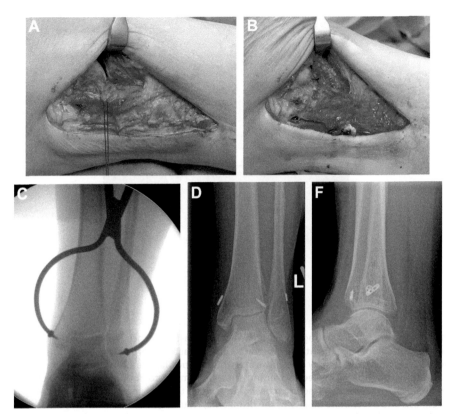

Fig. 3. (A) Intraoperative image of the same patient as in **Fig. 2** demonstrating rotational instability of the distal fibula and the displaced anterior tibial avulsion (marked with a suture). (B) The same situs following reduction of the distal fibula into the tibial incisura, syndesmotic stabilization with a suture-button implant and transosseous fixation of the anterior tibial avulsion with a suture anchor. (C) Intraoperative control of reduction with a pointed reduction clamp. (D, E) Weight-bearing radiographs one year after reconstruction showing a congruent and stable ankle mortise. The patient works full-time as a nurse with minimal residual pain.

tomography (CT) scans of 75 ankles of patients sustaining an ankle fracture with pure ligamentous syndesmotic injury were compared with 75 ankles of patients with bony avulsions of the syndesmotic ligaments. The syndesmoses sustaining a pure ligamentous injury were more shallow, more retroverted, and more disengaged (ie, with greater distance from tibia to fibula) than the controls. This was interpreted as a morphotype where ligamentous resistance is reduced in comparison to bone resistance.[24]

In another set of studies, the correlation between lateral malleolar fracture morphology and syndesmotic injury was observed. Choi and colleagues[25] analyzed the correlation between lateral malleolar fracture morphology and syndesmotic injury. They observed that more distal fibular fractures correlated with stable syndesmosis. In this group, the energy is dissipated through the bone of distal lateral malleolus. In similar oblique fractures, but located more proximally, syndesmotic instability was more common. In this group, the ligaments failed first and finally the energy was released through a more proximal path. Similarly, Cao and colleagues[26] analyzed

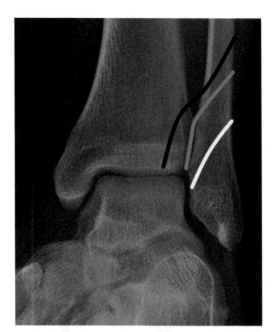

Fig. 4. The energy dissipating through the path of least resistance. With poor bone quality of the distal fibula and an intact syndesmosis, a low fracture morphology (*white line*) can be expected, whereas the gray line illustrates the fracture line resulting from a good bone quality at the lateral malleolus causing the syndesmosis to rupture first followed by a high fibular fracture.[27] A fracture morphology similar to black line indicates a resistant syndesmosis and a low bone quality of the distal tibia, resulting in the *locus minoris resistentiae* being located in the anterolateral distal tibia. The latter assumption may be supported by the fact that anterolateral distal tibia (anterior malleolar) fractures occur in elderly patients than ankle fractures without anterior malleolus involvement.[21]

148 SER stage 2 to 4 fractures. Among them, 41 (27.7%) had an unstable syndesmosis as assessed with an intraoperative Cotton test. Fracture height of the lateral malleolus at the posterior cortex (cutoff 40.4 mm) and peak height (cutoff 55.3 mm) were significant contributing factors. Fractures with an unstable syndesmosis were steeper and higher. The cutoff for the inclination angle was 55.6°.

A third set of studies considering bone quality documented that the fracture pattern preferentially affects less dense parts of bone. Choi and colleagues[25] investigated the bone density of the lateral malleolus in patients having sustained SER fractures. Two groups were identified: one where fracture of lateral malleolus coincided with syndesmosis rupture, in the other group of fractures, the syndesmosis was competent. They observed, that patients belonging to the stable syndesmosis group presented lower bone quality than patients presenting with unstable syndesmosis. They concluded that, in the setting of less resistant bone, the injury energy dissipated through the bone producing a low fibular fracture. In the group, with higher bone quality, the lateral malleolus remained intact and the injury tended to produce a ligamentous injury of the syndesmosis first. If eventually the fracture occurred, it would present more proximally. Warner and colleagues[27] analyzed the bone density in CT images of 67 operatively treated SER 4 type injuries. The group consisted of unimalleolar, bimalleolar, and trimalleolar fractures. Authors observed that patients sustaining soft tissue equivalent injuries presented with higher regional bone density assessed in Hounsfield units. In this group, the path of least resistance leads through the soft tissues. To the contrary, in the group with reduced bone quality, medial and posterior injuries more often presented as fractures. The authors also concluded that an increased number of malleoli fractured indicates reduced bone quality and suggested that this should prompt clinicians to use more robust fixation techniques in such patients.[27] These conclusions are supported by an increasing number of quadrimalleolar fracture patterns in elderly patients (**Fig. 5**).

The observation that fractures more often affect less-dense areas of bone offers another possible explanation to problems with recreating the Lauge-Hansen experiments.[11] His studies were performed during World War II in Denmark, and he based his studies on freshly amputated limbs.[6] Although the origin of specimens is not clearly described, it can be speculated, that in the setting of war, patients undergoing amputation were younger and had higher bone quality than more recent cadaver studies and the current, increasingly aged and multimorbid population sustaining ankle

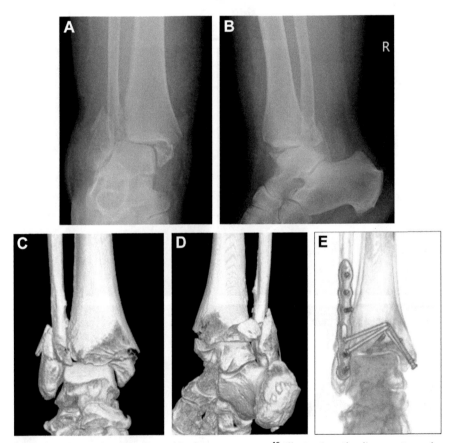

Fig. 5. (*A, B*) Quadrimalleolar ankle fracture pattern[46] illustrating the ligamentous ring injury. It is simultaneously indicative of a low bone quality. (*C, D*) CT imaging reveals the relatively small fragments from avulsions of the anterior and posterior syndesmosis as well as the deltoid ligament. (*E*) Fixation of each fracture fragment was performed without the need of additional indirect syndesmotic fixation.

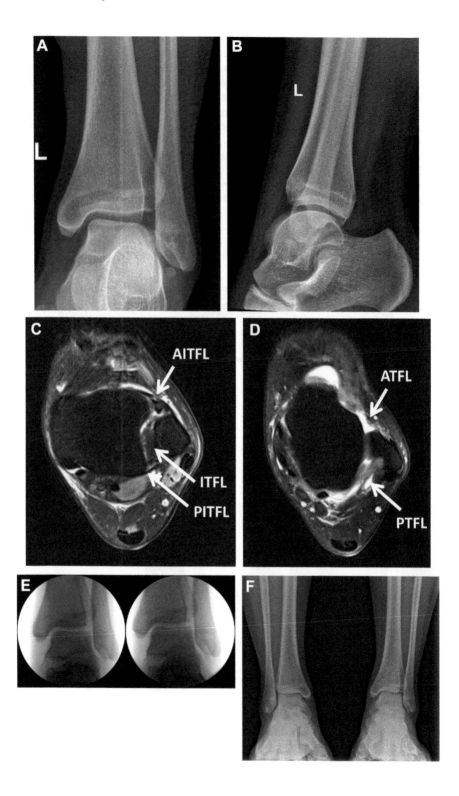

fractures. This would explain consistent ligamentous patterns of injury—indicative of good bone quality—observed by Lauge-Hansen and problems with recreating the results of his experiments in cadaver limbs nowadays. The interplay between the different acting forces and the local bone quality explains the highly variable morphology of malleolar fractures.

Predicting ligament injury and stability in ankle fractures

Incorporating a ligament-centered analysis explains the problems of predicting stability of ankle fracture and syndesmotic stability. It has been long documented that the application of the Lauge-Hansen classification is not able to predict syndesmotic stability of the fracture.[28–30] This is caused by the inability to deduce stability from the fracture morphology or displacement as has been reiterated most recently by Shahien and Tornetta.[31] Analysis of fracture morphology, especially lateral malleolus displacement, failed to predict stability of the fractures in 350 SER type fractures. In 15% of fractures that tested positive for instability in the external rotation test, the lateral malleolus showed no displacement at initial presentation.

Similarly, the ability of the Lauge-Hansen classification to predict ligamentous injuries is a matter of controversy. On one hand, Warner and colleagues[32] found a 94% concordance between Lauge-Hansen predictions and MRI and intraoperative findings in 300 operatively treated ankle fractures. This is in contrast to the findings of Gardner and colleagues[33] and Cabuk and colleagues.[34] In the latter study, the overall compatibility of the radiologic classification with the MRI findings was only 66.1% with the maximum compatibility for SER 4 accounting to be 77.3%. In the earlier stages of SER fractures, the deltoid injury was frequently underestimated in the radiographic analysis.[34] Similarly, several studies have shown that, in Maisonneuve fractures, the interosseous membrane is regularly not ruptured up to the level of the high fibular fracture.[1]

More effective were attempts of incurring stability based on morphology of the medial malleolar fracture. Ebraheim and colleagues,[35] in a study of 112 ankle fractures, observed that syndesmotic injury was positively correlated with a transverse medial malleolar fracture line. Similarly, Sanchez Morata and colleagues[36] observed that the chances of syndesmotic disruption were lower when the angle between the line perpendicular to tibial plafond and the tangent to the fracture line of medial malleolus was more than 60° indicating a more vertical fracture line. The combination of this angle, Lauge-Hansen classification and of tibiofibular clear space measurement was able to predict syndesmotic injury in 86% among 138 patients.

In contrast to x-ray-based imaging, MRI seems optimally suitable for assessment of the soft-tissue component of the injury. Various teams attempted to examine the added value of MRI for ankle fractures. When looking at 58 patients with syndesmotic ligament injuries confirmed by arthroscopy, Oae[37] found assessment of AITFL and

---

Fig. 6. (*A, B*) Radiographs of the right ankle of a 17-year-old female patient following a sleigh accident. She could not recall the exact mechanism of injury to her right foot. No acute fracture was seen. Note the slight talar tilt with the foot being in plantarflexion. (*C, D*) MRI 3 days after the injury revealed a rupture of both the AITFL and ATFL, which does not correspond to any of the proposed Lauge-Hansen stages. The ITFL and PITFL remained intact. (*E*) There was no relevant instability on external rotation stress under fluoroscopy. (*F*) Weight-bearing radiographs 1 week after the injury revealed a stable ankle mortise. The patient was treated in an ankle orthosis under full weight-bearing for 6 weeks.

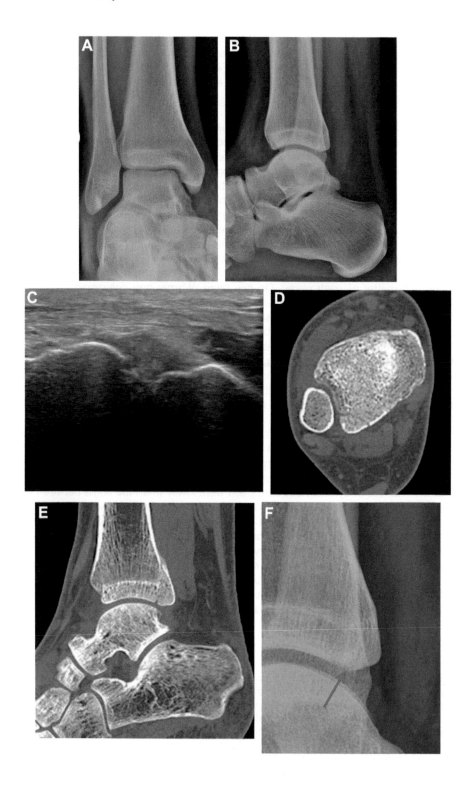

PITFL in MRI to be 100% sensitive. Hermans and colleagues[38] when analyzing the MRI of 44 patients noted that examination of syndesmotic ligaments was limited by its oblique orientation and relatively small size. This resulted in overestimation of the rate of injury to AITFL in 45% of patients and PITFL in 62% of patients in the standard horizontal planes. Adding oblique planes improved imaging accuracy to 100% (30/30 patients) with AITFL injury and 73% (11/15) for the PITFL.

MRI has been shown to provide less value in terms of predicting deltoid ligament stability. Bäcker and colleagues[39] analyzed MRI, gravity stress testing, and weight-bearing radiographs in 34 patients with SER–morphology fractures. The MRI assessment of deltoid ligament injury failed to predict medial clear space measurement in weight-bearing radiographs. Nortunen and colleagues[40] attempted to correlate MRI findings of deep deltoid rupture in SER-morphology fractures with external rotation stress radiographs. Among 61 patients with malleolar fractures, MRI identified some form of deltoid injury in all, whereas instability was confirmed in only 54% of these patients. However, the authors observed that the medial clear space increased with increasing severity of deltoid injury in MRI. Overall, while demonstrating a high sensitivity, MRI tends to overread deltoid ligament injuries and does not predict medial instability.

The ligament-centered analysis is incorporated into current methods of fracture stability assessment.

Traditionally the diagnosis was based on gravity stress test[41] supplemented by examination (mostly external rotation) under anesthesia. Current methods emphasize the role of weight-bearing radiographs—which considers the physiological stability reserve of the ankle under axial load and tests deltoid competence (**Fig. 6**).[42,43] Seidel and colleagues[44] analyzed 104 patients with ankle fractures of SER morphology. Patients without marked (>7 mm) medial clear space widening were assessed with gravity stress test and weight-bearing radiographs. The patients were indicated to nonoperative protocol based on nonwidening of the medial clear space in weight-bearing radiographs. In 44 of these cases, gravity stress radiographs were interpreted as unstable. Because all of these patients managed nonoperatively healed with a congruent ankle, gravity stress test was interpreted to overestimate the instability. Similarly good results in the group with weight-bearing stable ankle despite instability on stress testing were observed by Hoshino and colleagues.[45]

The above studies base their definition of stability on the ankle ring theory. This is in analogy to well-known pelvic ring theory. Similar to the pelvis, the ankle joint forms an osteoligamentous ring. As long as the ring is interrupted in one location, it remains stable, and when a double injury is present, the ring becomes unstable. These concepts, which have their origin in the ideas of Lauge-Hansen, have been revisited and expanded during the recent years.[46–48]

Fig. 7. (*A, B*) A case of importance of CT in detecting occult lesions. A 33-male sustained injury to the right ankle after fall from the bicycle. His preliminary radiographs including the whole lower leg did not reveal any bony injury. (*C*) Based on symptoms in external rotation testing and ultrasound documenting injury to AITFL, a high ankle sprain was diagnosed. (*D, E*) Residual complaints prompted CT imaging at 3 months, which revealed an undisplaced posterior malleolar fracture (Bartonicek/Rammelt type 2). (*F*) With the benefit of hindsight, the fracture may have been suspected in the enlarged image of the initial lateral radiograph (*red arrow*). Because of the completely undisplaced fracture, nonoperative treatment was continued in this case.

IMPLICATIONS FOR CLINICAL PRACTICE: CLINICS CARE POINTS

The observation that in ankle fracture the ligamentous component of injury is at least as important as the bony component has multiple implications for practice.

- First, avulsions are more important to fracture stability than their small size would suggest. They offer the chance of anatomical reduction and advantages of bone-to-bone healing rather than indirect syndesmotic fixation with a screw or dynamic implant.[49] When overlooked, they may interfere with anatomic reduction of the distal fibula into the tibial incisura, which is of prognostic relevance.[50]

- For this reason, even small avulsion fractures should be actively sought. This is especially important because plain x-rays notoriously fail to visualize them[51] (**Fig. 7**). Typically, this omission affects the anterior malleolus,[21] posterior malleolus[16] as well as anterior fibular avulsions.[52] These 3 translate to an incompetent syndesmosis.[49] For these reasons, CT imaging should be used more generously in the evaluation of ankle fractures.[49,53,54] It has been well proven that incorporation of CT into diagnostic setup may not only serve the purpose of better understanding the ankle morphology but will reveal small unexpected fractures as well.[55] This is particularly true for fractures involving the anterior or posterior tibial rim, syndesmotic disruption and inconruity, suspected intercalary fragments, or impaction of the tibial plafond.[51–58]

- Simultaneously, the size of the avulsed posterior (and anterior) fragment loses its relevance as the sole criterion for fixation. A long-honored value of 25% joint involvement for the fixation of posterior malleolar fractures[56] has been abandoned and replaced with individualized treatment recommendations classifications based on the 3D pathoanatomy of these fractures and their impact on ligament stability.[52,57,58]

- Finally, planning of operative treatment should no longer be based on global fracture morphology and supposed "mechanism" of fracture. This should be replaced by thorough analysis of each of the 4 ligamentous-osseous components forming the ankle joint complex.[46–48] The concepts of Lauge-Hansen that have been constantly challenged and refined during the last decades will continue to be useful for that purpose.

REFERENCES

1. Bartoníček J, Rammelt S, Tuček M. Maisonneuve fractures of the ankle: a critical analysis review. JBJS Rev 2022;10(2). https://doi.org/10.2106/JBJS.RVW.21. 00160.
2. Lauge N. Fractures of the ankle; analytic historic survey as the basis of new experimental, roentgenologic and clinical investigations. Arch Surg 1948;56(3): 259–317.
3. Bartoníček J, Rammelt S. History of ankle fractures in the German-speaking literature. Fuss Sprungg 2022;20(3):165–76.
4. Lauge-Hansen N. Fractures of the ankle. IV. Clinical use of genetic roentgen diagnosis and genetic reduction. Arch Surg 1952;64(4):488–500.
5. Lauge-Hansen N. Ligamentous ankle fractures; diagnosis and treatment. Acta Chir Scand 1949;97(6):544–50.
6. Lauge-Hansen N. Fractures of the ankle. II. Combined experimental-surgical and experimental-roentgenologic investigations. Arch Surg 1950;60(5):957–85.
7. Stiehl JB, Skrade DA, Johnson RP. Experimentally produced ankle fractures in autopsy specimens. Clin Orthop Relat Res 1992;285:244–9.
8. Michelson J, Solocoff D, Waldman B, et al. Ankle fractures. The Lauge-Hansen classification revisited. Clin Orthop Relat Res 1997;345:198–205.

9. Haraguchi N, Armiger RS. A new interpretation of the mechanism of ankle fracture. J Bone Joint Surg Am 2009;91:821–9.

10. Zahn RK, Frey S, Moritz M, et al. Die Supinations-Eversions-Verletzung des OSG in osteoporotischen Unterschenkelpräparaten. Unfallchirurg 2011;114(8):697.

11. Kwon JY, Gitajn IL, Walton P, et al. A cadaver study revisiting the original methodology of Lauge-Hansen and a commentary on modern usage. J Bone Joint Surg Am 2015;97(7):604–9.

12. Rodriguez EK, Kwon JY, Herder LM, et al. Correlation of AO and Lauge-Hansen classification systems for ankle fractures to the mechanism of injury. Foot Ankle Int 2013;34:1516–20.

13. Boszczyk A, Fudalej M, Kwapisz S, et al. Ankle fracture - Correlation of Lauge-Hansen classification and patient reported fracture mechanism. Forensic Sci Int 2018;282:94–100.

14. Boszczyk A, Fudalej M, Kwapisz S, et al. X-ray features to predict ankle fracture mechanism. Forensic Sci Int 2018;291:185–92.

15. Patton BK, Orfield NJ, Clements JR. Does the Lauge-Hansen Injury Mechanism Predict Posterior Malleolar Fracture Morphology? J Foot Ankle Surg. February 2022. https://doi.org/10.1053/j.jfas.2022.02.013.

16. Bartoníček J, Rammelt S, Kostlivý K, et al. Anatomy and classification of the posterior tibial fragment in ankle fractures. Arch Orthop Trauma Surg 2015;135(4):505–16.

17. Pankovich AM, Shivaram MS. Anatomical basis of variability in injuries of the medial malleolus and the deltoid ligament. II. Clinical studies. Acta Orthop Scand 1979;50(2):225–36.

18. Pankovich AM, Shivaram MS. Anatomical basis of variability in injuries of the medial malleolus and the deltoid ligament: I. Anatomical studies. Acta Orthop Scand 1979;50(2):217–23.

19. Cromeens BP, Kirchhoff CA, Patterson RM, et al. An attachment-based description of the medial collateral and spring ligament complexes. Foot Ankle Int 2015;36(6):710–21.

20. Nwosu K, Schneiderman BA, Shymon SJ, et al. A medial malleolar "fleck sign" may predict ankle instability in ligamentous supination external rotation ankle fractures. Foot Ankle Spec 2018;11(3):246–51.

21. Rammelt S, Bartoníček J, Kroker L. Pathoanatomy of the anterolateral tibial fragment in ankle fractures. J Bone Joint Surg Am 2022;104(4):353–63.

22. Kinghorn A, Finlayson G, Faulkner A, et al. Perilunate injuries: current aspects of management. Injury 2021;52(10):2760–7.

23. Boszczyk A, Kwapisz S, Krümmel M, et al. Anatomy of the tibial incisura as a risk factor for syndesmotic injury. Foot Ankle Surg 2019;25(1). https://doi.org/10.1016/j.fas.2017.08.003.

24. Boszczyk A, Kwapisz S, Krümmel M, et al. Correlation of Incisura Anatomy With Syndesmotic Malreduction. Foot Ankle Int 2017;39(3). https://doi.org/10.1177/1071100717744332. 1071100717744332.

25. Choi Y, Kwon S, Chung CY, et al. Preoperative Radiographic and CT Findings Predicting Syndesmotic Injuries in Supination-External Rotation-Type Ankle Fractures. J Bone Joint Surg Am 2014;96(14):1161–7.

26. Cao M-M, Zhang Y-W, Hu S-Y, et al. 3D Mapping of the Lateral Malleolus Fractures for Predicting Syndesmotic Injuries in Supination External Rotation Type Ankle Fractures. J Foot Ankle Surg 2022. https://doi.org/10.1053/j.jfas.2022.01.026.

27. Warner SJ, Gausden EB, Levack AE, et al. Supination External Rotational Ankle Fracture Injury Pattern Correlation With Regional Bone Density. Foot Ankle Int 2019;40(4):384–9.
28. Gougoulias N, Sakellariou A. When is a simple fracture of the lateral malleolus not so simple? how to assess stability, which ones to fix and the role of the deltoid ligament. Bone Joint Lett J 2017;99-B(7):851–5.
29. Delaney JP, Charlson MD, Michelson JD. Ankle Fracture Stability-Based Classification: A Study of Reproducibility and Clinical Prognostic Ability. J Orthop Trauma 2019;33(9):465–71.
30. Briet JP, Hietbrink F, Smeeing DP, et al. Ankle fracture classification: an innovative system for describing ankle fractures. J Foot Ankle Surg 2019;58(3):492–6.
31. Shahien AA, Tornetta P. Lack of displacement of the fibula is not a confirmation of ankle stability in supination external pattern ankle fractures. J Orthop Trauma 2022;36(1):e1–5.
32. Warner SJ, Garner MR, Hinds RM, et al. Correlation between the lauge-hansen classification and ligament injuries in ankle fractures. J Orthop Trauma 2015; 29(12):574–8.
33. Gardner MJ, Demetrakopoulos D, Briggs SM, et al. The ability of the Lauge-Hansen classification to predict ligament injury and mechanism in ankle fractures: an MRI study. J Orthop Trauma 2006;20(4):267–72.
34. Çabuk H, Çelebi F, İmren Y, et al. Compatibility of Lauge-Hansen Classification Between Plain Radiographs and Magnetic Resonance Imaging in Ankle Fractures. J Foot Ankle Surg 2018;57(4):712–5.
35. Ebraheim NA, Weston JT, Ludwig T, et al. The association between medial malleolar fracture geometry, injury mechanism, and syndesmotic disruption. Foot Ankle Surg 2014;20(4):276–80.
36. Sánchez-Morata E, Martínez-Ávila JC, Vacas Sánchez E, et al. Predicting syndesmotic injuries in ankle fractures: a new system based on the medial malleolar focus. Injury 2017;48(Suppl 6):S86–90.
37. Oae K, Takao M, Naito K, et al. Injury of the tibiofibular syndesmosis: value of MR imaging for diagnosis. Radiology 2003;227(1):155–61.
38. Hermans JJ, Beumer A, Hop WCJ, et al. Tibiofibular syndesmosis in acute ankle fractures: Additional value of an oblique MR image plane. Skeletal Radiol 2012; 41(2):193–202.
39. Bäcker HC, Vosseller JT, Bonel H, et al. Weightbearing Radiography and MRI Findings in Ankle Fractures. Foot Ankle Spec 2021;14(6):489–95.
40. Nortunen S, Lepojärvi S, Savola O, et al. Stability assessment of the ankle mortise in supination-external rotation-type ankle fractures: lack of additional diagnostic value of MRI. J Bone Joint Surg Am 2014;96(22):1855–62.
41. Nortunen S, Flinkkilä T, Lantto I, et al. Diagnostic accuracy of the gravity stress test and clinical signs in cases of isolated supination-external rotation-type lateral malleolar fractures. Bone Joint Lett J 2015;97-B(8):1126–31.
42. Dawe EJC, Shafafy R, Quayle J, et al. The effect of different methods of stability assessment on fixation rate and complications in supination external rotation (SER) 2/4 ankle fractures. Foot Ankle Surg 2015;21(2):86–90.
43. Weber M, Burmeister H, Flueckiger G, et al. The use of weightbearing radiographs to assess the stability of supination-external rotation fractures of the ankle. Arch Orthop Trauma Surg 2010;130(5):693–8.
44. Seidel A, Krause F, Weber M. Weightbearing vs Gravity Stress Radiographs for Stability Evaluation of Supination-External Rotation Fractures of the Ankle. Foot Ankle Int 2017;38(7):736–44.

45. Hoshino CM, Nomoto EK, Norheim EP, et al. Correlation of weightbearing radiographs and stability of stress positive ankle fractures. Foot Ankle Int 2012; 33(2):92–8.
46. Rammelt S, Bartoníček J, Kroker L, et al. Surgical Fixation of Quadrimalleolar Fractures of the Ankle. J Orthop Trauma 2021;35(6):e216–22.
47. Nicolai C, Bierry G, Faruch-Bilfeld M, et al. The concept of ring of injuries: evaluation in ankle trauma. Skeletal Radiol 2022;51(10):2027–37.
48. Joannas G, Arrondo G, Rammelt S, et al. Quadrimalleolar fractures of the ankle: Think 360°—A step-by-step guide on evaluation and fixation. J Foot Ankle Surg 2021;8(4):193–200.
49. Rammelt S, Boszczyk A. Chronic syndesmotic injuries: arthrodesis versus reconstruction. Foot Ankle Clin 2020;25(4):631–52.
50. Marx C, Schaser KD, Rammelt S. Early corrections after failed ankle fracture fixation. Z Orthop Unfall 2021;159(3):323–31.
51. Black EM, Antoci V, Lee JT, et al. Role of preoperative computed tomography scans in operative planning for malleolar ankle fractures. Foot Ankle Int 2013; 34(5):697–704.
52. Rammelt S, Bartoníček J, Schepers T, et al. Fixation of anterolateral distal tibial fractures: the anterior malleolus. Operat Orthop Traumatol 2021;33(2):125–38.
53. Rammelt S, Boszczyk A. Computed tomography in the diagnosis and treatment of ankle fractures: a critical analysis review. JBJS Rev 2018;6(12):e7.
54. Szymański T, Zdanowicz U. Comparison of routine computed tomography and plain X-ray imaging for malleolar fractures-How much do we miss? Foot Ankle Surg 2022;28(2):263–8.
55. Leung KH, Fang CXS, Lau TW, et al. Preoperative Radiography versus Computed Tomography for Surgical Planning for Ankle Fractures. J Orthop Surg 2016;24(2): 158–62.
56. Harper MC, Hardin G. Posterior malleolar fractures of the ankle associated with external rotation-abduction injuries. Results with and without internal fixation. J Bone Joint Surg Am 1988;70(9):1348–56.
57. Bartoníček J, Rammelt S, Tuček M. Posterior malleolar fractures: changing concepts and recent developments. Foot Ankle Clin 2017;22(1):125–45.
58. Rammelt S, Bartoníček J. Posterior malleolar fractures. A critical analysis review. JBJS Reviews 2020;8(8). e19.e00207.

Moving?

Make sure your subscription moves with you!

To notify us of your new address, find your **Clinics Account Number** (located on your mailing label above your name), and contact customer service at:

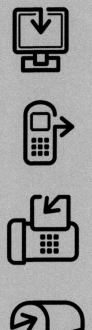

Email: journalscustomerservice-usa@elsevier.com

800-654-2452 (subscribers in the U.S. & Canada)
314-447-8871 (subscribers outside of the U.S. & Canada)

Fax number: 314-447-8029

Elsevier Health Sciences Division
Subscription Customer Service
3251 Riverport Lane
Maryland Heights, MO 63043

*To ensure uninterrupted delivery of your subscription,
please notify us at least 4 weeks in advance of move.

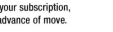